AFTER GOD

Morality and Bioethics in a Secular Age

After God

Morality and Bioethics in a Secular Age

by

H. Tristram Engelhardt, Jr.

ST VLADIMIR'S SEMINARY PRESS

YONKERS, NEW YORK

2017

Library of Congress Cataloging-in-Publication Data

Engelhardt, H. Tristram (Hugo Tristram), 1941–
   After God : morality and bioethics in a secular age / by H. Tristram Engelhardt.
    pages cm
   Includes bibliographical references.
   ISBN 978-0-88141-499-8 (pbk.) — ISBN 978-0-88141-500-1 (electronic)
   1. Bioethics. 2. Bioethics—History. 3. Philosophy and religion. 4. Applied ethics.
 I. Title. II. Title: Morality and bioethics in a secular age.
   QH332.E536 2014
   174.2—dc23

2014019778

ST VLADIMIR'S SEMINARY PRESS
575 Scarsdale Road, Yonkers, NY 10707
1-800-204-2665
www.svspress.com

ISBN 978-088141-499-8

PRINTED IN THE UNITED STATES OF AMERICA

To my wife
Susan Gay Malloy Engelhardt
in gratitude for a gay marriage, three children, and thirteen grandchildren.
Without her generous support, patience, and wise guidance,
I would have accomplished nothing.

Table of Contents

Acknowledgements

This book grew out of a half-century of reflections about God, morality, and what has become bioethics. This volume is the final common pathway of numerous chains of reflections and conversations in moral theory, the history of thought, ontology, bioethics, and theology. Only a few of the many friends and colleagues who joined me in these reflections, and from whom I learned immensely, are mentioned in the first chapter of this work. The people to whom I am in debt for the ideas, insights, and arguments that helped shape this volume are legion. I am under a very special debt to Professor Maurizio Mori (Turin), who generously and with much labor brought me to give a series of lectures in 2012: "Religion, Politics, and the State: Rethinking Morality in Modern Secularized Societies," Politeia, University of Milan, Milan, Italy, January 30; "Bioethics after Foundations: Feeling the Full Force of Secularization," Secularization and Bioethics, Centro Evangelico di Cultura "Arturo Pascal" and Consulta di Bioetica Onlus, Turin, Italy, January 31; "The Deflation of Morality: Rethinking the Secularization of the West," University of Salento, Lecce, Italy, February 1; "Autonomy, Medical Professionalism, and the Culture Wars," University of Naples Frederick II, Naples, Italy, February 3; "How Can an Autonomy-based Morality Get along with a Quasi-Religious Profession like Medicine?" Instituto Banco di Napoli, Naples, Italy, February 3; and "Religion, Politics, and the State in Modern Secularized Societies," Comune di Napoli, Naples, Italy, February 6. The lecture I gave at Turin appeared much transformed as "Bioethics and Moral Pluralism" in *Notizie di Politeia* 105 (June 2013): 7–21. As the lectures took shape, Prof. Mori was as always an insightful and engaging conversation partner.

These manuscripts began to grow into a book due in part to conversations with Prof. Kurt Bayertz and his colleagues, including the Rev. Kurt Schmidt (Zentrum für Ethik in der Medizin, Frankfurt/Main), when I was a Visiting

Fellow at the Centre for Advanced Study in Bioethics, Westfälische Wilhelms-Universität, Münster, in April 2012. Over the next ten months, all was recast to appear as *Dopo Dio: Morale e bioetica in un mondo laico* (Turin: Claudiana 2014). The text of this book was then in turn thoroughly reframed and substantially developed over the period of nearly a year. During this time, Thomas J. Bole III and Corinna Delkeskamp-Hayes with great generosity and patience read through numerous drafts of the evolving manuscript. Graham M. Valenta not only went through the manuscripts but copy-edited the page proofs and produced the index. Last but not least, I must acknowledge the intercession of my holy patron whose name I bear: St. Herman of Alaska. "The prayer of a just man availeth much" (James 5: 16).

Morality, Bioethics, and the Failure of the Enlightenment

We are after God. That is, the dominant secular culture is deaf and blind to God's existence. The result is that, in eschewing a God's-eye perspective, morality, bioethics, the state, and the meaning of life are all approached as if everything came from nowhere, were going nowhere, and for no enduring and ultimate purpose. This book examines the roots and implications of this full immanentization of all meaning within the dominant secular culture. What has happened is that the faith in secular rationality at the roots of the Western philosophical project born in Greece and then reborn in Western Christianity in the early second millennium has been shown to be unjustified. The aspirations of the Enlightenment of Immanuel Kant (1724–1804) have been deflated as well: reason has not been able to substitute for God.

As the term bioethics was re-engaged in 1971 (Reich 1994), John Rawls (1931–2007) had just published *A Theory of Justice* (Rawls 1971). Many saw Rawls as having vindicated moral philosophy's universalist claims to providing the basis for a philosophically-grounded canonical account of justice, along with a canonical bioethics of health care allocation (Daniels 1985). The creation and success of bioethics appeared to vindicate Enlightenment hopes for secular moral rationality. Bioethics was full of Enlightenment expectations. Reason would triumph and on the basis of sound rational argument establish a canonical secular morality and bioethics. Bioethicists with a faith in philosophy could thus help realize the Enlightenment dream: morality would be anchored in rationality, the authority of the state would be secured in moral rationality, and all persons would be recognized as members of a single, all-encompassing, moral community. There would be a rationally justified bioethics to direct society in navigating the dizzying pace of biomedical progress. However, in the same year that Normal Daniels published *Just Health Care* (1985), his bioethics of health care allocation, Rawls confessed his recognition of the impossibility of giving a moral-theoretical or -metaphysical justification for an account of justice and therefore for a bioethics of health care allocation (Rawls 1985). Rawls had begun to face post-modernity. What had seemed so certain and so firm a foundation for bioethics, and for morality generally, had been brought into question. Although this volume is about moral foundations as such, it gives a special focus to health care and therefore to bioethics. Bioethics provides some of the most important battles in the culture wars.

Bioethics confronts a major intellectual and cultural failure of core expectations. It is now clear that there is no bioethics or morality that philosophy can establish as canonical. There is no final secular view regarding the nature of the right, the good, and the virtuous. The Western moral-philosophical project begun in ancient Greece and re-embraced in the Western Middle Ages and in the Enlightenment is now being acknowledged as a failure. As Judd Owen summarizes, "Today, belief in the comprehensive philosophic teaching of the Enlightenment appears to lie in ruins, and few hope that any other comprehensive philosophy could successfully replace it. This despair is, to a considerable extent, due to a radical critique of reason as such" (Owen 2001, p. 1). The very sense and meaning of morality and bioethics must be rethought. As G. W. F. Hegel (1770–1831) appreciated, and as Richard Rorty (1931–2007) emphasized, it is impossible for secular moral reflection to establish a canonical content for morality, because "there is no way to step outside the various vocabularies we have employed and find a metavocabulary which somehow takes account of *all possible* vocabularies, all possible ways of judging and feeling" (Rorty 1989, p. xvi). As the interminable debates regarding the moral status of homosexual acts, reproduction outside of marriage, abortion, health care allocation, and euthanasia demonstrate, we do not agree when it is licit, forbidden, or obligatory to have sex, reproduce, transfer property, or take human life. It is even impossible to secure a neutral philosophical standpoint that through sound rational argument can show that one should always act from the moral point of view. Among other things, there is no neutral moral point of view. The confrontation with such disappointments is the force of post-modernity. The West entered modernity and the Enlightenment with the expectation that its new, fully secularized reason would establish a canonical morality. Bioethics did the same in the 1970s. The intellectual supports sought for this hope have turned out to be non-existent.

At the inception of the moral-philosophical project two-and-a-half millennia ago, many saw that the project was flawed: one cannot by philosophical argument establish a particular morality as canonical, because one must always grant particular background assumptions in order to establish the bases for what one seeks to prove. Any particular moral philosophy always presupposes particular controverted basic premises in order to secure the particular conclusions it wishes to demonstrate. The insurmountable challenge is to determine by sound rational secular argument which premises should at the outset be conceded so as to get the moral argument started that one supports. Recognizing this difficulty, "Protagoras [fl. 5th century B.C.] was the first to maintain that there are two sides to every question, opposed to each other, and he even argued in this fashion, being the first to do so" (Diogenes Laertius 1979, vol. 2, p. 463, IX.51). The Sophists have received bad press, but they openly faced the impossibility of the secular moral project that Socrates, Plato, and Aristotle had begun: rationally establishing a canonical morality. By the time of the early Christian Fathers, the failure of the Greek philosophical project was widely acknowledged, as Agrippa (1st century A.D.) and Clement of Alexandria (*c*. 150–*c*. 215) attest. Post-modernity is the admission of what was always true, and which had already been recognized in ancient Athens. Philosophy cannot pull the rabbit of a canonical morality out of the magic hat of philosophical argument. Secular bioethics, morality, and public policy, so this book argues, must be considered anew.

Why did the secular culture, in particular bioethics, expect so much more from secular moral rationality than it could ever deliver? The culture of the West as it took shape in the early second millennium was marked by a dialectic of *fides et ratio*, of faith and reason rooted in the early second millennium's rebirth of faith in the moral philosophy of the Greeks. There was a faith that reason could, in the area of morality, establish what faith also taught. After the Reformation, the West's Christian faith was shattered into a plurality of denominations locked in bloody conflict. Following the religious wars of the 17th century, there arose the hope, indeed the faith, that at least reason would not fail, much less lead to bloodshed, as faith in faith had done. There would be one secular morality justified by one canonical view or account of what secular moral rationality ought to be that would replace the multiplicity of views regarding God and His commands. Reason, it was thought, would guide all to a single morality and thus to a single canonical bioethics. However, this faith in reason has proved false. Reason failed. There is no one secular sense or understanding of the morally rational. As a consequence, there is an intractable diversity of secular moralities and bioethics. There is no single account of moral rationality and/or of the politically reasonable to substitute for a God's-eye perspective. Moreover, secular reason led not to perpetual peace, but to the French Revolution's Reign of Terror, and eventually to the slaughter of tens of millions by the secular, rationalist regimes of Joseph Stalin, Mao Zedong, and Pol Pot, all in pursuit of a supposedly philosophically justified moral vision that had its own secular bioethics.[1]

Within the horizon of the finite and the immanent, how could one have ever thought that it would be possible to lay out a view from nowhere that could neutrally and canonically guide morality, bioethics, and public policy? Nevertheless, it was a general conceit. Immanuel Kant, for instance, had fed this vain hope by appealing to a rational impartial observer [*ein vernünftiger unparteiischer Zuschauer*] (*The Foundations of the Metaphysics of Morals*, AK IV.393) so as to establish and give substance to his moral point of view. But there is no such impartial rational point of view. There is no view from nowhere. For a rational observer or decision-maker to guide, in order for it to make a principled choice or decision, it must already possess a moral sense or thin theory of the good. It cannot be impartial, but must instead at the outset be partial to a particular sense of the morally rational. It must have a particular moral content. But which moral content ought to be selected to guide? Which moral sense, thin theory of the good, or view of the morally rational ought the rational observer, decision-maker, or hypothetical contractor to embrace? How ought one, for example, to rank such cardinal human goods as liberty, equality, prosperity, and security, and why? Depending on how one ranks these goods, one will affirm a particular morality, bioethics, and health care policy such as that of a social democracy or instead that of a one-party capitalist oligarchy as in Singapore. Without begging the question, arguing in a circle, or engaging in infinite regress, there is no way to identify the correct ranking. There is no argument to establish one view of the morally rational as canonical without already conceding particular background basic premises and rules of evidence, and so on forever. *Pace* the promise of Plato's *Euthyphro*, there is no rational substitute for a God's-eye perspective. A morality with a bioethics that is rationally compelling to all is purchased at the price of content. Universal moral principles are empty: "Do the good," but what is the good? Content is purchased at the price of universality. Any morality or bioethics with content is particular, and therefore one in contrast to a plurality of others. Secular morality and bioethics are as a consequence intractably plural.

But there are even more radical implications that follow from an honest assessment of the state of affairs within which morality and bioethics find themselves. Once everything is placed within the horizon of the finite and the immanent, and God is no longer recognized as the anchor for morality, and once morality is recognized as unable to provide a canonical surrogate, what had been moral choices become mere life-style choices. The meaning of morality and bioethics changes radically. There is no perspective from which to hold that choices contrary to what one's moral and bioethical point of view determines to be obligatory are in fact wrong in the sense of violating the canons of the good, the right, and/or the virtuous that all rational persons should endorse. Such a canonical moral standpoint cannot be secured. There is no one actual or hypothetical canonical moral community. *Pace* Rawls (1971), there is no one canonical original position. Secular moral and bioethical pluralism is as a result intractable. We are confronted with a principled moral and bioethical chaos. Worse yet, it is now clear that the moral point of view cannot rationally be shown to trump concerns of prudence and self-interest. For example, if one no longer recognizes the existence of God and of a God's-eye perspective, and therefore one is left in an apparently ultimately meaningless universe, why rationally ought one always to support the greatest good for the greatest number rather than one's own good and/or that of one's family and associates? Is it irrational to act immorally but for high stakes, as did Alexander the Great and Julius Caesar? What particular sense of rationality ought one to endorse and why ought it always to govern? Again, once all is placed in a context after God, everything, including morality, becomes without ultimate meaning.

At stake is not just God as an object of religious devotion, but God as a point of final and ultimate, epistemic, and axiological reference. Without God in this minimal sense, all non-transient meaning is gone. For example, virtue and vice, love and hate, kindness and cruelty will all be equally forgotten in an ultimately meaningless universe. Even Kant, who was an atheist, acknowledged the impossibility of morality as it had come to be understood since at least the beginning of the second millennium, in the absence of an enforceable God's-eye perspective. This postulate was not needed in order to motivate moral behavior, but to ensure its binding rationality. As a consequence, Kant affirmed an as-if God for empirical reflection, and for morality the postulates of God and immortality. He recognized that without God and immortality, the sense of morality and of political authority that had defined the West for centuries was without coherent foundations. In a secular culture after God and immortality, bioethics and morality are fundamentally transformed.

The contemporary dominant culture, contrary to Western modernity and Kant, is increasingly framed by a morality and bioethics after God and in the absence of even Kant's theistic moral postulate. After Christendom, after a morality that had been traditionally anchored in a transcendent framework that gave morality ultimate meaning, everything, including bioethics, must now be rethought down to its roots. Already in 1802 Hegel saw this when he talked of the death of God. He recognized that the secular morality of the West could only have an immanent, sociohistorically conditioned meaning. Now clearly without an anchor in being or moral rationality, secular morality had to be approached fully anew within the horizon of the finite and the immanent. We can now see the consequences of a culture after God even more starkly than Hegel was willing to acknowledge. We are confronted with morality, bioethics, and public authority relocated within a culture shaped by an agnostic methodological postulate, so that one is invited to proceed as if all ultimately came from nowhere, was going nowhere, and for no final reason. Secular morality, bioethics, medical professionalism, and public authority must also be articulated in the face of intractable moral pluralism and absent any enduring meaning. Secular morality and bioethics must come to terms with post-modernity. They must recognize the failure of its Enlightenment expectations.

This state of affairs is ever more widely conceded. Rorty admits this without a blush. The great cultural cleft separating traditional Christian and secular senses of morality and bioethics is defined by the latter being anchored in a culture after God: "To say, with Nietzsche, that God is dead, is to say that we serve no higher purposes" (Rorty 1989, p. 20). As a consequence, after God there is not only no unifying common sense of morality, but no common sense of humanity or of why we should be moral, whatever that means. "There are no problems which bind the generations together into a single natural kind called 'humanity'" (Rorty 1989, p. 20). Not only is God dead, but man is dead as a foundation for the humanities or for a common moral vision. The implications of not recognizing God and a God's-eye perspective are radical. Everything is changed. Human rights are without foundations. There is no basis for secular claims about human dignity. This book confronts this state of affairs and its implications for secular morality and bioethics. It offers a reassessment of the meaning and significance of bioethics through an encompassing reconsideration of the meaning of morality and bioethics after God.

The first chapter examines the emergence of a post-Christian culture bereft of ultimate meaning. It recalls how the remaining framework of public Christian culture, a relic of Christendom, rapidly collapsed at the end of the 20th century, just as bioethics was being established as an academic field and as the praxis of clinical ethics was being launched. This chapter also introduces the perspective from which this volume is written: the philosophical recognition that modernity is over, and the Enlightenment project has failed, all as a consequence of recognizing that secular morality is after God. "The Demoralization and Deflation of Morality and Bioethics", the second chapter, examines in detail why, since there is no canonical secular moral perspective, much of what had once been authentically matters of morality and bioethics are now reduced to life-style choices—hence the demoralization of morality and bioethics. *In vitro* fertilization with embryo wastage, the use of donor gametes in third-party-assisted reproduction, physician-assisted suicide, and euthanasia become mere life- and death-style choices. This chapter lays out as well why there is no general moral-philosophical argument to show that the moral point of view should always trump prudence and self-interest. As a consequence, morality and bioethics are themselves deflated into macro life-style choices. Secular morality is reduced to personal choices, not objectively binding norms in the sense of norms grounded in narrative independent obligations. The secular moral landscape within which morality and bioethics find themselves is substantially other than what had been expected.

The next chapter, "More on Secularization, Thoughts on Sex, and the Authority of the State", places developments within the phenomenon of secularization in terms of the dominant secular culture's transformation of the significance of sex and reproduction, as well as the legitimacy of the state. Against the background of the demoralization and deflation of morality, the force and sweep of contemporary secularization are magnified. These wide-reaching changes in the appreciation of morality have become part and parcel of a transformed everyday life-world, within which sexual relations, reproduction, and abortion have lost any moral gravitas. As the chapter shows, how and with whom one has sex, whether one reproduces outside of marriage, whether one within marriage uses donor gametes, and whether one has an abortion have lost any particular moral meaning within the bioethics and morality that the secular, post-Christian life-world sustains. A whole sphere of what had once been moral issues is now beyond morality. In addition, within this context, political structures are without any grounding in a canonical moral rationality or sense of the politically reasonable. The state, medical law, and health care policy reflect political life-style choices, political arrangements that constitute at best a *modus vivendi*, an arrangement with which one is willing to live for at least the time being. The meanings of secular morality, bioethics, and health care policy are being fundamentally transformed because it has become clear that morality and political authority have no canonical rational warrant.

The fourth chapter examines in greater depth why the West engendered such unsecured hopes for a canonical secular morality and bioethics, which aspirations were then followed by their collapse. "*Fides et ratio*, the Western Medieval Synthesis, and the Collapse of Secular Bioethics and Morality" explores the ethnocentric character of the roots of the contemporary dominant morality and bioethics, highlighting the particular developments within the Christianity of the Western Middle Ages that led to the rebirth of the Greek moral-philosophical project. Medieval Western Europe in re-embracing the Greek moral-philosophical project took a philosophical turn with momentous consequences for the West and for the world. This chapter addresses both the cultural peculiarities of this Western Christian moral-philosophical synthesis, as well as how differently things turned out in the Muslim cultural sphere because of Mohammed al-Ghazali (1058–1111). Al-Ghazali appreciated what the Christian Apostles and

Fathers such as St. Paul and St. John Chrysostom had seen, and what post-modernity would rediscover: the Greek moral-philosophical project of establishing moral norms as canonical apart from God cannot succeed. There cannot be a canonical secular morality or bioethics without reference to God. As a consequence, the contrast between the dominant bioethics of Europe and the Americas contrasts starkly with that within the Muslim cultural sphere. The dominant culture and bioethics of Muslim countries tend to be religious, while that of the contemporary secular West, with its morality and bioethics, is being brought into question because of the collapse of the rational foundations for which it had hoped.

One is left with a deeply rooted basis for bioethical conflict: the incompatibility of claims made by the contemporary secular state about what should count as proper medical professional conduct and those claims grounded in the demands of God. The fifth chapter, "Bioethical Conflicts: Obligations to God versus Obligations to the Secular State", explores the irresolvable character of the tensions between the consciences of believing health care professionals, on the one hand, and the legal and health care public policy requirements of the secular state on the other. Here it is important to recognize that the contemporary secular state has become a secular fundamentalist state in the sense that a particular secular ideology, along with its secular morality and bioethics, has been established in a fashion similar to the establishment of a religion, along with its morality and bioethics, in a religious fundamentalist state. Because the differences between the moral and bioethical claims of believers and those of the secular state are so different in content and justification, there is no place for compromise. The gulf is unbridgeable because what is at stake is incommensurable: obligations to God versus obligations grounded in particular health-profession norms for conduct required by a particular secular state shaped by a particular secular narrative. A somewhat similar gulf, though not as deep, divides a Kantian morality and its bioethics from what is now demanded by the secular state after the collapse of its foundations. Kant still held there was a canonical morality, although it had no actual transcendent anchor. Faced with these gulfs in meaning, how ought health care professionals with religiously-based obligations to regard their conflicts with the secular state? In particular, how are these conflicts to be appreciated when the secular state has lost any canonical moral or political authority, becoming only a *modus vivendi*, whose law and public policy reflect one among a plurality of freestanding accounts, none of which is anchored in being or in a canonical account of moral rationality? How is one to understand the authority of the canons of proper health-professional conduct established by a state, after the secular moral authority of the state has been radically deflated? Against this background, one can recognize the depth of the moral and bioethical battles in the culture wars and the reasons for their persistence.

Special attention is given in the sixth chapter to Tom Beauchamp and James Childress's account of bioethics and their claims regarding an underlying common morality. Although Tom Beauchamp appears to have qualified his views (Beauchamp 2004), the claim of a common morality is already advanced in their first edition of *Principles of Biomedical Ethics* (1979, p. 34), the most influential textbook in the field. However, their assertion of a common morality collides with the actual intractable plurality of moral visions and of bioethics, so that their version of bioethics in the *Principles* is clearly untenable. But how is this state of affairs, this principled chaos and plurality of secular moralities and bioethics, to be understood, given the international success of health care ethics consultation? Indeed, what should one make of bioethics in general? On the one hand, one again confronts secular morality's crisis of foundations, along with the consequence that academic bioethics in principle fails to provide a canonical moral vision or a guiding foundation for the field. Theory in bioethics, as even Tom Beauchamp acknowledges, has been brought radically into question. Secular theoreticians of bioethics are reduced to serving as geographers of our ongoing controversies, unable to give any canonical moral guidance. They are like mapmakers or tour guides who can show us alternative moral and bioethical destinations, but who cannot tell us what destination one ought to choose, where one should go on the map. On the other hand, health care ethics consultation has succeeded world-wide, despite moral and bioethical pluralism. The reason for this success in the face of moral pluralism is that health care ethics consultants and clinical ethicists generally do not function as moral experts but as quasi-lawyers. They have succeeded as experts, not about morality in general, but as experts about that particular morality that in a particular locale happens to be established in medical law and public policy. Hence, there is not just an

American, but a Californian and a Texan clinical ethics, not to mention Chinese, German, and Italian clinical ethics. Health care ethics consultants have done so well because they provide useful quasi-legal advice and services. Matters have turned out quite differently from what the bioethics of the 1970s and early 1980s, with its Enlightenment aspirations, had expected.

In order to appreciate more fully where we find ourselves, the book returns to addressing our religious-cultural context. Chapter seven explores how the vast changes in mainline Western Christianity during the 19th and 20th centuries, and particularly in Roman Catholicism following Vatican II, led to the birth of the secular bioethics of the 1970s. To engage the language of Thomas Kuhn, because of Vatican II there was a paradigm change in how Roman Catholicism conceived of itself, along with its liturgical and ascetic life, as well as its academic theology. This paradigm change set aside a three-hundred-year-old medical moral manualist scholarly tradition, including the medical-moral manuals it had produced. This dramatic change created a new socio-moral environment that supported the appearance of the new secular bioethics. "Common Ground as Battleground: Seeking an Anchor in God" examines the idiosyncrasies of the Western Christianities that produced secular bioethics and established the tone and character of the culture wars within which contemporary bioethics emerged. This chapter further develops the picture of the cultural geography within which contemporary bioethics must be understood. Building on the account given in the first three chapters, this chapter looks at how in the late 20th and early 21st centuries much of dominant Western Christianity entered into a state of theological and moral transformation, if not chaos, setting the stage onto which the contemporary secular bioethics of the 1970s entered. Vatican II not only ended a centuries-old paradigm of medical-moral reflection, which had produced a considerable literature on medical ethics, but it produced a new medical ethics: the bioethics that was confected at Georgetown University. It is impossible to appreciate the situation within which bioethics is now located, absent a recognition of the foundational disputes and changes within Western Christianity that lie at the roots of the dominant culture of the 21st century. The statements of Pope Francis, including *Evangelii Gaudium* (Francis 2013), suggest that further developments are underway within Roman Catholic moral theology with implications for the general culture and the character of the culture wars. Roman

Catholicism appears to be moving to adopt a weak theology stance that will subtly demoralize its morality and bioethics of sexuality, reproduction, and end-of-life decision-making, while affirming a populist social justice of health care resource allocation. This chaos at the heart of Western Christianity, as well as its fragmentation into a plurality of sects, threatens to bring the very plausibility of Christianity and Christian bioethics into question. As this chapter explains, the way out lies in Orthodox Christianity, whose theology, moral norms, and bioethics are rooted in the Christianity of the first millennium: a Christianity unfragmented and without novel doctrines. To have access to a canonical God's-eye perspective, one will need a veridical direct experience of God, which experience is at the core of Orthodox Christian theology. The existence of Orthodox Christianity ensures that the moral and bioethical battles in the culture wars between Christianity and the dominant secular culture will continue, even after this dominant culture is fully after God.

The last chapter returns to the nature of morality and bioethics, once they are set within the horizon of the finite and the immanent. Hegel's post-religious and post-metaphysical view of secular culture has triumphed. Morality and bioethics cannot be what were once expected: canonical secular moral guideposts for behavior are unavailable. Rorty in a Hegelian key recognized the consequences of what has occurred, including the unjustifiability of "the Kantian vocabulary of 'inalienable rights' and 'the dignity of man'" (Rorty 1991, p. 198). What happens now? How will people behave when within the dominant secular culture it becomes clear that "there is no human dignity that is not derivative from the dignity of some specific community, and no appeal beyond the relative merits of various actual or proposed communities to impartial criteria which will help us weigh those merits" (Rorty 1991, p. 197). For secular thought, the character of morality, bioethics, medical professionalism, medical law, and the appreciation of reality is set fully within the dominant, completely immanent conceits of the day. These are, as Hegel recognized, not anchored in being or reason, but in the parochial, indeed ethnocentric "realities" and rationalities of diverse socio-historically-conditioned communities. The chapter closes by examining the latter-day secular celebration of this outcome by Alexander Kojéve and Francis Fukuyama in their recasting of morality (and therefore of bioethics) in terms of a humanity reduced to the desires of post-human animals.

We are left in a social context that may not be fully stable. We are confronted with the core concerns and passages of life: sexuality, reproduction, suffering, dying, and death. But there is no agreement about how properly to live, have sex, reproduce, and die. As we have seen, in the dominant secular culture, possible decisions in these areas are reduced to life- and death-style choices, with morality itself becoming only a particular macro life-style choice and the state to being merely a *modus vivendi*, a political life-style choice. Is a society with such a "weak" account of morality, bioethics, and political authority sustainable? Are such morality, bioethics, and political authority sufficient to the task of maintaining social stability and public governance? What happens when most realize that any particular secular morality or bioethics reflects only one among a plurality of clusters of intuitions nested in one among a plurality of freestanding moral accounts, each floating within the horizon of the finite and the immanent without any ultimate meaning? What happens when all secular moral commitments are recognized as merely contingent? What will things be like when the authority and legitimacy of the state are appreciated as no more than expressions of the state's hegemony of public propaganda, seduction, manipulation, and power? In a culture after God, where there is no legitimacy for the state other than being *pro tempore* better than civil strife, unrest, and/or civil war, will secular morality, bioethics, and public policy be able effectively to guide? Will the state be able to govern? Is a society after God actually governable over the long run? Is a society fully without God livable? And if so, in what sense? Who knows? God knows, these are very troubling questions. With these puzzles this book concludes, certain that traditional Christians will remain and with them the culture wars.

So we end where we began: looking at the place of morality and bioethics in the culture wars, encountering a secular morality and bioethics lacking any anchor in being or in a canonical moral rationality. We find bioethics as both an academic field and a clinical praxis embedded in a culture marked by rapid change, profound dispute, and without a point of ultimate orientation. The very sense of what it is to have a secular ethics that bioethics can engage or apply has been brought into question. The epistemological and metaphysical roots of contemporary morality and therefore of bioethics that many thought were available through an anchor in being or in moral rationality, turn out not to exist. Once one abandons God, once one attempts to live after God, as if all were without ultimate meaning, one is set adrift within the horizon of the finite and the immanent. Secular morality and therefore bioethics cannot be what many had presumed. This volume examines these complex and wide-ranging changes in the appreciation of what secular morality and its bioethics can be. It recognizes also that the substance of bioethics will still be known by traditional Christians to be anchored in the will of God. This knowledge will perpetuate the culture wars. The content and the significance of religious morality and bioethics contrast with that of secular morality and its bioethics. The conflicts will not abate. As this book shows, in this culture after God, God's powerful presence will endure in Orthodox Christianity.

Notes

[1]The moral diversity of medical ethics, bioethics, and medical law takes many forms. This diversity is illustrated *inter alia* by the different development, content, and significance of medical law and bioethics as they existed in the Soviet bloc, given a Marxist-Leninist justification and framework. Already in 1972 a conference had been held in the German Democratic Republic (October 1–4) addressing ethical problems in molecular biology (Geissler et al. 1974). For other examples of Marxist-Leninist bioethics, see Ehmann and Löther 1975; Syrnew and Tschikin 1975; Thom and Weise 1973; and Winter et al. 1979.

References

Beauchamp, Tom L. 2004. Does ethical theory have a future in bioethics? *Journal of Law, Medicine, and Ethics* 32: 209–217.

Beauchamp, Tom L. & James F. Childress. 1979. *Principles of Biomedical Ethics*. New York: Oxford University Press.

Daniels, Norman. 1985. *Just Health Care*. New York: Cambridge University Press.

Diogenes Laertius. 1979. Protagoras, in *Lives of Eminent Philosophers*, trans. R. D. Hicks. Cambridge, MA: Harvard.

Ehmann, Günter & Rolf Löther (eds.). 1975. *Sozialismus—Medizin—Persönlichkeit*. Berlin: Akademie für Ärztliche Fortbildung der Deutschen Demokratischen Republik.

Francis, Pope. 2013. *Evangelii Gaudium*. Vatican City: Vatican Press.

Geissler, E., A. Kosing, H. Ley, & W. Scheler (eds.). 1974. *Philosophische und ethische Probleme der Molekularbiologie*. Berlin: Akademie Verlag.

Owen, J. Judd. 2001. *Religion and the Demise of Liberal Rationalism*. Chicago: University of Chicago Press.

Rawls, John. 1985. Justice as fairness: Political not metaphysical, *Philosophy and Public Affairs* 14.5 (Summer): 223–251.

Rawls, John. 1971. *A Theory of Justice*. Cambridge, MA: Harvard University Press.

Reich, Warren. 1994. The word "bioethics": Its birth and the legacies of those who shaped its meaning, *Kennedy Institute of Ethics Journal* 4: 319–336.

Rorty, Richard. 1991. *Objectivity, Relativism, and Truth*. New York: Cambridge University Press.

Rorty, Richard. 1989. *Contingency, Irony, and Solidarity*. New York: Cambridge University Press.

Syrnew, W. M. & S. J. Tschikin. 1973. *Krankheit Arzt und Dialektik*, trans. H. Breyer. Berlin: Verlag Volk und Gesundheit.

Thom, Achim & Klaus Weise. 1973. *Medizin und Weltanschauung*. Leipzig: Urania-Verlag.

Winter, Kurt, Alfred Keck, Rolf Löther, & Horst Spaa (eds.). 1979. *Philosophische Schriften von Marx, Engels und Lenin und ihre Bedeutung für die Medizin heute*. Jena: Gustav Fischer Verlag.

CHAPTER ONE

Living in the Ruins of Christendom[1]

I. Reality, Morality, and Bioethics after God[2]

Christendom has fallen. What it built has been broken. It is more than in ruins. Stone no longer lies upon stone. A new orthodoxy has been established, and it is secular. We have entered an age resolutely set "after God." The contemporary dominant culture[3] of the West is committed to acting as if God did not exist. The implications of this culture without God are vast. They include, as we shall see, morality and bioethics being rendered into micro life-style choices, the loss of the authority of the moral point of view, and the loss of the moral legitimacy of the state, leaving the state as a mere *modus vivendi*. Morality, bioethics, and political authority within this new culture generally need to be thoroughly reconsidered. Without a God's-eye perspective, without an ultimate point of moral orientation, meaning, and enforcement of morality, what once seemed so secure is set adrift. Secular claims for morality, bioethics, and political authority can now rest only on particular clusters of intuitions and practices that constitute more or less coherent freestanding positions supported by particular narratives floating within the horizon of the finite and the immanent without any anchor in being. Much, if not most, of what had been taken for granted about morality, bioethics, and political authority is left unsecured. The very meaning of morality and bioethics must be critically reassessed.

We are in radically new cultural and moral territory. As Thomas Nagel realized, the differences between recognizing or failing to recognize God are dramatic. "If there were a god who was responsible for the existence of the universe and our place in it, the sense of everything would depend on him, but if there is no god, there is nothing by reference to which the universe can either have or lack sense" (Nagel 2010, p. 7). The full implications of a loss of a God's-eye perspective are only now becoming clear. Never before has there been a large-scale, politically established culture that explicitly acted as if God did not exist, as if all were without ultimate meaning. No culture like this existed before the 20th century. Even the First French Republic (22 September 1792–1801) on the 7th of May (18 Floréal) 1794 under Maximilien Robespierre forbade atheism and established *le culte de l'Être supreme*. The contemporary dominant secular post-Christian culture, including that of the European Union and the United States, has taken up, albeit in softer agnostic forms, the atheist commitments of the October Revolution (26 October 1917, 7 November new style). This secular culture not only removes public mention of Christ, but it also removes God from the public space. To clear the ruins of Christendom, there is to be a thorough exorcism by the secular culture of any hint of ultimate meaning.

The now-dominant culture eschews any point of transcendent orientation. Officially, all is approached as if there were no ultimate significance. All is to be regarded as if ultimately coming from nowhere, going nowhere, and for no enduring purpose. Within the now-dominant secular culture, one is to approach morality, bioethics, law, public policy, and ordinary life guided by an atheistic, or at least an agnostic, methodological postulate. That is, one acts according to the postulate that God does not exist. The public forum, as well as discourse within the public space, has been relocated fully within the horizon of the finite and the immanent, so that all mention of the transcendent is ruled out of order. A new fabric of public cultural reality now dominates. The recognition of sin has been erased from the public square. Any recognition of God has been erased. This volume explores this radically new cultural territory and its implications for morality, bioethics, and political authority.

Now I must attempt to forestall at least some possible misreadings of this volume. In recognizing the recent watershed change in the character of the dominant culture due to its loss of a God's-eye perspective, I am not claiming that, before this change, there was cultural unanimity, uniformity, or agreement. Pluralism has always characterized the fallen human condition. I am not claiming that there was no great sin. However, without a recognition of sin, repentance is now impossible. What is new is that the dominant culture, that culture established at law and in public policy, is now secular in the radical sense of being after God. Moreover, this dominant, now-secular culture is being confronted with a recognition of its post-modern character: that its ethics and bioethics have no ultimate anchor and are from the perspective of sound rational argument plural nouns. This intractable pluralism has always been a part of the fallen human condition. However, the Western moral-philosophical project, as we will see, was framed by an unfounded faith that this was not the case, that secular rationality could establish *the* canonical ethics and bioethics. This faith in secular rationality induced many, if not most, to ignore the intractability of secular moral and bioethical pluralism. Post-modernity involves the recognition of a truth modernity sought to deny: there is no canonical secular moral rationality or vision. This book explores the historical roots and the implications of this recognition of the ultimate groundlessness of the ethics and bioethics of the dominant secular culture. It is as if one had awakened one morning in a second-floor apartment and found there was no first floor, while many living in the other apartments were firm in holding that this did not matter. Again, this is not to deny that the world in the past was replete with agnostics and atheists. However, they did not define the dominant culture.

A world explicitly without a God's-eye perspective constitutes a novum in a way that some post-modernists such as Stanley Fish (1938–) will not fully admit. He claims, for example, that

> the unavailability of an absolutely objective vantage point, of a god's eye view, doesn't take anything away from us. If, as postmodernists sometimes assert, objective standards of a publicly verifiable kind are unavailable, they are so only in the sense that they have always been unavailable (this is not, in other words, a condition post-modernism has caused), and we have always managed to get along without them, doing a great many things, despite the fact that we might be unable to shore them up in accordance with the most rigorous philosophical demands (Fish 2008, p. 140).

Pace Fish, what constitutes post-modernity is not intractable moral pluralism or the absence in secular culture of a rationally justifiable God's-eye view (as Fish underscores, such has always been the case), but the recognition of this intractability and of the absence of any rationally justified secular ultimate meaning. Fish fails to appreciate that in the dominant secular culture we were able to "manage", as he puts it, by embracing a position similar to that of Immanuel Kant's (1724–1804), that is, by acting as if God existed (*Critique of Pure Reason* A685=B713f) and/or by embracing the equivalent of Kant's practical moral postulates of God and immortality (*Critique of Practical Reason* AK V.133), or at least by not frankly facing the consequences of being "after God."[4] It is the position taken by Marcello Pera, Pope Benedict XVI's agnostic friend who invites us "to act *velut si Deus daretus*, as if God existed" (Pera 2008, p. 160). However, once morality and bioethics are explicitly set within a reality widely regarded as ultimately meaningless, the character of morality and political legitimacy changes substantially. Morality and bioethics are demoralized and deflated.

The character of the dominant secular culture is so altered after the recognition of the absence of foundations that even Richard Rorty admits that liberal moral and constitutional commitments are merely a function of a particular ethnocentrism. He hopes nevertheless that his ethnocentrism can prevail by being open

> to encounters with other actual and possible cultures, and to make this openness central to its self-image. This culture is an *ethnos* which prides itself on its suspicion of ethnocentrism—on its ability to increase the freedom and openness of encounters, rather than on its possession of truth (Rorty 1991, p. 2).

An ethnocentrism remains an ethnocentrism. Given Rorty's view of morality, the force of his "strategy" rests on empirical socio-political claims regarding the strategy's promised future success. However, the strategy does nothing to erase the consequences of the loss for morality and political legitimacy of any ultimate anchor and meaning. One should also note that these observations regarding the loss of a God's-eye perspective do not involve a claim that the content of all or even most theologically anchored moralities and bioethics is better than that of the morality or bioethics framed apart from a God's-eye perspective (this volume defends only the norms of Orthodox Christianity). The claim is quite different. The claim is that, *contra* Stanley Fish, if one faces what it means to be without a God's-eye perspective, then the meaning of morality, bioethics, and political legitimacy is radically altered, in the sense of being demoralized and deflated. Moreover, the dominant secular culture is now beginning to face the consequences of being "after God." The next seven chapters develop and defend this claim.

This book is not an autobiography. However, in this chapter and at the beginning of the next, the arguments and analyses are located with reference to some events in my life and the beginning of contemporary bioethics. This is not done because these events have any importance in themselves, but in order more concretely to situate the arguments. In part, this is meant in an illustrative fashion to shed an introductory light on the immense cultural changes of the latter part of the 20th century, which are a focus of this volume. This is also done in order to avoid what might otherwise appear to be an unbridgeable divide between my early work and my later work, differences that have posed a serious and unintended puzzle for some readers.[5] In particular, autobiographical reflections are used to locate the arguments developed in *The Foundations of Bioethics* (Engelhardt 1986, 1996a) in terms of what I argue in subsequent work (Engelhardt 2000).

Previous works examined why sound rational argument cannot supply canonical foundations for a rationally justified secular morality or secular bioethics (Engelhardt 1986, 1991a, 1996a). However, I have never comprehensively addressed how this state of affairs is tied to the now-dominant secular culture's severance from God, although the question was in the background of *The Foundations of Bioethics* and *Bioethics and Secular Humanism*. Even *Viaggi in Italia: Saggi di bioetica* (Engelhardt 2011a) addresses only piecemeal and tangentially what it means to live without God, without ultimate meaning. None of these volumes lays out the full enormity of the cultural changes that we face, given the dominant culture's commitment to acting as if God did not exist, as if all were ultimately surd. Nor did I sufficiently address the roots of this now-dominant secular culture, as well as why, cut loose from a recognition of God, the establishment of atheism or at least agnosticism constitutes such a startling and devastating cultural novum.

This present volume shoulders these tasks. It explores the now-dominant secular culture's severance from God: its foundations (and lack thereof) and its implications of its forsaking God for morality, bioethics, public policy, law, and political structures. This volume shows why in the absence of a God's-eye perspective there is a demoralization and deflation of morality and bioethics, along with a delegitimization of the state. This volume also looks at how this secular culture is in tension with traditional Christianity,[6] and why, when a culture's morality and bioethics are after God, they are radically different from a culture, morality, and bioethics organized around an experience of ultimate meaning. Finally, this volume asks if this new culture's morality, bioethics, and political structure are stable and sustainable. Do we face a major crisis in the secular culture with important implications for how we can understand bioethics? Can the project of morality with bioethics continue without foundations, while prescinding from ultimate meaning? Is society sustainable when set fully within the horizon of the finite and the immanent? This book ends with this puzzle.

II. Meine italienischen Reisen: The Road that Led to New Rome[7]

This work is tied to Italy. It was in Italy in the 1980s that I finally and fully faced the implications of a life-world without God. More particularly, the core of this volume, an ancestor of which appeared in Italian (Engelhardt 2014), grew out of a series of six lectures on bioethics delivered in Italy in 2012 from January 30 in Milan to February 6 in Naples, with presentations in Turin on January 31, in Lecce on February 1, and two presentations in Naples on February 3. These lectures followed the publication of *Viaggi in Italia: Saggi di bioetica*, a volume of papers on bioethics delivered in Italy or published in Italian (Engelhardt 2011a). *Viaggi* presents some twenty years of scholarly connections with Italy, from 1991 through 2010. This present volume (and all my past work) is also in many ways indirectly tied to Italy. Anyone who has been a Roman Catholic has been connected at least implicitly with Italy. With a Roman pontiff and his administrative offices claiming universal jurisdiction, the perspective of Rome and Italy touches everything Roman Catholic. In addition, I have from my youth had many particular and pleasant connections with Italy.[8]

Public conversations with Italian scholars about bioethics began with a conference held in Milan on November 8–10, 1991, which had a major focus on the Italian translation of the first edition of *The Foundations of Bioethics* (1991b). Because the volume denied that moral philosophy could by sound rational argument severed from God identify universal canonical content-full bioethical and moral norms, it was incompatible with Roman Catholic views of the capacities of moral philosophy. *The Foundations* was at a white-hot point of collision between a Roman Catholic and a post-Christian Italy so that it engendered a controversy that reached into the public media. With the pope and the curia in Rome, the capital of a secular republic, disputes about the proper character of Italian mores, law, bioethics, and public policy carry theological implications. *The Foundations* had become enmeshed in these debates. These public scholarly controversies and the discussions they engendered were driven by an intimation of what it might mean to live and do bioethics "after God."

Private discussions in Italy and elsewhere in Europe preceded these public lectures and debates. They forced me to recognize that public morality and bioethics had been severed from their taken-for-granted moorings. At the time I was still Roman Catholic, indeed a practicing Roman Catholic increasingly attending Tridentine Latin masses whenever possible. Although my family and I were never officially associated with the Society of St. Pius X, the Society provided masses at least in part anchored in tradition and in a commitment to Roman Catholic orthopraxis in contrast to the prevailing liturgical and theological chaos (Hull 2010). From 1984 to 1990, in association with the Steering Committee of the Study Group of Bioethics of the International Federation of Catholic Universities, with which I was involved from 1984 and officially a member from 1987 to 1990, I took part in discussions on bioethics and moral theory with Roman Catholic scholars, including the late Carlo Cardinal Martini of Milan (1927–2012). I was for the first time immersed in the intellectual culture and controversies of Roman Catholicism, bringing me into contact with theologians such as Bruno Schüller of Münster (1925–2006), Klaus Demmer of Rome (1931–), and John Mahoney, S.J., of London (1931–), as well as the Catalan bioethicist Francesc Abel, S.J. (1933–2011) and the bioethicist Paul Schotsmans (1950–). As a result of these conversations, I was forced to face the question of what it meant to be a Christian, even what it meant to acknowledge the existence of God.

Cardinal Martini was a warm, personable, dynamic, and charming intellectual who wished to be pope. Because the time of the next papal election is unknown (unless as in the Middle Ages one has planned to accelerate a pontiff's appearance before the dread judgment seat of Christ, or bring the reigning pope to retire), one is forced to proceed with circumspection and patience.[9] Martini was cautious and in public spoke with discretion. I found myself engaged by, and engaging in, well-informed discussions about Roman Catholicism, European culture, morality, bioethics, and the remnants of Christendom. He had a particular interest in bioethics and health care policy. At times the possibilities were discussed for significantly liberalizing Roman Catholicism beyond what had been realized by Vatican II. The airs of aggiornamento were still blowing through the halls of theological reflection in ways that were often disorienting for clerics, theologians, and the laity.[10] Cardinal Martini himself wished to recast Roman Catholicism in a much more post-traditional mode.[11] During these discussions with Cardinal Martini and those with whom I had become associated, remarkably little to no attention was directed to the collapse of Western Christianity, in particular of Roman Catholicism, that had occurred since Vatican II. There was no discussion of whether the aggiornamento that had just occurred lay at the roots of clergy and congregants deserting Roman Catholicism. Discussions with the Steering Committee took place not only in Milan and Rome, but also in Barcelona, Maastricht, and Vienna. Although focused on Roman Catholic bioethics, these conversations usually also involved general matters of theology. They touched on Western culture generally, which in the 1980s still bore salient marks of Roman Catholicism.[12] These meetings proceeded against the backdrop of foundational theological reflections that raised challenging questions about the nature of theology and its relationship to philosophy but did not directly confront the dramatic decline of mainline Christianity. They never faced the unjustifiable moral-philosophical foundation supposedly undergirding the phenomenon of bioethics.

I was confronted with puzzles. They were foundational puzzles about the roots of bioethics and of morality generally. Prominent among these questions were what it means to acknowledge the existence of God, and what difference the acknowledgement of God does or should make in how one lives one's life. I was also brought to face the issue as to which church is the Church of the Apostles and the Fathers. For that matter, there was the puzzle of how a religion that arose in Palestine and was guided by Councils held in Constantinople and the Near East ever became Western Christianity. As I reflected, it became ever clearer that Roman Catholicism had created a new and distinct theological and liturgical project as it emerged from Orthodox Christianity and became a separate denomination in stages between the 9th and the 13th centuries. In the process, it had wedded itself to the Greek moral-philosophical project—from the 5th century before Christ—of rationally grounding morality and eventually bioethics. Indeed, it became evident to me that Roman Catholicism was not the Church of the Apostles and the Fathers, but instead a Western religion shaped by the cultural concerns that came to dominate Western Europe toward the end of the first millennium and the beginning of the second millennium. It also became clear that the West had recast what is involved in the traditional Christian pursuit of theology.

Within Western Christian theology, God was regarded ever more as a philosophical idea, rather than the Person of the Father, Who begets the Son, and from Whom alone the Holy Spirit proceeds. God as the most personal of all was obscured through a theology with a robust philosophical overlay that rendered the theological approach to God primarily one of scholarship, not of prayerful ascetical struggle. My discussions in association with the Steering Committee about the foundations of bioethics had forced me to examine, indeed often for the first time seriously to consider, the nature of Christian theology, worship, and asceticism. These discussions also disclosed the unsecured character of the moral-philosophical claims framing the phenomenon of bioethics.

These reflections came to a head when I was a Fellow at the Institute for Advanced Studies in West Berlin (1988–1989), finishing a volume that examined secular bioethics and secular humanism, but that also at least tangentially explored the history of Western Christianity (Engelhardt 1991a). I had the opportunity of extended conversations concerning the history of early Christianity with Prof. Martin Hengel (1926–2009), who was also a Fellow that year and was completing a book on St. John's Gospel (Hengel 1989).[13] Over the Christmas break I had gone with my family to the University of Istanbul and Marmara University to give lectures. Through grace, not through any clear choice of mine, I was brought to the source of all Christianity, the Christianity that is the Church of the Councils: the Orthodox Church. With my wife and two younger daughters, I took a taxi across Constantinople from the Sheraton in Beşiktas via the Galatea Bridge, over the Golden Horn to the "Romans." After all, in Istanbul it is the "Romans" (i.e., the Orthodox) who are the local Christians, the original *Rōmaíoi*, the old Roman citizens. They are those who are true to the second

Rome; they are Chalcedonians, non-monophysites. In that taxi that morning, we were going home at last to the ancient Roman Catholics. The result was that on Christmas, 1988, we stood in the Cathedral of St. George in the Phanar of Constantinople at our first Orthodox Liturgy, with Demetrios I, the Ecumenical Patriarch, the successor of St. Peter, presiding. Unwittingly, my involvement with the International Study Group on Bioethics and with Cardinal Martini had sent us on a journey that was, and indeed still is, inconceivable.[14]

After that Christmas, I was forced to reconsider everything. I resigned from the Steering Committee of the Study Group of Bioethics and from Roman Catholicism in September, 1990, at a meeting in Maastricht, an old Roman city, standing at that moment on a stone floor that had been laid in the 9th century when the West was still Orthodox. The symbolic force was quite clear. I was in the remnants of a structure dating from the time of united Christianity, both East and West. As I tendered my resignation, I dimly recognized the unity that had once existed. Even so, I could barely envisage my Great Saturday baptism that would follow in 1991. I had no clear understanding until the beginning of Lent, 1991, about what it was to convert. And I am still learning.

As of that September, 1990, I had begun in full earnest my journey from Old Rome to New Rome, from the Vatican to Constantinople, from Roman Catholicism to Orthodoxy (Engelhardt 2012a). I was brought from a philosophically structured theology to the recognition of the 4th-century adage that "if you are a theologian, you will pray truly. And if you pray truly, you are a theologian" (Evagrios 1988, vol. 1, p. 62). I was confronted with the most disturbing truth for an intellectual, namely, that good arguments and well-crafted books do not save; only true repentance, achieved through grace in a ceaseless prayer of repentance, can bring one to salvation. I came to appreciate theology anew, especially that theology is not merely an academic undertaking, but rather that in the strict sense theology involves an encounter with God. My reflections leading to this philosophical and theological aporia had been greatly enriched by my discussions, indeed debates, with Italian and other Roman Catholic scholars. Most importantly, they helped me to take God and Christianity seriously. They forced me to consider everything anew, including bioethics. To all of these, my former colleagues, my debt is eternal. My debt is particularly profound to a marvelous Catalan, the Jesuit Francesc Abel (1933–2011), who, along with John Collins Harvey, had persuaded me to join the Steering Committee.

To my amazement, on Great Saturday in 1991 in Texas, and in a monastery no less, I resolved to repent from a life of profound self-love and many other grievous sins, including the besetting sin of most philosophers, namely, the unfounded presumption that through my own philosophical reflection I could argue my way to the right norms for life and the true goals of human existence. On that day my daughters Christina and Dorothea followed me in baptism. Then the hieromonk sacramentally married me to Susan, who had been my wife for twenty-five years. On Pascha in 1991 I found myself in the Church from which Roman Catholicism itself had departed nearly a millennium beforehand. I was in a place unlike any place I had been before. I had not even imagined that this place existed. Everything had changed. All that had taken place had led me to a turning point, to an encounter through Orthodoxy with holiness. In a half century of my life, I had met good people, indeed some very good people, but before I came to Orthodoxy I had never met holy people. I had never encountered holiness. The awesomeness, the joyous fear of such encounters brought me to write *The Foundations of Christian Bioethics* (Engelhardt 2000). As a scholar, I was forced to examine everything anew.[15] I saw bioethics from what was a radically new perspective. I had come to encounter and to concede a highly politically incorrect truth: the one, holy, catholic, and apostolic Church is Orthodox Christianity.

III. Roman Catholicism, the Moral-Philosophical Project, and Bioethics

The Foundations of Christian Bioethics (2000, 2003, 2005, and 2007) addresses issues in morality, political theory, and bioethics that are raised but cannot be adequately treated within the limits of secular thought. *The Foundations of Christian Bioethics* lays out the character of moral and bioethical norms grounded in God, the moral norms that traditional Christians share as moral friends.[16] In different ways, *The Foundations of Bioethics* and *The Foundations of Christian Bioethics* show that the inabilities of a secular morality and a secular bioethics are the result of not possessing a God's-eye perspective. This involves a cardinal paradox. In order to establish a canonical morality and bioethics, one needs a canonical perspective, not just one moral perspective among a plurality of moral perspectives. A canonical secular view of human flourishing and of proper human conduct cannot adequately be envisaged without reference to God. This is not a religious point, but a philosophical one with broad bioethical implications. One needs a definitive, socially and historically unconditioned moral perspective, not just one among a multiplicity of webs of moral intuitions affirmed by a particular moral narrative floating within the horizon of the finite and the immanent. One needs a moral perspective that is not one among a multiplicity of socio-historically constituted perspectives. A secular morality thus presupposes what it cannot have: the objectivity of a God's-eye perspective.

In the early third millennium, two books took shape. One, *Allocating Scarce Medical Resources: Roman Catholic Perspectives* (Engelhardt & Cherry 2002), was underwritten through the generous aid of a foundation that had supported the Steering Committee of the International Study Group of Bioethics of the International Federation of Catholic Universities. It subvened meetings held in Schaan, Liechtenstein (August 30–September 1, 1997), Houston, Texas (February 7–10 and October 24–27, 1998), and near Dublin, Ireland (May 13–16, 1999). Even though I was an apostate from Roman Catholicism, the foundation nevertheless generously subvened this major research project in bioethics, because I was willing to endorse traditional Christian morality and to recognize that Christ had risen from the dead. By the time the book was published, my co-editor had converted as well. This foundation also supported my role in establishing the Southeast Asian Center for Bioethics, University of Santo Tomas, Manila, Philippines (site visits March 22–27, 1987, and August 8–20, 1989, with contact continuing until October, 1993), also enabling me to conduct intensive courses for Roman Catholic scholars from the Philippines, India, Indonesia, Brazil, and Europe (May 10–29, 1987, May 29–June 5, 1990, July 29–August 9, 1991, and May 17–28, 1993). The foundation's generous help remained strong for my work for a number of years before and after my conversion. Among other things, these contacts allowed me to have a better appreciation of the difficulties besetting Roman Catholicism. Orthodox Jewish colleagues, who participated in some of the conferences, were both amazed and disheartened by what they encountered. At one meeting in Barcelona in the early 1990s, a Jewish scholar began to groan.

The organizers asked if he were all right. He said he was, but they were not, and that they should take some minimal advice from a grandson of the Pharisees, namely: Do not throw away all God's commands! The meetings also confirmed through the international scholars who participated that bioethics is intractably plural (Alora & Lumitao 2001).

The second volume, *Global Bioethics: The Collapse of Consensus* (Engelhardt 2006b), explicitly examined the possibility of a universal morality. The book took shape with the aid and support of Liberty Fund, drawing participants from America, Europe, and the Pacific Rim, for meetings held in Houston, Texas (October 2001), Palermo, Sicily (January 2003), and near Dublin, Ireland (June 2004). The discussions at the meeting in Sicily were especially fruitful, laying bare the limits of the moral-philosophical project. Italy thus again played an important role. So did an Italian Brazilian intellectual, Fr. Leo Pessini, who by securing a Portuguese translation of *Global Bioethics* (Engelhardt 2012b) led to my further encounters in Brazil and Portugal with the collapse of the façade of a global morality and a global bioethics. All over, there were signs of a cultural earthquake. After the publication of *The Foundations of Christian Bioethics* (Engelhardt 2000) and Iltis and Cherry's study of this work (Iltis & Cherry 2010) in Romanian (Engelhardt 2005; Iltis & Cherry 2011), with subsequent honorary doctorates from the University of Medicine and Pharmacy "Gr. T. Popa" in Iasi on November 9, 2005, and from the faculty of theology of "1 Decembrie 1918" University of Alba Iulia on May 6, 2011, I had come fully home to Orthodoxy, which had no illusions regarding the moral-philosophical project. These events to some extent said grace over the second edition of *The Foundations of Bioethics* (Engelhardt 1996a). I now saw bioethics from outside of the Western moral-philosophical project.

Viaggi in Italia (2011a) asks, focusing on bioethics, whether generally recognizable moral and political authority makes sense after an acknowledgement of God's existence is lost. The volume confronts the consequent loss of a hoped-for foundation for bioethics, morality, and political authority in sound rational argument. From Aristotle through Kant, an appeal to a God's-eye perspective had been evoked, which promised an unconditioned point of reference. In the now-dominant secular culture, all has changed and foundations are gone. Moral-philosophical reflection could not secure an unconditional point of reference. *Viaggi* addresses the core philosophical difficulties underlying the capacities, or rather incapacities, of secular moral reflection to secure foundations for its claims and the bioethics it promised. However, *Viaggi* does not sufficiently address the remarkable change in the dominant culture of the West as a result of its becoming a culture after God. The full force of the loss of ultimate meaning, of transcendent orientation, still remained to be spelled out. Yet, it is this cultural novum that defines the now-dominant secular public mores, secular bioethics, public policy, law, and the state. It is the focus of this present volume.

In his preface to *Viaggi*, Maurizio Mori notes that my work is in tension with the commitments of Roman Catholicism, because it is the defender of a supposedly global ethics and bioethics secured through sound rational argument (Mori 2011). In the late 1980s as I was about to be appointed to the Steering Committee, I was denounced for heresy by a person I knew well. He was a prominent American Roman Catholic bioethicist who did not want me to have any influence on the Steering Committee, because he considered me (falsely) to be much more post-traditional than he. The accusations were discounted when I responded to a committee appointed to review the issue, and which had apparently been preselected to vindicate me. I explained that I understood *The Foundations of Bioethics* (1986), and my work in general, to have explored *only* that which can be known by reason unaided by grace. I presumed that my defense was accepted not because of its merits (my response was not sufficient within the framework of Roman Catholicism and Roman Catholic bioethics), but because those backing me took me to be an extreme theological liberal. They wanted me for what they held to be my liberal theological, moral-philosophical, and bioethical perspective, which they saw confirmed *inter alia* by my role as chairman of the Advisory Panel "Infertility: Medical and Social Choices" of the Office of Technology Assessment of the United States Congress (1986–1989). My supporters had mistaken my recognition of the incapacities of moral philosophy for a commitment to recast moral theology, along with traditional Roman Catholic bioethics. Of course, my position was threatening because without moral philosophy Roman Catholic moral theology and bioethics collapse.

My views of the inadequacy of moral philosophy were by no means a rebirth of the 13th-century view of the double truths of philosophy and theology, but a judgment of the inadequacy of the claims of secular reason. In defense, I pointed out that *The Foundations* stated:

> The differences between the conclusions in this volume and those offered by traditional natural law theory, such as that of St. Thomas Aquinas, will lie in the limitations of reason that this volume will acknowledge. If one cannot establish through reason alone the great body of Judeo-Christian precepts, there will be, as we shall see, a sharp contrast between secular ethics and the ethics of particular moral communities that rely on special traditions or special revelations. The gulf between church and state will widen, and one will find oneself living a moral life within two complementary but distinct moral perspectives (Engelhardt 1986, p. 13).

My position rested on a recognition of the radical limitations of moral philosophy. In a footnote I had added:

> Classically, there was a distinction made between what can be concluded by natural reason, by reason unaided by grace and revelation, and what can be known through revelation. As St. Thomas stated, "It was therefore necessary that, besides the philosophical disciplines investigated by reason, there should be a sacred doctrine by way of revelation" (*Summa Theologica* I, art. 1. *The Basic Writings of Saint Thomas Aquinas*, Anton C. Pegis (ed.), vol. 1 (New York: Random House, 1945), p. 6 (Engelhardt 1986, p. 15).

However, Roman Catholicism does not recognize such radical limitations on moral philosophy. By the late 20th century, the Roman Catholic faith in reason had if anything become more desperate in its attempts to secure bioethics and health care policy positions by reason alone. My defense was no longer, and actually had never been, sufficient for Roman Catholicism. I was again denounced after a presentation in Hannover, Germany, at the Forschungsinstitut für Philosophie on the 13th of July, 1989. But by the time this came to be a problem, the matter was moot. I was on the way to becoming Orthodox.

    With the appearance of the Italian translation of the first edition of *Foundations of Bioethics* (Engelhardt 1991b),[17] the distinction I offered between what could be established through philosophical reason and what theology supplies was not only not accepted, but had become provocative, even though I was no longer Roman Catholic. On this point, one should underscore again that the Orthodox and the Roman Catholics are separated *inter alia* not just by incompatible understandings of theology, indeed of reality and morality, but of the foundations of bioethics as well. The limits to moral philosophy that I described made perfect sense to the Orthodox but were repudiated by Roman Catholics. My work received a condemnation in *La Civiltà Cattolica* (Editorial 1992). Some Roman Catholic critics even regarded *The Foundations of Bioethics* as taking a utilitarian position, *mirabile factu*, similar to that of Peter Singer (Mori 2011, p. 12). My Italian Roman Catholic critics did not realize, or if they did realize, they did not take seriously, that I had embraced what should have been characterized by them as a Christian, albeit from their perspective a heretical Christian, position. I had in fact become an apostate—not for having abandoned Christianity, but for having embraced through baptism the Christianity of the Fathers. In any event, I was surely not a utilitarian, as I had been described by Elio Cardinal Sgreccia, as well as by others.[18]

For many Roman Catholics, it was hard to imagine that, while still remaining a traditional Christian, one could reject moral philosophy's project of establishing through discursive moral reasoning objective moral truths along with the Roman Catholic account of natural law, bioethics, and social justice. For them, the bond between faith and reason, which forged medieval Christianity, creating Roman Catholicism, was still strong enough to fashion a life-world within which my views were impossible. Our points of reference were radically different. Their "traditional" Christianity is a Christianity born of the Western European medieval synthesis, not the Christianity of the first centuries. As a consequence, St. Basil and St. Gregory the Theologian look exotic to Roman Catholics, while Thomas Aquinas, at least until recently, was taken for granted as "current." Even dissident Roman Catholic theologians tend to employ discursive philosophy as core to their theology and surely live in a paradigm startlingly apart from Orthodox Christians. Even if the moral-philosophical project has collapsed, and with it Roman Catholic moral theology and bioethics, this bad news has not yet arrived for most Roman Catholics.

As clear as yesterday, I can remember sitting with a distinguished, fairly liberal Roman Catholic theologian at Leahy's Bar in the Morris Inn at Notre Dame after having given the 1992 Clarke Lecture on March 20th, "The Moral

Inevitability of a Two-Tier Health Care System" (Engelhardt 2008). She was aghast at my presentation. It was not simply that she disagreed with the conclusions, and she surely did disagree, for among other things my presentation was critical of the Roman Catholic vision of social justice and bioethics. More fundamentally, the lecture was framed in terms of the failure of moral philosophy to deliver a canonical secular account of the proper allocation of medical resources, a failure rooted in the false expectations of the medieval moral-philosophical synthesis. This failure of the moral-philosophical project seemed to her to be impossible, because moral philosophy, especially in various forms of new natural-law theory that are cut free of an experience of the transcendent God,[19] had become one with Roman Catholicism (Finnis 1980 and 1983; Grisez 1965). To bring into question the moral-philosophical project was to bring into question the moral viewpoint Roman Catholicism had created.

Given the circumstance that moral philosophy cannot establish canonical moral norms, including canonical secular norms for justice in health care, and given that in secular moral terms the state cannot be shown to be more than a *modus vivendi*, we do not possess a canonical secular account of justice that can require a single one-tier system from which one could be morally obliged not to buy out by purchasing better basic health care (Engelhardt 1986). When she finally realized that I did not credit Roman Catholicism's account of natural law's or moral philosophy's supposed capacities to establish a canonical content-full moral understanding of justice in health care, in exasperation she accused me of being an atheist, not of being a fideist, but an atheist.[20] Although she knew I had converted to Orthodox Christianity, for her it was inconceivable that one could be a Christian, indeed a believer, without recognizing the claims of moral philosophy that undergird Roman Catholicism. Again, this reaction is fully understandable. In 1992 we were living in entirely different life-worlds framed by radically different paradigms. I had rejected the moral-philosophical paradigm that has fashioned Roman Catholicism and been at the roots of Western Christian theology and culture for a millennium. Instead, I had embraced the paradigm within which the Christianity of the first centuries lived and within which Orthodox Christianity still lives. I had entered a life-world that Western Christians had not enjoyed for a thousand years. Everything, including bioethics, looked different.

IV. The World after God

This sliver of an autobiography is meant concretely to introduce how the complex cultural transformations that resulted from the collapse of Christendom and from the recognition of the future of the Western moral-philosophical project framed the contemporary dominant culture.[21] The recognition of the failure of the Western moral-philosophical project is a cultural event as momentous as the Renaissance and the Reformation. The aspiration had been to provide the modern secular state with a secular moral authority secured by reason through philosophical arguments that could be recognized by all persons as conclusive. The secular state would then enjoy a canonical moral authority, as well as a canonical account of secular constitutionalism. The faith in moral philosophy that lies at the roots of Roman Catholicism also lies at the roots of contemporary secularism. As Sajó asserts, "The sovereignty of a people exercising its faculty of reasoning is the essence of the constitutionalism that necessitates secularism" (Sajó 2008, p. 621). Moreover, all would be shown to be members of one, universal, rationally justified, moral community. This undertaking promised a political and canonical moral and bioethical vision of commonly justifiable values, human dignity, and human rights that could be expressed in terms recognizable as rationally binding on all. This project, not to mention the Western Christian project of grounding theology in philosophy, has proved to be without general rational justification. The full force of what has occurred has not yet been adequately appreciated. Even now, there still remain powerful but unfounded philosophical expectations regarding the existence of a generally secularly justifiable morality, bioethics, and political authority that persist as remnants from the *via antiqua* of the Western Christian Middle Ages.[22]

Intellectually, the break from Christendom and from an orientation toward the God of the Christians had been affirmed with the Enlightenment, yet the illusion that moral philosophy can deliver on its promises of a canonical morality and bioethics after God still lingers on. Enough cultural residue remains from Western Christendom and the Enlightenment that many people, bioethicists included, do not yet see how starkly different life is once it is lived after God, after metaphysics, and after foundations. The demoralization and deflation of morality and bioethics, as well as the delegitimization of political authority deprived of a God's-eye perspective, are only beginning adequately to be recognized. This volume explores the collapse of the moral-philosophical illusion and its consequences for bioethics. Most significant is the severance of morality, bioethics, and state authority from any hint of ultimate meaning. Because the contemporary dominant secular culture is after God, secular moral reflection must approach everything as if it came from nowhere, were going nowhere, and existed for no ultimate purpose. The point is not simply that in a godless universe there is no necessary retribution for immense, unrepented-for acts of evil. More fundamentally, all in the end is simply ultimately meaningless. At various levels, many already appreciate some of the implications of the absence of foundations for the now-dominant secular culture. As Judd Owen observes:[23]

> Today, belief in the comprehensive philosophic teaching of the Enlightenment appears to lie in ruins, and few hope that any other comprehensive philosophy could successfully replace it. This despair is, to a considerable extent, due to a radical critique of reason as such (Owen 2001, p. 1).

The full and consummate force of this surdness is still adequately to be gauged and acknowledged. This volume takes a step in that direction. It explores the geography and implications of this quite new moral, bioethical, and political terrain in all its God-forsakenness.

Even though Christendom has fallen and lies in ruins, Christianity still has its partisans living in its rubble, struggling to maintain the integrity of Christian subcultures. They are loyal to norms embedded in the will of God. In the ruins of Christendom, traditional Christians will continue to wage cultural guerilla wars of resistance against the dominant secular culture and the secular fundamentalist states that this secular culture supports (Engelhardt 2010a, 2010b). The issues of bioethics are central to the battles in these culture wars (Hunter 1991). The chapters that follow explore the character, significance, force, and implications for morality and bioethics of the now-dominant culture. They explore our contemporary post-Christian culture. They explore a culture that is after God.

Notes

[1] An ancestral version of this chapter, "Religion, Politics, and the State in Modern Secularized Societies," was delivered for the Comune di Napoli in Naples on February 6, 2012, where I was honored with an award "cantore della diversità morale e della tolleranza". I am in deep debt to Naples for its flawless and generous hospitality, as well as for the fruitful discussions that marked my time there.

[2] The phrase "after God" is used to indicate that the now-dominant secular culture has set itself apart from God by ignoring the question of the existence of God, the existence of ultimate meaning. Obviously, not all would fully agree with the view advanced in this volume. See, for example, Sinott-Armstrong 2011. "After God" is employed to indicate that the absence of a canonical God's-eye perspective radically changes the force and meaning of morality and bioethics.

[3] In this volume, the term *culture* is invoked, recognizing all its ambiguity. The etymology of *culture* ties tilling the soil with worshipping God (*cultus*). The Latin *cultus* embraces both agricultural cultivation and religious reverence, as does the noun *cultor*. By the time of Cicero (106–43 B.C.), *cultura* had come to compass not just agricultural cultivation, but also the refinement exemplified by philosophy and manners at court. Culture here will be used with an additional Hegelian valence to identify the dominant spirit or *Geist* of the time so that culture is compassed in *Geist*. What all is embraced by this notion of spirit will become clearer in chapter eight, where Absolute Spirit is the intellectual self-apprehension, self-consciousness of a culture. Here it is enough to observe that a culture frames and sustains what is at any time the dominant view of reality and morality.

[4] Save for references to the first *Critique*, which identify passages from the first edition (1781) as A and the second edition (1787) as B, pagination is given to the Preussische Akademie der Wissenschaften edition (Berlin: de Gruyter, 1902 and subsequently published volumes) as AK followed by the volume indicated in Roman numerals and the page in Arabic numerals.

[5] To illustrate the puzzle regarding my early and my late work, one university in Europe has held a course on Engelhardt 1 versus Engelhardt 2.

[6] In this volume, the terms *traditional Christian* and *traditional Christianity* identify that Christianity at one with the Church of the first seven Councils.

[7] My friend Maurizio Mori, co-editor of *Viaggi in Italia*, chose the title to make allusion to Johann Wolfgang von Goethe's (1749–1832) autobiographical *Italienische Reise*, which chronicles Goethe's artistic rebirth in Italy, and to indicate the important role Italy has played and continues to play in my flourishing as a scholar. Goethe's *Italienische Reise* was a work that spanned most of Goethe's lifetime, beginning with a simple diary for Charlotte von Stein as indicated in his letter to her of 14 October 1786, to a work revised and expanded in 1816/1817 following his travels through Italy in 1815, and which was then given its final form in three volumes in 1829. Italy was for Goethe a place of recovery, rebirth, and transformation. Mori recognized that it was the same for me.

[8] As a young man, I loved Italy. During my first papal audience in the summer of 1958, as the name of the diocese of Galveston-Houston was read out in St. Peter's, I gave out a loud

"yahoo!" The aging Pope Pius XII (1876–1958, elected 1939) turned to me and smiled while he blessed me.

[9] The death of Pope John Paul I (26 August 1978–28 September 1978) is an intriguing puzzle. Some consider him to have been murdered.

[10] Aggiornamento has had a generally deleterious impact on Roman Catholicism, engendering confusion and conflict. "In the United States, . . . Catholic subculture has been quite impressive right up to the very recent past. The trouble with opening windows is that you can't control what comes in, and a lot has come in—indeed, the whole turbulent world of modern culture—that has been very troubling to the Church" (Berger 1999, p. 5). Conservative Roman Catholics have attributed the major decline in church attendance not just to the doctrinal and liturgical chaos, but also in part to the "dumbing down" of the Roman Mass.

Why has Church attendance dropped despite the introduction of a "more accessible" Mass? It is because people are *not* stupid! They see Father ad-libbing the re-presentation of Jesus on Calvary and presume it is no more than a religious show. When one walks into a modern Catholic church, instead of being drawn to God by beautiful artwork, vestments, and music, the individual is confronted with the same worldliness seen in everyday life (Iannacone 2012, p. 33).

Among other things, Roman Catholicism lost faith in itself. For example, Professor Ruiping Fan (City University of Hong Kong), while a graduate student, was shocked by his initial encounter with Western Christianity, especially Roman Catholicism. He offers the following account.

In the fall of 1992, I took a plane from the People's Republic of China to accept a graduate fellowship in philosophy at Rice University, Houston, Texas. At the time, I never dreamt I was about to encounter at least some remnants of Christianity: a mystical faith that claims access to the true God and would, if it could, baptize every available pagan, including myself. Prior to that event, I had only episodic encounters with Christians, most of whom were nominal at best. They either were embarrassed to be called Christian, rejected the categorization outright, or reduced its meaning to a matter of cultural taste. Still, in my home town in Inner Mongolia, I recall a Christian teacher who, when asked to confess that Mao Tse-tung was better than Christ, refused and died for her commitment during "the cultural revolution" in the late 1960s. This seemed to me even then when I was a child to indicate a courage and a wholeheartedness of belief that I came to find was deep and admirable. Then in 1989 I had the opportunity to visit West Germany, a nominally Christian country with two established Christian religions. At the conference, an ordained Lutheran minister, now a professor of philosophy, took pains to invite members of the Chinese delegation, male and female, to the pleasures of a mixed nude German sauna. It was only later that I recognized that such behavior was at odds with traditional Christianity, as well as with the faith to which the woman was committed who died in my Inner Mongolian town. Initially, it seemed quite clear that the Christianity I was encountering played largely a cultural or aesthetic role. . . . In our attempt to

become better acquainted with the local culture [in Houston, Texas], my wife and I
proceeded to the neighboring Roman Catholic church for Christmas services and
received their communion, noticing that among the priests handing out communion
to a long and anonymous stream of visitors was a fellow graduate student at Rice.
This seemed pleasantly inclusive and culturally enriching. My wife and I enjoyed
exploring American Christianity, which at least in most of its forms presented itself
in a non-judgmental fashion that affirmed people as they were.

It was only later that I asked if one of the co-editors of *Christian Bioethics* would
be so kind as to allow me to visit his Orthodox church. Though my wife and I had
visited a number of Christian churches, we had not fully anticipated the difference.
To begin with, these people took extended worship quite seriously, spending some
three hours in the endeavor each Sunday morning. Their God is for them a very serious matter. In addition, unlike the other churches, they took painstaking efforts to
make sure that no one who was not an Orthodox Christian in good standing came
close to participating in what they referred to as their Mysteries. First, their church
bulletin announced that no one should dare come up for their Eucharist who was not
Orthodox and who had not kept their fast. Also, they positioned a half-dozen robust
gentlemen in the altar area, who seemed to watch the communicants and guard
the approach. Finally, the priest appeared to know everyone by name. As I came to
recognize over time, the elaborate ceremonies so much cherished by the Orthodox
Christians had their roots in a piety drawn from the ancient Jewish temple services.
In a Christendom generally bland, ecumenical, and all-embracing, the Orthodox
Christians were loving but persistently intent on both excluding those beyond the
faith and converting everyone who showed interest in their religion. When invited
to receptions in their parish hall, I was quite clear that, if my wife and I showed the
slightest interest, they would be more than pleased to submerge us under water three
times. Though mainstream Western Christendom may have generally evaporated
in a vague cosmopolitan social gospel, this Christianity was unembarrassed in its
sectarian commitments. . . . After a number of bioethical discussions with Roman
Catholic thinkers, quite a few took pains to assure me that they considered me not
a pagan, but an anonymous Christian. As I came to appreciate, this was an expression of the ecumenism of the West as well as the particular influence of the Jesuit
theologian Karl Rahner, who opined that "the Christian will regard the non-Christians as anonymous Christians who do not know what they really are deep down in
conscience, by grace and by a possibly very implicit yet true realization of what the
Christian too realizes" (Rahner 1966, p. 357).

How could it be that these people would accuse me of being an anonymous
Christian? First, it was clear that not all Christians would make such a claim. The
Orthodox Christians, for their part, would take great pains to remind me to keep
distant from their Mysteries until I in fact converted. Indeed, prior to conversion,
in their more pious monasteries Orthodox Christians were quite willing, lovingly
but firmly, to exclude all not able to participate in their Mysteries from standing in

the main part of the church. If one took seriously the significance of their belief in the power of baptism, this all made excellent sense. The easiest way to understand the allegation of Western Christians about my anonymous Christian status was to recognize that they had come to equate being a good person or perhaps being a good philosopher with being a Christian, at least in an anonymous mode. That is, if one could discern and affirm the general lineaments of secular morality, which constitute the general lineaments of Western Christian morality, one was indeed affirming the core of Western Christianity. In part, they could use the term 'anonymous Christians' with such ease because they had become radically secularized. Indeed, in this secularity they were willing to embrace a diversity of religious perspectives. In this robust ecumenism and syncretism, they embraced an authentically pagan position: all gods are in some sense the manifestation of a deeper reality. Once I saw this, I knew what I needed to tell them: I thanked them for having called me an anonymous Christian but told them that, with a few exceptions, they were anonymous pagans. This seems to me to be the destiny of Western Christianity (Fan 1999, pp. 232–233, 235, 236).

[11]Because these conversations with the cardinal were private, I will let the past obliterate their content, while noting what others have recorded concerning Cardinal Martini's commitments. With regard to fornication and concubinage, the cardinal stated:

Today no bishop or priest is unaware of the fact that physical intimacy before marriage is a fact. We have to rethink this if we wish to protect the family and promote marital fidelity. Nothing will be gained by unrealistic positions or prohibitions. I have learned from friends and acquaintances how young people go on holidays together and sleep in the same room. It has never occurred to anyone to hide this or to consider it a problem. Should I be commenting on this? That is difficult. I cannot understand everything, although I feel that here, perhaps, a new respect for one another, a mutual learning and a strong generational togetherness is emerging. This benefits both old and young and does not leave anyone unsupported in their questions about love and loneliness. I will follow this development with good will, with interest, and with prayer (Martini & Sporschill 2012, p. 96).

As to homosexuality, Sporschill recorded that Martini circumspectly advanced his view of changing Roman Catholicism's position concerning homosexual acts.

The Bible judges homosexuality with strong words. The background to this is the problematic practice in the ancient world, when men would have boys and male lovers alongside their families. Alexander the Great is a famous example. The Bible wants to protect the family, the wife, and the children's space. . . . The deepest concern of the Holy Scriptures, however, is the protection of the family and a healthy space for children—something now seen among homosexual couples. As a result, I am already leaning toward a hierarchy of values in these matters and basically not towards equality. I have now said more than I should have said (Martini & Sporschill 2012, p. 98).

The cardinal did concede that Orthodox Christianity, the Church at one with the Church of the Councils, cannot accept homosexual relations (Martini & Sporschill 2012, p. 98).

[12]The term *mainline Christianity* was first used in the United States to designate the American Baptists, members of the Congregational Church, Disciples of Christ, Episcopalians, Evangelical Lutherans, Presbyterians, and United Methodists. The notion of mainline Christianity grew out of and around the journal *The Christian Century*. See Coffman 2013. This group, the so-called Seven Sisters, was set in contrast with the evangelical, fundamentalist, and/or charismatic Protestants. As Gary Dorrien observes,

> The mainline churches assumed a leadership role in American society, they built a large stock of cultural capital, they crafted a persuasive rhetoric about modern Christianity and America, they built an ecumenical national church, they were (and still are) overrepresented in the corridors of power, and they served as guardians of America's moral culture (Dorrien 2013, p. 27).

In this book, I employ the term *mainline Christian* to identify those Christian bodies of a liberal-theological commitment that through their social prominence attempt to influence the polities in which they find themselves. In this fashion, I use *mainline Christian* to identify by implication such Christian groups as the Evangelische Kirche Deutschlands (EKD) and the Roman Catholics.

[13]Among other things, through my conversations with Martin Hengel, it became clear that the claims advanced by Walter Bauer (1964) and Elaine Pagels (1979) regarding the absence of an orthodox Christianity from the beginning were false. The Gospel of John fell within the true lineage of Christianity, not one that was developed by the Gnostics under the influence of Greek philosophy. Here I must also acknowledge my years of conversation with Hans Jonas (1903–1993).

[14]For my wife's account of her conversion, see Susan Engelhardt 1996 and 1995.

[15]For a sense of my coming to work as an Orthodox Christian scholar, compare Minogue et al. 1997 with Iltis & Cherry 2010.

[16]Moral friends are persons who share sufficient basic moral premises and understandings of what counts as moral evidence, and/or a common understanding of who is in authority to resolve moral disputes, so that all substantive moral disagreements can in principle be brought to closure.

[17]The first edition of *The Foundations of Bioethics* (1986) appeared in Japanese, Italian, and French (Engelhardt 1989, 1991b, 2015). The second edition appeared in Italian (1999), Chinese (1996b, 2006a), Spanish (1995), and Portuguese (1998).

[18]Cardinal Sgreccia remained a strong defender of the Roman Catholic faith in reason, in particular in philosophy, which he has developed within the paradigm of personalism. His well-known *Manuele di Bioetica* has appeared in an English translation (Sgreccia 2012).

[19]It should be noted that by the 16th century it was quite clear that natural law on the one hand was supposedly embedded in natural reason and knowable without a life of right worship and right belief, while the law of God on the other hand established prohibitions such as those against fornication and lying not justifiable through reason alone. See, for example, Francisco de Vitoria (1492-1546), Relection of the distinguished master Friar Francisco de Vitoria *On Dietary Laws* delivered in Salamanca, A.D. 1539: On Self-Restraint, Second Conclusion (Vitoria 1991, p. 221).

[20]Orthodox Christians understood my position not as fideist, but as grounded in the non-sensible, empirical, noetic knowledge of Orthodox Christianity.

[21]The term *Western moral-philosophical project* is used in realization of the complexity and heterogeneity of Western moral philosophy and its multiple agendas. The term *Western moral-philosophical project* is nevertheless engaged to identify a major intellectual undertaking that emerged in Athens in the 5th century before Christ and that in different ways was embraced anew in the West in the second millennium. The project of justifying morality sought to anchor morality and political authority in being and/or reason through philosophical arguments, including importantly natural-law arguments. This project has failed.

[22]In this volume, reference is made to both the *via moderna* and the *via antiqua*. In the 14th century, the *via antiqua* identified the Scholasticism of Thomas Aquinas and his followers which was characterized by a confidence that philosophy could by reason justify the core of the moral life. Because Aquinas was a Dominican, the *via antiqua* became associated with the Dominicans. In the 14th century, the term *via moderna* was used to identify a train of thought that has roots in Duns Scotus (ca. 1266–1308) and took full form with William of Ockham (ca. 1287–1347), and which was critical of the views of Thomas Aquinas. Because Scotus and Ockham were Franciscans, this approach to philosophy was associated with the Franciscans.

[23]Judd Owen provides a masterful overview of the consequences of the loss of foundations for contemporary culture with a special focus on the work of Stanley Fish and Richard Rorty. Owen himself embraces a form of liberalism.

> The principle of religious freedom aims to provide an unparalleled liberty to seek out and discover the truth for oneself in the needed conversation with the contending parties. The true religion is one's own only when it is embraced in full awareness of its truth. And liberalism is ennobled when the human capacity thus to embrace the truth is affirmed. At the core of the freedom to seek out the truth for oneself is a recognition that human dignity is seated ultimately in the dignity of the mind (Owen 2001, p. 172).

Owen with apparent approval quotes Thomas Jefferson's prophecy in a letter to Benjamin Waterhouse dated 26 June 1822: "I trust that there is not a young man now living in the United States who will not die a Unitarian" (Owen 2001, p. 170; Pangle 1988, p. 83). As Pangle summarizes, "Jefferson goes on to indicate doubts, however, as to whether any core of religious truth can be discovered. He speaks as if there is nothing but irresolvable diversity of opinion in religious matters" (Pangle 1988, p. 82). Owen himself observes:

> It is tempting to dismiss Jefferson's predictions about the spread of Unitarianism as manifest folly. Unitarianism remains a tiny sect. Transformation, however, is not quite the same as conversion. In assessing Jefferson's prediction, therefore, it is necessary to take a somewhat broader view of Unitarianism. Unitarianism places little importance on doctrine, creed, and theology, and a very high importance on toleration. By that standard most Presbyterians and Methodists, for example, are much closer to the Unitarians of Jefferson's day than to the Presbyterians and Methodists

of Jefferson's day. Ask a typical Methodist what the important doctrinal differences are between him and a Presbyterian that lead him to profess Methodism, and he will likely have very little to say. It seems that Jefferson's scheme has largely, if not entirely, succeeded (Owen 2001, p. 197).

Owen appears to join Jefferson in approving of this transformation of mainline Christianity.

References

Alora, Angeles Tan & Josephine M. Lumitao (eds.). 2001. *Beyond a Western Bioethics: Voices from the Developing World*. Washington, DC: Georgetown University.

Altizer, Thomas. 2006. *Living the Death of God: A Theological Memoir*. Albany: State University of New York Press.

Bartholomew, Patriarch. 1997. Joyful light; address at Georgetown University, Washington, DC, October 21.

Bauer, Walter. 1964 [1934]. Rechtgläubigkeit und Ketzerei im ältesten Christentum. Tübingen: Mohr.

Berger, Peter L. (ed.). 1999. *The Desecularization of the World*. Washington, DC: Ethics and Public Policy Center.

Caputo, John & Gianni Vattimo. 2007. *After the Death of God*. New York: Columbia University Press.

Coffman, Elesha. 2013. *The Christian Century and the Rise of the Protestant Mainline*. New York: Oxford University Press.

Dorrien, Gary. 2013. America's mainline, *First Things* 237 (November): 27–34.

Editorial. 1992. "Chi" è persona? Persona umana e bioetica, *La Civiltà Cattolica* IV: 547–559.

Engelhardt, H. T., Jr. 2015. *Les Fondements de la bioéthique*, trans. Jean-Yves Goffi. Paris: Les Belles Lettres.

Engelhardt, H. T., Jr. 2014. *Dopo dio: Morale e bioetica in un mondo laico*. Turin: Claudiana.

Engelhardt, H. T., Jr. 2012a. A journey to the east: Coming to right worship and right belief, in *Turning East: Contemporary Philosophers and the Ancient Christian Faith*, ed. Rico Vitz, pp. 211–240. Yonkers, NY: St. Vladimir's Seminary Press.

Engelhardt, H. T., Jr. 2012b. *Bioética Global: O colapso do consenso*. São Paulo: Paulinas.

Engelhardt, H. T., Jr. 2011a. *Viaggi in Italia: Saggi di bioetica*, eds. & trans. Rodolfo Rini & Maurizio Mori. Florence: Le Lettere.

Engelhardt, H. T., Jr. 2011b. Orthodox Christian bioethics: Some foundational differences from Western Christian bioethics, *Studies in Christian Ethics* 24.4 (November): 487–499.

Engelhardt, H. T., Jr. 2010a. Political authority in the face of moral pluralism: Further reflections on the non-fundamentalist state, *Notizie di Politeia* 26.97: 91–99.

Engelhardt, H. T., Jr. 2010b. Religion, bioethics, and the secular state: Beyond religious and secular fundamentalism, *Notizie di Politeia* 26.97: 59–79.

Engelhardt, H. T., Jr. 2008. The moral inevitability of two tiers of health care, in *Medical Ethics at Notre Dame*, eds. Margaret Monahan Hogan & David Solomon, pp. 111–129. Notre Dame, IN: Notre Dame Center for Ethics and Culture.

Engelhardt, H. T., Jr. 2007. *ΤΑ ΘΕΜΕΛΙΑ ΤΗΣ ΒΙΟΗΘΙΚΗΣ*, trans. Polyxeni Tsaliki-Kiosocloy. Athens: Harmos (translation of Engelhardt 2000).

Engelhardt, H. T., Jr. 2006a. *The Foundations of Bioethics*, 2nd ed., trans. Ruiping Fan. Beijing: Peking University Press.

Engelhardt, H. T., Jr. (ed.). 2006b. *Global Bioethics: The Collapse of Consensus*. Salem, MA: Scrivener Publishing.

Engelhardt, H. T., Jr. 2005. *Fundamentele bioeticii creștine*, trans. Mihail Neamțu, Cezar Login, & Ioan I. Ică Jr. Sibiu: Deisis (translation of Engelhardt 2000).

Engelhardt, H. T., Jr. 2003. *Fundamentos da bioética cristã ortodoxa*, trans. Luciana Moreira Pudenzi. São Paulo: Edições Loyola (translation of Engelhardt 2000).

Engelhardt, H. T., Jr. 2000. *The Foundations of Christian Bioethics*. Salem, MA: Scrivener Publishing.

Engelhardt, H. T., Jr. 1999. *Manuale di bioetica*, 2nd ed., trans. Stefano Rini. Milan: Il Saggiatore.

Engelhardt, H. T., Jr. 1998. *Fundamentos da Bioética*, 2nd ed., trans. Jose A. Ceschin. São Paulo: Edições Loyola.

Engelhardt, H. T., Jr. 1996a. *The Foundations of Bioethics*, 2nd ed. New York: Oxford University Press.

Engelhardt, H. T., Jr. 1996b. *The Foundations of Bioethics*, 2nd ed., trans. Ruiping Fan. Changsha, China: Hunan Science and Technology Press.

Engelhardt, H. T., Jr. 1995. *Los fundamentos de la bioética*, 2nd ed., trans. Isidro Arias, Gonzalo Hernández, & Olga Domínguez. Barcelona: Ediciones Paidos.

Engelhardt, H. T., Jr. 1991a. *Bioethics and Secular Humanism*. Philadelphia: Trinity Press International.

Engelhardt, H. T., Jr. 1991b. *Manuale di bioetica*, trans. Massimo Meroni. Milan: Il Saggiatore.

Engelhardt, H. T., Jr. 1989. *The Foundations of Bioethics*, trans. Hisatake Kato & Nobuyuki Iida. Tokyo: Asahi Publishers, Inc.

Engelhardt, H. T., Jr. 1986. *The Foundations of Bioethics*. New York: Oxford University Press.

Engelhardt, H. T., Jr., & Mark J. Cherry (eds.). 2002. *Allocating Scarce Medical Resources: Roman Catholic Perspectives*. Washington, DC: Georgetown University Press.

Engelhardt, Susan. 1996. From Rome to home, in *Our Hearts' True Home*, ed. Virginia Nieuwsma, pp. 61–71. Ben Lomond, CA: Conciliar Press (Chesterton, IN: Ancient Faith Publishing).

Engelhardt, Susan. 1995. Bless me, St. Patrick, I'm coming home, *Again* 18 (June): 18–19.

Evagrios the Solitary. 1988. On prayer, in *The Philokalia*, 3 vols., eds. Sts. Nikodimos & Makarios, trans. G.E.H. Palmer, Philip Sherrard, & Kallistos Ware, vol. 1, pp. 55–71. Boston: Faber and Faber.

Fan, Ruiping. 1999. The memoirs of a pagan sojourning in the ruins of Christendom, *Christian Bioethics* 5.3: 232–237.

Finnis, J. 1983. *Fundamentals of Ethics*. Washington, DC: Georgetown University Press.

Finnis, J. 1980. *Natural Law and Natural Rights*. Oxford: Clarendon Press.

Fish, Stanley. 2008. *Save the World on Your Own Time*. New York: Oxford University Press.

Gomez-Lobo, Alfonso. 2002. *Morality and the Human Goods: An Introduction to Natural Law Ethics*. Washington, DC: Georgetown University Press.

Grisez, Germain. 2001. Natural law, God, religion, and human fulfillment, *The American Journal of Jurisprudence* 46: 3-46.

Grisez, Germain. 1965. The first principle of practical reason: A commentary on the *Summa Theologiae* 1-2, Question 94, Article 2, *Natural Law Forum* 10: 168-201.

Hengel, Martin. 1989. *The Johannine Question*, trans. John Bowden. London: SCM Press.

Hull, Geoffrey. 2010. *The Banished Heart: Origins of Heteropraxis in the Catholic Church*. London: T&T Clark.

Hunter, James Davison. 1991. *Culture Wars*. New York: Basic Books.

Iannacone, Timothy A. 2012. American perseverance within the Catholic Faith, *Latin Mass* 21.2 (Fall): 31–33.

Iltis, Ana & Mark J. Cherry (eds.). 2011. *La temeliile bioeticii creştine: Eseuri critice asupra gândirii lui H. Tristram Engelhardt jr*, trans. Maria Aluaş, Cezar Login, Dumitru Vanca. Cluj-Napoca: Renaşterea (translation of Iltis & Cherry 2010).

Iltis, Ana & Mark J. Cherry (eds.). 2010. *At the Roots of Christian Bioethics: Critical Essays on the Thought of H. Tristram Engelhardt, Jr.* Salem, MA: Scrivener Publishing.

Martini, Cardinal Carlo & Georg Sporschill. 2012. *Night Conversations with Cardinal Martini*, trans. Lorna Henry. New York: Paulist Press.

Minogue, Brendan, Gabriel Palmer-Fernández, & James Reagan (eds.). 1997. *Reading Engelhardt: Essays on the Thought of H. Tristram Engelhardt, Jr.* Dordrecht: Kluwer.

Mori, Maurizio. 2011. Prefazione, in H. T. Engelhardt, *Viaggi in Italia*, pp. 9–31. Florence: Le Lettere.

Owen, J. Judd. 2001. *Religion and the Demise of Liberal Rationalism.* Chicago: University of Chicago Press.

Pagels, Elaine. 1979. *The Gnostic Gospels.* New York: Vintage Books.

Pangle, Thomas L. 1988. *The Spirit of Modern Republicanism.* Chicago: University of Chicago Press.

Pera, Marcello. 2008. *Why We Should Call Ourselves Christians*, trans. L. P. Lappin. New York: Encounter Books.

Peterson, Daniel J. 2005. Speaking of God after the death of God, *Dialog: A Journal of Theology* 44.3: 207-26.

Rahner, Karl. 1966. *Theological Investigations*, vol. 5, *Later Writings*, trans. K. H. Kruger. London: Darton, Longman & Todd.

Robinson, John A. T. 1963. *Honest to God.* Philadelphia: SCM Press.

Rorty, Richard. 1991. *Objectivity, Relativism, and Truth.* New York: Cambridge University Press.

Sajó, András. 2008. Preliminaries to a concept of constitutional secularism. *I•CON* 6.3–4: 605–629.

Sgreccia, Elio Cardinal. 2012. *Personalist Bioethics: Foundations and Applications*, trans. John di Camillo & Michael Miller. Philadelphia: National Catholic Bioethics Center.

Sinott-Armstrong, Walter. 2011. *Morality Without God?* New York: Oxford University Press.

Vitoria, Francisco de. 1991. *Political Writings,* eds. Anthony Pagden & Jeremy Law-
    rance. New York: Cambridge University Press.
Williams, Robert W. 2012. *Tragedy, Recognition, and the Death of God: Studies in
    Hegel and Nietzsche.* Oxford: Oxford University Press.

CHAPTER TWO

The Demoralization and Deflation of Morality and Bioethics[1]

I. The End of an Age

It was 1954. I had arrived in Europe for the first time, indeed in Genoa. In that early June, bright with flowers, a joy for my mother, I entered a world that was a universe apart from the Europe of the second decade of the 21st century. The moral and metaphysical texture of the then-dominant life-world was radically different. There was a pronounced folk piety. Italy's streets were full of young priests and children. Everywhere there were grey and black friars. Italy was young, generally pious, and dynamic (although side chapels were at times marked by signs bearing an astonishing warning: *Vietato urinare*). The churches were not empty. These observations are not meant to deny the presence even then of the roots of the now-dominant secular culture.[2] Italy had its full share of agnostics and atheists. However, Italy was then just before, but still surely before, a major and dramatic cultural tipping point. Vatican II (1962–1965), the sexual revolution of the late 1960s, the student protests beginning in 1968, and the general impact of the Frankfurter Schule[3] would soon precipitate a comprehensive secularization. However, this transformation had not yet taken place. I was in a cultural lull before widespread turbulence and change. It was not yet a culture after God.

There surely have been other periods when Italy was just before an immense, thoroughgoing, and largely unanticipated change. In A.D. 395 when the Eastern and Western portions of the empire were divided following the death of Emperor Theodosius (349–395), most Romans could not have imagined that

in fifteen years the City would fall to Alaric and his Goths.[4] In 1954 I could not
have envisaged that by 1969 as a Fulbright post-doctoral scholar working in
Bonn with Klaus Hartmann (1924–1991) and Gottfried Martin (1901–1972), as
well as long-distance with Thomas Luckmann (associated with the Frankfurt
School) on a manuscript by Alfred Schutz (Schutz & Luckmann 1973) and on
my first book (Engelhardt 1973), I would be in a completely different Europe, a
Europe in which my second daughter Christina would be born. The Europe I
was experiencing in 1954 would have disappeared. Even in 1965 when I was in
Italy and Germany, the full scope of the changes would have been hard to anticipate. The major shift in the dominant public culture that was about to occur
involved a radical change in what constituted matters of guilt, shame, and public
embarrassment. As with any tipping point, all of a sudden the changes became
dramatically apparent. Within a half century, affirmation of traditional Western
morality, of traditional Christianity, and of God's existence became off-color. In
1954 this great transformation had not yet occurred. One could still recognize
that one was living in a Christian culture that took itself to be anchored in the
very heart of reality.

Now Italy is different. Italy has aged, young priests are rare, there are far
fewer children. Sitting in the Piazza Navona at an open-air restaurant with a
gaggle of young grandchildren, we now look quite out of place. My granddaugh-
ters Macrina and Theodora, as well as my grandson Stefan, ask why Italy is
so post-Christian. They can feel the difference. A similar question came from
my grandsons Duncan, Keegan, and Aidan, as we toured the empty mainline
churches of Frankfurt. Italy and Germany are not like Texas or Alaska, where
there are large flourishing fundamentalist Christian communities and Orthodox churches. My grandchildren can sense that Europe is a world apart from
where they live. Most significantly for this volume, the dominant culture of Italy,
indeed of the West, is now profoundly secular. It is framed as if God did not exist.
It is not just that the public space is robustly after Christendom. In addition, the
dominant secular culture makes no claim to be anchored in the transcendent
order of things. Or to put matters more starkly, the dominant secular culture
positively eschews any grounding in the transcendent. Indeed, there is no public
reflection on, much less a recognition of, the importance of the transcendent.
The dominant culture is without foundations. Europe and Italy have a public

life-world that is different in kind from Italy and Europe of 1954. In that June of 1954 I had entered into a way of life about both to be undone and to be radically marginalized. The public moral assumptions were substantively other than the Europe of the first decade of the third millennium. It was a world where even within the public square one could still speak of sin. From today's perspective, it all seems so different. From the perspective of the now-dominant culture, it all seems so patriarchal, heterosexist, and Christian. It was a world where, within the public square, one could still speak of offenses against God. In terms of the now-dominant political correctness, it now all seems so wrong.

The Italy of the 1950s was an Italy that could not have conceived that there would soon be serious debates regarding the possibility of Roman Catholic priestesses and homosexual marriages, not to mention the propriety of third-party-assisted reproduction with donor gametes, abortion, physician-assisted suicide, and euthanasia. This is not to say that in the 1950s there was no abortion, fornication, adultery, active homosexuality, and even physician-assisted suicide. There surely was. However, the official culture expected repentance for such acts, or at least the tribute of hypocrisy. Such activities were still publicly appreciated, even if often insincerely, as sinful. Indeed, they were generally illegal. Those who engaged in such behavior recognized the collision of their moral commitments with the then dominant culture, which was then still a Christian culture. After all, the Roman Catholic Church was Italy's legally established church. The cardinal difference between then and now turns not just on a difference regarding certain norms, but much more on a change in the very nature of public morality. It turns not just on the force and meaning of norms, but on the contemporary requirement that the public square must be free of any mention of God. As a consequence, public moral discourse had a very different character. In the dominant culture of the West, and of Italy in particular, one could still be publicly judgmental regarding the morality, or better regarding the immorality, of abortion, fornication, adultery, homosexual acts, and physician-assisted suicide. Such adverse judgments were taken to have foundations, to be anchored in reality, in being itself. Moreover, one could publicly mention God. The culture I experienced in the 1950s was a world in deep contrast with what one encounters today in the public space of the West, even in that of Texas.

To engage Thomas Kuhn's (1922–1996) metaphor, the dominant moral paradigm of Italy, indeed of Europe and the Americas, has changed (Kuhn 1962, 1970). The traditional Christian moral paradigm of the West no longer governs. Instead, the dominant culture has embraced a secular moral vision. The previous dominant cultural-moral paradigm has been replaced. Here, I employ Thomas Kuhn's metaphor of paradigm, as it was somewhat recast by Margaret Masterman (1910–1986) (Masterman 1970), in order to indicate the depth and scope of the transformation that has taken place in the culture of the West, radically reconforming the cultural context in which morality and bioethics find themselves. Our experience of reality is shaped by our commitments regarding the deep ontology of things, the character of being, how one knows reality, who the expert knowers are, and, in the case of morality and bioethics, what the cardinal goods are, and in what ranking. These commitments provide the framework of our life-worlds. With regard to the place of God and Christianity in the dominant culture, there has been a change in taken-for-granted ontology, moral epistemology, sociology of moral experts (in 1954 it had included theologians), and axiology. There has been a transformation of the public cultural understanding regarding that about which one should feel guilt, shame, and/or embarrassment. This foundational recasting had been developing for more than two centuries, and in the last half-century it came thoroughgoingly to define public discourse. The very life-world of Western Europe and the Americas has changed. The texture and character of the two life-worlds (1954 and the present) are literally worlds apart.

The then-dominant traditional morality claimed a metaphysical anchor in natural law, in being as it is in itself. The now-dominant culture in contrast asserts moral claims based on moral intuitions that are held to be self-evident, at least within its narrative, which intuitions are claimed to be as good as the revelations of God. The secular moral narrative is ultimately foundationless. The once-dominant Western Christian culture was framed by moral claims that guided sexual activity, reproduction, and how one should face death in terms of century-old normative understandings, all supposedly secured by sound rational moral-philosophical argument. The now-dominant culture has abandoned these expectations and has transformed these once moral matters into life-style and death-style choices, which are to be appreciated fully within the horizon of the finite and the immanent. Since I first walked the streets of Italy in 1954, a thoroughgoing change has occurred: immanence has triumphed and the transcendent has been exorcized. The discourse of sin has become politically unacceptable. Even Christian democratic parties no longer speak of Christ or God, but only vaguely of "Christian values." It is a life-world apart from that of the mid-1950s and from traditional Christianity. Of course, the same changes have also occurred in Texas, but at home I experienced the changes gradually, day by day. Moreover, the changes in Texas have not even yet been as far-reaching as in Europe. We still know that God exists, and we still have our guns (Luke 22:36).

II. The Great Rupture: The End of Christendom and the Marginalization of Christianity

Ours is a new age. There has been a profound rupture from the Christian past. The dominant culture of the West, as one finds it in contemporary law and public policy, is not just disconnected from its Christian past: the contemporary secular culture is aggressively setting its Christian past behind it, as if it had been an evil temptation. As Octavio Paz correctly observes, the modern age is better characterized as beginning with a "breaking away from Christian society" (Paz 1974, p. 27). Modernity involves a separation from Christianity. Post-modernity involves a separation from God, from any ultimate anchor , along with a fracturing of modernity's hopes and understandings.[5] The Enlightenment had wanted its own paganism. As Peter Gay correctly puts it:

> The philosophes' experience . . . was a dialectical struggle for autonomy, an attempt to assimilate the two pasts they had inherited—Christian and pagan—to pit them against one another and thus to secure their independence. The Enlightenment may be summed in two words: criticism and power. . . . I see the philosophes' rebellion succeeding in both of its aims: theirs was a paganism directed against their Christian inheritance and . . . a *modern* paganism, emancipated from classical thought as much as from Christian dogma (Gay 1966, p. xi).

In having severed itself from any transcendent point of orientation, the contemporary dominant culture of the West is an age resolutely after Christ as Messiah and God. St. Peter answers Jesus' question, "Who do you say that I am?" (Mt 16:15), with "You are the Messiah, the Son of the Living God" (Mt 16:16). In contrast, the dominant secular culture gives at best secular reductive accounts of Jesus as "a marginal Jew who came to be regarded not only as the messiah but as a god."[6] The answer must be in fully atheistic, or at least agnostic terms. The dominant secular culture means to constitute itself not just as a culture after Christendom, but as a culture beyond any acknowledgement of Christ as God and the Messiah of Israel. It is a culture beyond God.[7] The contemporary culture is even after deism.

St. Peter's response is the core commitment of Christendom. In contrast, the denial of St. Peter's response is at the core of our contemporary culture. In the West, the Enlightenment project,[8] which produced the strong laicist response of the French Revolution, but now without deism,[9] has transformed the dominant culture. As noted in chapter one, there has never been any time quite like it before. It is an age "after God". Until the 20th century, there never before had been a major culture that was resolutely after God, that was articulated without any reference to spiritual powers, without any acknowledgement of the transcendent, which sought to frame its view of reality and human flourishing apart from any transcendent anchor, as if all were in the end ultimately meaningless. In the case of Eastern Europe, aside from Russia and its associated states, the post-Christian and post-deist commitments of the now-dominant ethos of the European Union have come to substitute for the official atheism of the previous communist regimes.

The dominant secular culture, as a result, is clearing away not just the remnants of Christendom, but of any public recognition of God.[10] Given the background circumstance that European culture for a millennium and a half has been defined by Christendom, this secularization involves a dramatic rearticulation of public discourse and public institutions. Modernity had attempted to preserve Christian morality without Christianity and without Christ, but usually with some form of deism. There is now a fully post-Christian, post-deist laicist age whose increasingly secular fundamentalist, post-Christian culture is aggressively after God. It is also a post-modern age if one means by *post-modern* the recognition that a single, secular, and canonical moral rationality and view of reality cannot be identified as canonical by sound rational argument. Directed by an atheistic practical postulate, a fully atheistic or at least agnostic culture and bioethics have been established. Now after the fall of the atheist communist regimes in Eastern Europe, the European Union and the United States have emerged as the vanguard of a secular public culture that is fully committed to shaping a global culture as if God did not exist.

Although it is clear that we are in a new age, the contours and implications of this new state of affairs are far from clear. A distinctly new dominant culture is in place. There are substantive points of conflict between the now-dominant secular culture and the culture of Christendom it displaced. Those already transformed by the now-dominant secular culture may have already forgotten how they once felt, thought, experienced, and lived, so that the radical character of the changes is often obscured or at least ignored. However, those still embedded in traditional Christian communities live in the Christian culture that was previously dominant, and that the now-dominant secular culture seeks fully to set aside. Traditional Christians can but regard the now-dominant secular culture and its bioethics as misdirecting, perverse, and indeed evil.[11] The contrast between the two cultures is stark and evocative of bitter cultural and political conflicts. In this new context, Richard Rorty could but regard devout traditional Christians as crazy (Rorty 1991, pp. 187, 190f).

The secularist agenda is broad. The public forum, and as far as possible the public space, are not just to be rendered innocent of the obvious, direct, or even indirect control of the church, but to be purged as well of all acknowledgements of the existence of God. Public discourse has come to eschew any reference to the transcendent, as well as to focus resolutely on the immanent. The depth and compass of this secularization are still adequately to be appreciated. The very general outlines can now be recognized not simply in terms of a removal of religious considerations from the public forum and a removal of religious discourse and images as far as possible from the public space, but in terms of the marginalization of religious discourse into an ever-shrinking sphere of privacy. All is to be placed within the horizon of the finite and the immanent. If one is to speak of spirituality as one speaks of various views of wellness, one must be sufficiently vague and reduce what is at stake to immanent considerations.

We are somewhat like people at the end of the Middle Ages. We know a vast change is taking place, but we are not quite sure how adequately to describe it, much less to gauge its full implications. We can at least in part see how our cultural context is significantly different from that of even a half-century ago. At the end of the Middle Ages, in the shadow of a period of excess and decadence in which Rodrigo Borgia (1431–1503) after he became Pope Alexander VI (elected 1492) had his bastard daughter Lucrezia married in the Vatican on June 12, 1493, following the precedent of Pope Innocent VIII (1432–1492, elected 1484), who had his bastard son married in the Vatican, there was a feeling of change.[12] Those at the end of the Middle Ages could sense that, especially with the fall of Constantinople, the Renaissance had been further fueled by scholars and manuscripts from Byzantium. The dominant culture had begun to take on a new character. By 1469, the term *media tempestas* had been employed, and by 1518 *media aetas* and by 1604 *medium aevum* were used to indicate that a new age had dawned that was distinct from the Middle Ages that had just been rendered past (Brunner et al. 1978, vol. 4, p. 98; Edelman 1939).[13] After Luther tacked his 95 theses to the Schlosskirche in Wittenberg (31 October 1517), Western Christendom became rapidly and dramatically rent, and the Western empire fell into war within itself. In 1543, Andreas Vesalius (1514–1564) had brought the time-honored anatomy of Galen (130–200) into doubt, and Nicolaus Copernicus (1473–1543) had done the same with respect to Ptolemy's (†A.D. 168) astronomy (Vesalius 1543; Copernicus 1543). By the mid-17th century, this new age was no longer looking primarily to the past achievements of Greece and Rome as the Golden Age. It had instead turned its gaze to the future. The Golden Age was yet to be achieved through human reason and energies. Rather than regarding Greco-Roman civilization as the highest human achievement, the focus began to turn to the future through confidence in scientific, technological, and cultural progress.[14] By the mid-17th century, it was clear that one had entered into a new life-world shaped by new realities and new expectations. Yet, again, most of what had taken place was not very clear until at least the Enlightenment. Even for us it is difficult to comprehend and articulate what is occurring and reshaping our life-world at the beginning of the 21st century.

The rupture from Christendom first became salient with the French Revolution and the events it engendered. The French Revolution was tantamount to a revolution against Christianity (Latreille 1948; Vovelle 1991). It involved the bloody slaughter of men, women, and children especially in the Vendée because they were resolutely traditional Christians(Secher 2003), as well as the establishment of a state-run church under the authority of the Civil Constitution of the Clergy (12 July 1790). This was followed by the establishment of the Cult of Reason, along with the Feast of Reason in the Notre Dame Cathedral (9 November 1793) (Mathiez 1977 [1904]; Latreille 1948). At times the French Revolution had the character of an almost theatrical, but at the same time violent, assault on Roman Catholicism. One might think of Napoleon's 1796 invasion of the papal states, the proclamation of a Roman Republic (1798), and the kidnapping of Pope Pius VI (1775–1799, born 1717), who was taken to Valencia where he died. One should also note the Reichsdeputationhauptschluss of 22 August 1802, through which the Western empire, the Holy Roman Empire of the German Nation, under pressure from the French authorized the dissolution of the remaining Roman Catholic episcopal principalities,[15] and the seizure of properties, to be used as compensation for German sovereigns who had lost holdings on the west bank of the Rhine, and to provide spoils for allies (Hofmann 1976, pp. 329–358).[16] The Secularization involved not just a political change (the dissolution of Roman Catholic episcopal sovereignties), but also the obliteration of systems of Christian education and charity with roots in the Middle Ages. Institutions embedded in Christendom were replaced by secular institutions.[17]

This theater of secularization continued when Pope Pius VII (1742–1823, elected 1800) was induced to come to Paris to crown Napoleon, who proceeded to crown himself on December 2, 1804, and proclaim his new code. Then on the Feast of the Transfiguration, the sixth of August, 1806, the last emperor of the Holy Roman Empire, Francis II, abdicated after his defeat by Napoleon, so that Europe was symbolically transfigured into a secular empire with Napoleon as its self-crowned emperor. These dramatic changes were further highlighted through Napoleon's seizing the Papal States. The pope was then in 1809 again transported, this time becoming a prisoner in Savona and later in Fontainebleau. All of this was part of a political and cultural drama that underscored that Christendom had fallen and that Christianity had been displaced. A new age along with its post-Christian culture had been established.

In the 19th and 20th centuries, the laicism born of the French Revolution developed strength, became entrenched, and attempted to render society affirmatively secular. The culture that was emerging was marked by an anger against God reflected in the work of such as Charles Baudelaire (1821–1866), especially in *Les Fleurs du Mal* (1857), and Arthur Rimbaud (1854–1891). This anger against God is striking in the poetry of the Franco-Uruguayan Jules Laforgue (1860–1887).

> The stars, it is certain, will one day meet,
> Heralding perhaps that universal dawn
> Now sung by those beggars with caste marks of thought.
> A fraternal outcry will be raised against God (Laforgue 1958, p. 203).

This struggle between Christendom and a post-Christian France led at times to bloody clashes. One must recall that it was Napoleon III (1808–1873, reigned 1852–1870) who protected Rome with a garrison of French troops, along with Roman Catholics who had come from across the world to protect the Vatican and Rome. They remained until the war with Germany began, while Pope Pius IX (1792–1878, elected 1846) during Vatican I was being proclaimed infallible. On September 20, 1870, Italian troops finally entered through a breach in the Porta Pisa, and Rome was declared the capital of Italy on June 30, 1871. On May 1, 1871, the law of papal guarantees had been issued, granting the Vatican, the Lateran, and Castel Gandolfo extra-territorial status. The papal states were reduced to a symbolic residuum of what had come into existence through the first Donation of Pepin in 754, and fully so with the second Donation of 756. The intellectual cultures of both Italy and France were transformed.

In France the transformation was dramatic. In the vacuum created by the defeat of Napoleon III, the Paris Commune established itself on March 18, 1871 (Gildea 2008). In the end, laicism reshaped French society, as for example when Émile Combes (1835–1921) as prime minister of France completed the secularization of French education inaugurated by Jules Ferry (1832–1893). By 1905, *laïcité* was imposed by law separating church and state, so that French primary and secondary schools were rendered secular (Reclus 1947). This laicism largely succeeded in removing Christianity from the public forum of France. These events were a harbinger of the secularization that would become general in the West by the end of the 20th century.

In the United States, an analogous transformation occurred primarily over the last three-quarters of a century. The United States into the 20th century had been *de facto*, indeed *de jure* Christian.[18] After all, the First Amendment only forbade a federal establishment of a particular religion, where this was understood as the establishment of a particular Christian denomination. The United States comprised a Christian people[19] and forthrightly supported Protestant Christianity.[20] Until the middle of the 20th century, Christianity was the established religion of the United States. However, in both the European Union and the United States, the dominant culture is now secular, after Christianity and after God, a point that has been made by the European Court of Human Rights.[21] In France, as just noted, the process of secularization occurred in fits and starts beginning with the French Revolution. In countries such as the United Kingdom where there is still an established church, secularization has been more complex, marked primarily by a decline in engaged congregants and an increasing perception of the established church's primarily cultural rather than religious significance (Leigh & Haydon 2009). The result is that many persons who are members of the Church of England do not know that Christ has risen from the dead.

At the beginning of the 21st century, we see the truth of G. W. F. Hegel's observation in 1802 regarding "the feeling that 'God Himself is dead,' [as that feeling] upon which the religion of more recent times rests" (Hegel 1977, p. 190; Hegel 1968, p. 414).[22] The 19th century saw the death of God in Protestant Europe and in England. As A. N. Wilson summarizes in his book *God's Funeral*:

> As Dostoevsky made so clear in that terrible prophecy, and as Thomas Hardy and Leslie Stephen and Morrison Swift would probably all in their different ways have agreed, the nineteenth century had created a climate for itself—philosophical, politico-sociological, literary, artistic, personal—in which God had become unknowable, His voice inaudible against the din of machines and the atonal banshee of the emerging egomania called The Modern. The cohesive social force which organized religion had once provided was broken up. The nature of society itself, urban, industrialized, materialistic, was the background for the godlessness which philosophy and science did not so much discover as ratify (Wilson 1999, p. 12).

For countries that were a part of the Soviet bloc, which lived through the Lenin-ist-Marxist regimes' commitment to an atheist secular state, the encounter with the laicism of the European Union represented a second wave of secularization, which reflects the now thoroughly secular culture of the West.

Given this dominant secular cultural framework, and given the worldwide dominance of the West, the dominant culture of the world can be described as secular, post-modern, post-Christian, after God, and after foundations. This culture is increasingly characterized by a robust laicism that seeks to define not just the public forum, but also the public space in strongly secular terms so as to banish any reference to the transcendent, in particular to God, from public acts and public discourse (Cumper & Lewis 2012; Zucca 2012). Religious symbols from the past, if they cannot easily be removed, are to be evacuated of religious meaning. They are only allowed to stay if they are reduced to rel-ics of a cultural and national heritage. One might think of how the European Court of Human Rights first forbade Italy from displaying crucifixes in its public schools, as had occurred in Germany, where the display of crucifixes could no longer be required (BVerfGE 93, 1—Kruzifix [16. Mai 1995]; Wiedemann 2012). Similar developments occurred in Romania (Andreescu & Andreescu 2010, pp. 56–57). In Italy after a major struggle, crucifixes were allowed to remain through interpreting their presence as a mere cultural phenomenon. Their religious sig-nificance had been set aside. There had been a cultural translation and reduc-tion of the religious (Andreescu & Andreescu 2010; Puppinck 2012; Puppinck & Wenberg 2010).

Against this background, one can understand the strident conflicts between the remnants of Christian Europe and the now-regnant post-Christian West regarding any public acknowledgement of Christianity and its importance (Kallscheuer 1996; Marauhn 2004; Rendtorff 1975; Schreiber 2012). A good example is offered by the debates regarding the treaty proposed in 2004 to serve as a constitution for Europe. The treaty was produced by a committee chaired by the former president of France, Valéry Giscard d'Estaing, with the support of the then-president of France Jacques Chirac. A dispute arose because the treaty omitted any reference to Christianity's role in the development of Europe. The first two paragraphs of the Preamble to the proposed European constitutional document read:

DRAWING INSPIRATION from the cultural, religious and humanist inheritance of Europe, from which have developed the universal values of the inviolable and inalienable rights of the human person, freedom, democracy, equality and the rule of law,

BELIEVING that Europe, reunited after bitter experiences, intends to continue along the path of civilisation, progress and prosperity, for the good of all its inhabitants, including the weakest and most deprived; that it wishes to remain a continent open to culture, learning and social progress; and that it wishes to deepen the democratic and transparent nature of its public life, and to strive for peace, justice and solidarity throughout the world,

CONVINCED that, while remaining proud of their own national identities and history, the peoples of Europe are determined to transcend their former divisions and, united ever more closely, to forge a common destiny,

CONVINCED that, thus 'United in diversity', Europe offers them the best chance of pursuing, with due regard for the rights of each individual and in awareness of their responsibilities towards future generations and the Earth, the great venture which makes of it a special area of human hope . . . (British Data Management Foundation 2004, p. 10).

Although a non-specific religious inheritance was mentioned, the accent fell on rights, including nothing that was particularly Christian. The language of rights, human rights, and even social justice has after all no deep roots in Christianity.[23] In such a central document, laicists did not allow any mention of Christianity, even if only to acknowledge Christianity as a cultural residuum, as a mere historical connection. After all, the European Union as a secular political project was beginning anew. It claimed an identity born *de novo* of the Enlightenment. It was to be the universal nation. The distinctiveness of Europe was to be found in its post-religious moral commitments to the supposedly non-ethnocentric, universal canonical norms of human dignity and human rights, not to an ethnocentric or religiocentric history. For example, András Sajó in his defense of "democratic constitutionalism" asserts that "Democratic constitutionalism recognizes only one source of power, and this is the power of the people over itself. . . . Popular sovereignty means that all power in the state originates from people, therefore it cannot originate from the sacred" (Sajó 2008, p. 627). Europe's particular identity was to be found in its supposedly secular, rational, non-particular roots, in its commitments to universal moral and democratic norms. This commitment to universal norms ruled out reference to particular religious roots.

The nominally Protestant, largely secular northern European nations were at home with omitting reference to the Christian roots of Europe, although this omission was criticized by Pope John Paul II and by predominantly Roman Catholic nations, such as Poland and Lithuania.

> The Vatican and some other scholars . . . propose[d] a Christian foundation to the European polity. The idea is that Europe grew into a secularized set of states without ever shaking off its Christian roots. At the basis of European morality lie Christian values, which are the necessary building blocks and glue that keep all Europeans together (Zucca 2012, p. 194).

A similar position has been endorsed by the agnostic friend of Pope Benedict XVI, Marcello Pera, a defender of Christianity as the cultural cement of Europe and the West (Pera 2011). These disputes regarding the proposed constitutional document for Europe and the failure of its ratification engendered wide-ranging discussions about the place of Christianity and "Christian values" in a proper understanding of the European Union. What went largely unnoticed was that the language of "values" that many employed in defending a recognition of Christianity reflects the secularization of religion in the West. Traditional Christians and Jews, for example, do not have "values" but a God Who commands ("teaching them to obey everything I have commanded you"—Matthew 28:20). The language of values that is now engaged suggests that there exists a *lingua franca* available without a recognition of the God Who lives and commands. The language of values reduces religion to its cultural significance.[24] The proposed Constitution was rejected by referenda in France (2005) and the Kingdom of the Netherlands (2005) on grounds other than the omission of a reference to Christianity. Although this proposed Constitution was abandoned, the controversies engendered reflected a backlash against the goal of establishing a robust post-Christian identity for Europe (Bernstein 2003; Cvijic and Zucca 2004; Sajo 2008; Weiler 2003 and 1999; Zucca 2009).[25]

The new Western European secular self-consciousness involves a profound, and at times passionate, disassociation from Christianity. The now-dominant, contemporary, secular Western European morality and culture with their law and public policy, with the exception of Hungary, which in its 2011 Constitution recognizes the role of Christianity in preserving nationhood (Uitz 2012), are retreating from the Christianity that for a millennium and a half defined Europe. The dominant culture has cut itself loose from any anchor in God. The result is an unprecedented genre of secularity with laicist passions to remove every remaining, albeit minor, public non-reduced or non-culturally-recast reference to God. Again, this state of affairs constitutes a cultural novum and seeks to be a cultural novum. The agenda is to create a public culture for Europe that is cut from Europe's Christian past so that Europe's Christian past is not even a part of contemporary Europe's past, so that the new European culture can be appreciated *ab initio* without not just Christ, but without God. This laicism seeks to render Christianity in particular, and other religions in general, but especially fundamentalist monotheistic religions, into a past that is not even to be recognized as an element of the past of this new secular culture. Traditional Christianity, it should be conceded, is fundamentalist in requiring that its commitments trump the claims of secular moral rationality and the secularly politically reasonable.[26] The secular culture can only be fully understood through its contrast with, and its repudiation of, Christendom and God.

III. Framing a Culture without a God's-eye Perspective

God is important for reasons other than worship. God provides a meaning and final perspective outside of, and independent of, particular, transient, socio-historically conditioned communities and their narratives. Indeed, without a God's-eye perspective, there is in principle no vantage point from which to consider one morality to be canonical, that is, as anything more than one among a plurality of socio-historically conditioned moral vantage points. From Aristotle (384–322 B.C.) through Descartes (1596–1650), Spinoza (1632–1677), Leibniz (1646–1716), and even Kant (1724–1804), reference was made to God not for religious, but for ontological and epistemological reasons. God was recognized as the reference point for non-socio-historically-conditioned truth.[27] The perspective of God, the existence of a God's-eye perspective, in principle secured objectivity and prevented moral relativism. As we will see, this role of God is also important for Kant, who appreciated that he was constrained to affirm the practical moral postulates of God and immortality in order to maintain the traditional objective force of morality. Friedrich Nietzsche (1844–1900) and Fyodor Dostoyevsky (1821–1881) in different ways recognized that after God everything appears radically different. However, it was, and still is, unclear what the full scope and force of the consequences are, or will be, of denying the existence of God and of a God's-eye perspective.

In particular, how should one think of morality and bioethics when one approaches reality as ultimately meaningless? What are the consequences of no longer even in principle having an ultimate point of reference? Among other things, secular morality becomes intractably plural. One lacks, even in principle, a final perspective that can transcend the plurality of competing moral views and establish a particular morality as canonical. Unlike what Plato, Aristotle, Thomas Aquinas, and Immanuel Kant had promised, moral philosophy does not agree about the content and force of the good, the right, and the virtuous. Instead, moral pluralism prevails. We do not agree when it is licit, obligatory, or forbidden to have sex, reproduce, transfer property, lie, or take human life. We disagree regarding the moral significance of homosexual acts, abortion, third-party-assisted reproduction, the welfare state, and physician-assisted suicide. Even if it were the case that all humans valued the same goods, simply placing these goods in a different order would constitute a different morality. Different rankings of cardinal human goods provide the basis for different visions of what should count as a morally proper way of life and the character of a proper or reasonable political structure.

If one gives priority first to liberty (e.g., as expressed in democratic civil liberties), then to fair equality of opportunity, and then only afterward to prosperity, insofar as that prosperity redounds to the benefit of the least-well-off class, one will have embraced that moral rationality, as well as that sense of the politically reasonable, that lies at the foundations of the social-democratic state. One might think of John Rawls's account of justice (1971), as well as of his view of the politically reasonable (1993). If, however, one first gives priority to security and then to familial prosperity, focusing on the bonds that maintain the cohesion of the family rather than on fraternity among isolated individuals, giving accent to liberty only insofar as it is compatible with security, prosperity, and the flourishing of the family, one will have embraced the moral rationality and sense of the politically reasonable that form the foundations of Singapore's dominant morality and bioethics, along with its vision of the politically reasonable (Lim 2012 and 2004; Fan 2011 and 2010). Given the central importance of elites, those persons who most crucially contribute to the socio-economic stability of a country (i.e., groups with a significant vested interest in and insight regarding the stability and flourishing of a society, such as lawyers, physicians, and successful businessmen), one will also affirm an authoritarian, one-party, familist, capitalist state (Li & Wang 2012; Fan et al. 2012). Unlike what follows if one grants John Rawls's moral-political vision, a Singaporean view of the morally rational and politically reasonable contrasts with social-democratic morality, bioethics, and political views and instead supports a one-party capitalist oligarchy.[28] This view of the morally rational and/or the politically reasonable will discount concerns with liberty and equality, and require rejecting the pursuit of fair equality of opportunity because it is incompatible with the centrality of the family (Alora & Lumitao 2001). After all, Rawls correctly observes that "the principle of fair opportunity can be only imperfectly carried out, at least as long as the institution of the family exists" (Rawls 1971, §12, p. 74).[29]

As Steven Smith put it, there is no unbiased perspective that can guide: "the quest for neutrality . . . is an attempt to grasp an illusion" (Smith 1995, p. 96). Despite the Kantian aspiration at the core of the Enlightenment, there is no "rational impartial observer [*ein vernünftiger unparteiischer Zuschauer*]" (Kant 1959, p. 9, AK IV.393). In the absence of a canonical standard, a morality becomes nothing more than a particular cluster of moral intuitions supported by one among a plurality of moral narratives. A secular canonical moral standard cannot be established, because to establish one normative standard as canonical one needs a further background normative standard. To secure as canonical a particular thin theory of the good, a particular view of a properly disinterested moral judge, observer, decision-maker, or hypothetical contractor, a proper moral rationality or canonical moral sense so as to be able to pick out one view as canonical, one needs a further background standard by which canonically to order basic right-making conditions, cardinal moral values and goods, etc.

A purely disinterested observer or decision-maker cannot make a principled choice without a guiding canonical standard. However, one cannot establish particular basic guiding moral premises and rules of moral evidence for such a standard without already having accepted a further particular background view of morality and moral rationality. Attempts through sound rational argument to establish a particular morality or moral rationality as canonical as a consequence beg the question, argue in a circle, or engage in infinite regress.

This impasse can thus be shown to be in principle unavoidable by pointing out that any concrete claims involve guiding background standards. That is, in order to establish a canonical thin theory of the good, or a canonical notion of rational choice, moral rationality, or game-theoretic rationality, or a canonical account of preferences, one must already know how one ought properly to rank values, correct preferences, and compare rational versus impassioned preferences, in addition to knowing God's discount rate for preferences over time. One must already know the correct way to compare goods and/or pleasures in order to identify or articulate the correct approach. But which standard should one choose in order to get the entire process started? And if one hopes instead to proceed by balancing different moral appeals, what balance ought one to use, and how does one compare competing possible balances? To choose the right background standard or balance, one will need a further background standard or balance and so on forever.

If one appeals to morality as a natural phenomenon that developed with the evolution of humans, this will not help either. This is the case because in order to secure normative conclusions one must specify the "goals" of evolution and the character of the reference environment. If the goal is reproductive fitness, then those males who love their neighbors, while getting their neighbors' wives pregnant, possess inclusive biological fitness in many environments. But is this good, right, or virtuous? To make a moral judgment, one needs a standard. Yet once again, which standard should one use? In each case, the choice presupposes selecting a set of basic premises and rules of evidence. The question remains: which basic premises and rules of evidence should one affirm? If one takes an evolutionary point of view, one needs first to specify a particular environment and the goals at stake (is the goal simply inclusive fitness?). Again, one confronts the same problem. In giving an answer, one imports a particular point of view.

Given different environments, different moral dispositions, which appear to be pleomorphic, along with different balances among those who act morally, act hypocritically, or act immorally, will maximize group adaptation and survival, as well as help realize other goals. However, to secure guidance from the empirical facts of the matter, one needs a standard; one needs to specify the environment and the goals of adaptation one should endorse. But which are they?

One is returned to the problem of securing canonical secular moral guidance. The difficulty is that, within the horizon of the finite and the immanent, all standards are socio-historically conditioned and ethnocentric. As a consequence, as Judd Owen summarizes with reference to Richard Rorty and Stanley Fish, all immanent standards rest on particular, conditioned perspectives, on particular socio-historically embedded views from somewhere.

> Both Rorty and Fish repeatedly criticize attempts and aspirations to apprehend and demonstrate timeless truths, which they regard as truths that necessarily appear the same from each of the infinite variety of historical human perspectives. . . . We could recognize a timeless truth only from a vantage point outside of time—from a "God's eye view" —a vantage point that no human being can occupy or even imagine. All descriptions of the world and all alleged political and moral principles are irreducibly historical. The awesome variety of conflicting human opinions about the whole cannot be transcended toward a universal knowledge. Fish's shorthand expression for this situation is "irreducible difference" (Owen 2001, p. 12).

The result, given a plurality of different basic premises and rules of inference, is clear: secular morality and bioethics are irreducibly plural. Appeals to nature or evolution will not help. The pluralism is intractable.

The core difficulty is that there is no canonical sense of morality or even of the politically reasonable, much less one sense of the morally rational. Again, we do not possess a common view of when it is forbidden, allowable, or obligatory to have sex, reproduce, transfer property, or take human life. Moreover, it is impossible to secure a philosophical foundation that can anoint as canonical one account of morality or bioethics, or even one view of the politically reasonable in the fashioning of law and public policy. To make the point yet again: the Western moral-philosophical project born in ancient Greece, reborn in Western Europe in the 12th–13th centuries, and recast in increasingly post-Christian terms during the Enlightenment, fails. Unless one can invoke the true God's-eye perspective, one cannot establish one view of the morally rational or of the politically reasonable as canonical.

One surely did not need to wait for the 21st century to recognize that moral philosophy cannot through sound rational argument establish a particular morality or a particular bioethics as canonical. The fact of intractable moral pluralism was acknowledged by many in the ancient world. Clement of Alexandria (A.D. 155–220), for example, appreciated that rational argument by itself cannot deliver binding conclusions unless one first grants initial background premises. "Should one say that Knowledge is founded on demonstration by a process of reasoning, let him hear that first principles are incapable of demonstration; for they are known neither by art nor sagacity" (Clement of Alexandria 1994, *The Stromata*, Book 2, §IV, p. 350). The limits of philosophical argument were also famously limned by the third-century philosopher Agrippa in his *pente tropoi*, his five ways of indicating that controversies, such as those regarding the canonical content of morality and bioethics, as well as canonical political authority, cannot be resolved by philosophy, that is, by sound rational arguments. Philosophy cannot deliver a canonical justification for any concrete philosophical position, including morality and bioethics, in that those in dispute argue from disparate perspectives that must themselves be justified and therefore (1) argue past each other, (2) beg the question, (3) argue in a circle, or (4) engage in an infinite regress. Beyond that, by the time of Agrippa, (5) eight hundred years of philosophical analysis and argument had proven inconclusive.[30] There is no neutral secular moral perspective that can determine the moral facts of the matter, that can establish through sound rational argument a conclusion regarding the necessary content of a canonical secular morality, bioethics, or account of the politically reasonable. Post-modernity triumphs.

IV. The Demoralization and Deflation of Traditional Morality and Bioethics

The intractable plurality of morality and bioethics has been largely hidden by the Western medieval faith in reason. This faith in reason, born of the Western

Middle Ages, anointed philosophy (the *via moderna* notwithstanding) as the taken-for-granted source of a universally valid rational account of reality, morality, and bioethics. In particular, moral philosophy was considered competent to comprehend the nature of the good, the right, and the virtuous so as to be able to give concrete canonical rational moral guidance. Western Christian, in particular Roman Catholic thought embraced the assumption that moral-philosophical reasoning without a reliance on God could ground morality. However, such attempts at an anchorage in being and in a canonical moral rationality were brought into question in the wake of David Hume's (1711–1776) critique of claims of access to reality as it is in itself (Engelhardt 2010c). After Hume, it could no longer plausibly be denied that philosophy had proven unable to secure grounding for the moral guidance that it had promised. Recognition of this state of affairs led to the demoralization and deflation of the traditional morality of the West.

Here, demoralization of morality refers to the rendering of what had been considered to involve universally governing considerations of the right, the good, and the virtuous into mere life-style preferences about which moral judgments are now held to be inappropriate. The term demoralization is used to recognize that what had once been issues of morality in the sense of involving norms defining how, *ceteris paribus*, persons are obliged universally to act in order to be praiseworthy, worthy of happiness, or indeed productive of good consequences, have been reduced to life-style choices. This demoralization occurs because after God there are no universal, canonical, secular norms that can establish what is necessary for persons to be worthy of happiness, to be good persons and/or to be virtuous persons, rather than merely persons with alternative life-styles. What had involved moral judgments have become non-moral matters of life-style and death-style choices.

The deflation of morality refers to the loss of a secular, rational basis for the claim that one as a rational agent must always act from a universal perspective, from the so-called moral point of view, regarding the right, the good, and the virtuous, rather than from a particular viewpoint such as a family-centered bias that gives priority to the flourishing of one's own family. The deflation of morality identifies the circumstance that it is impossible to establish that one ought rationally to accept the moral point of view of pursuing what is right in general (whatever that might mean) and beneficial for persons generally, rather than, say, a family-centered point of view in terms of which one judges the right, the good, and the virtuous from the perspective of what is beneficial for one's family. As a consequence, the traditional significance and force of secular morality, as Richard Rorty and Gianni Vattimo (1936–) have insisted, cannot be sustained. As we have seen, no particular secular morality can be shown to be *the* moral rationality that persons as such should affirm. No particular morality can be shown to have a canonical claim on persons. This is the case, as Hegel and later Rorty appreciated, because one cannot "step outside the various vocabularies we have employed and find a metavocabulary which somehow takes account of *all possible* vocabularies, all possible ways of judging and feeling" (Rorty 1989, p. 59). Once one has lost a God's-eye perspective, there is no neutral vantage point from which a particular morality and bioethics can in general secular terms be established as canonical for all persons as such. Each moral narrative stands on its own, sustaining its own intuitions along with its own view of proper action. A polytheism of secular moral viewpoints becomes unavoidable. Morality that had been putatively grounded in an unavoidable vision of moral rationality anchored in being-as-it-is-in-itself is now adrift.

The threat of the demoralization and deflation of morality led Kant to develop his mature account of moral philosophy. Kant saw that Hume left morality as at best grounded in contingent sympathies and sentiments held together by equally contingent habits. If Hume were right, moral sentiments and proclivities would then be mere facts of the matter, and could always be otherwise. They could not secure a moral standpoint that was canonically morally normative. Given the plurality of moral sentiments and proclivities, morality cannot be shown to be grounded in a framework justified by rational, moral-philosophical reflection as universally binding on all persons as such. In the absence of a canonical standard, a God's-eye perspective that can definitively order the various human goods, secular moral rationality remains intractably plural. There can be neither a necessary nor a canonically normative content for morality or bioethics. The dominance of any particular morality or bioethics represents at best the contingent valorization of one among many competing moralities and bioethics. Hume led to the view that morality as it had once been understood, as compassing universal norms binding on all persons, cannot be established by sound rational argument, because morality turned out to be grounded in sympathies, not in reason. Sympathies are heterogeneous and often in tension, if not incompatible. As an example of a normative perspective that is not that of the traditional Western moral point of view, consider the injunction of the chief Norse god Odin (alias Wotan). "He should early rise, who another's property or life desires to have. Seldom a sluggish wolf gets prey, or a sleeping man victory" (Sigfusson 1906, #58, p. 35).

Kant therefore recognized that, without God, a grounding of morality in canonical rationality would not be possible. It would not be enough to forward various natural-law or human-rights claims in order to counter the response by the "immoralist" that it is *not* always rational to act morally. One needed both a God's-eye perspective, as well as God as the guarantor that in the end persons will be happy in proportion to their worthiness to be happy. Both conditions were essential to maintain the traditional coherence of morality. Without God it would not always be rational to act in accord with Kant's categorical imperative, Kant's norms for the universalizing morality of rational agents. Kant, who was likely an atheist,[31] nevertheless affirmed the need for a God's-eye perspective, as well as for immortality, in order to preserve the rationality of canonical content and force that Western European morality had promised. Kant placed God centrally as the lynchpin of his account of the kingdom of ends,[32] arguing that the existence of God and immortality had to be affirmed as postulates of practical reason in order to ensure a canonical content for morality, to maintain a rational coherence of the right and the good, as well as to secure the priority of morality over prudence.[33] In conformity with the Western Christian philosophical project, Kant sought to ground morality in a moral rationality congruent with a God's-eye perspective so as to vindicate a canonical morality anchored in being through moral philosophical argument. At stake is not fear of God's punishment as a motivation to be moral, but God as the source of the ultimate significance for morality, the rational coherence of the right and the good, and the necessary priority of moral choices over prudent choices. In the absence of these conditions being met, Kant understood that morality would cease to have a unique canonical content and an unqualified rational binding force or priority over non-moral normative concerns.

Kant recognized that if he failed in his project, the meaning of traditional Western European morality would be radically recast, with its claims receiving a different extension and intension. He recognized that without a God's-eye perspective the categorical claims of traditional morality would not be rational.

Kant anticipated G. E. M. Anscombe (1919–2001), who also recognized that a morality after God is so radically changed in its meaning as to deserve to be articulated in fundamentally different, non-moral terms. Anscombe argued that after God traditional Western morality was so changed that the term "moral" should if possible be abandoned. She held, for example, that "the concepts of obligation, and duty—*moral* obligation and *moral* duty, that is to say—and of what is *morally* right and wrong, and of the *moral* sense of 'ought,' ought to be jettisoned if this is psychologically possible" (Anscombe 1958, p. 1). Anscombe wished to undermine the illusion that after God, morality could still be morality as it had been beforehand in the Christian West. Western Christian morality through the dialectic of faith and reason had placed the commands of God within a philosophical framework, which still required a God's-eye view to sustain it. Kant's response in the Second Critique was to require that one affirm the practical postulates of God, free will, and immortality.

Kant also anticipated what Anscombe would recognize, namely, that, without God and immortality, a person who acts immorally would be somewhat like a person who would be termed a criminal, "if the notion 'criminal' were to remain when criminal law and criminal courts had been abolished and forgotten" (Anscombe 1958, p. 6). "Acting immorally" would be radically deflated in its force and significance in a fashion analogous to what it would mean to claim that someone acted illegally in the absence of any police, courts, or prisons to define, identify, and punish illegal acts. After all, the immoralist could always respond to the claim that he acted immorally with the riposte that, in an ultimately meaningless universe, the assertion of his will to pursue his own goals is as authoritative as any among the plurality of other normative points of view. On this point, the affirmation of the postulates of God and immortality, as mere postulates, by the atheist Kant do not provide a justified solution to the threat of the demoralization and deflation of morality, as well as bioethics. Kant's affirmation of his postulates was a cry of metaphysical desperation. As a consequence, in these circumstances, aside from a morality actually being established at law and in public policy, morality's force is substantively deflated, a point to which we will return in the next section of this chapter.

The loss of a God's-eye perspective, along with the consequent demoralization and deflation of morality, which now frames the dominant culture of the West, reflects the failure of Kant's project, indeed of the moral-philosophical project in general, to provide an adequate secular justification for traditional morality. With no anchor in being-in-itself, in a canonical moral rationality, or in a God's-eye perspective, morality now in the plural floats free, nested only within diverse narratives set within the horizon of the finite and the immanent. David Hume (1711–1776), Denis Diderot (1713–1784), and Baron Pierre-Henri d'Holbach (1723–1789) saw this. They also aided in undermining the illusion that moral philosophy could establish a canonical morality. The post-Christian world they helped establish was dramatically different from that which had just passed. As Karl Löwith appreciated, "[T]he break with tradition at the end of the eighteenth century . . . produced the revolutionary character of modern history and of our modern historical thinking" (Löwith 1949, p. 193). It was a culture within which everything looked different as ultimate meaning was evacuated.

> If the universe is neither eternal and divine, as it was for the ancients, nor transient but created, as it is for the Christians, there remains [after Christendom] only one aspect: the sheer contingency of its mere "existence." The post-Christian world is a creation without creator, and a *saeculum* (in the ecclesiastical sense of this term) turned secular for lack of religious perspective (Löwith 1949, pp. 201–202).

Everything was now to be regarded as ultimately contingent.

A culture after God became a central feature and a prominent characteristic of the West following the French Revolution. Within a generation after the French Revolution, the vanguard philosophers of this post-Christian age recognized the emergence of a way of life after God. It is for this reason that Hegel, already in "Glauben und Wissen" in 1802, spoke of the death of God. For many, this did not mean that Christianity needed to be set aside, only transformed. Hegel was content with a Christianity deprived of transcendent significance and reduced to being no more than a cardinal cultural adornment. Hegel could live as a Lutheran without a transcendent God, and with only the immanent God of a post-metaphysical philosophy as the default God's-eye perspective.[34] Hegel embraced the collapse of traditional morality and metaphysics, which Hume had threatened. Hegel articulated a post-metaphysical account through which he recognized that the moral-philosophical project of maintaining a canonical secular morality with the content of traditional Christian morality through rational argument could not succeed.[35]

Again, because reason cannot supply for secular morality an ahistorical metaphysical grounding, or anchorage, the moral-philosophical project born of the secularization of Greece in the 5th century before Christ,[36] which was re-embraced in the Western Christian Middle Ages, fails to provide canonical moral content. It became a rationality that was to function within a God's-eye perspective, and then was *inter alia* recast by Kant. Even Kant's attempt to establish a unique, historically unconditioned, canonical content for morality as a fact of reason cannot succeed.[37] One always presupposes a particular background view of how to rank cardinal human values, a particular set of basic premises and rules of evidence. Absent God and absent a canonical, content-full moral standard, the intellectual core of European culture is after God[38] and after metaphysics. It must be seen as it is, namely, as ethnocentric, as socio-historically conditioned and contingent.[39] In this circumstance, the content and substance of morality come from neither reason nor God's commands, but from a particular socio-historical context whose content is contingent and ethnocentric. As Hegel understood, any concrete secular morality can only be recognized as one socio-historically conditioned, contingent morality among a multitude of others, as one among a plurality of *Sittlichkeiten*.[40]

V. Morality and Bioethics Demoralized and Deflated: A Further Exploration of the World after Hegel

Given the West's historical bond to the moral-philosophical project, the secularization of the West is associated with the complex phenomenon of post-modernity. If modernity is understood as the attempt to orient oneself and one's culture to a guiding canonical understanding of rationality as a substitute for a reference to the one and only God, post-modernity involves the recognition that secular moral rationality and indeed even the politically reasonable are inextricably plural and without ultimate significance. As a result, it is now clear that no one secular moral narrative can be *the* universal narrative. In post-modernity, as Jean-François Lyotard observes, "The grand narrative has lost its credibility, regardless of what mode of unification it uses, regardless of whether it is a speculative narrative or a narrative of emancipation" (Lyotard 1984, p. 37). G. Elijah Dann makes the same point in slightly different terms by arguing for the "privatization" of religion or any other ultimate standpoint "because there is no epistemological vantage point, philosophical or theological, whereby grandiose proclamations about Reality can be made and then used to measure against the truthfulness of our other beliefs" (Dann 2011, p. 54). We are faced with numerous and incompatible views of the right, the good, the virtuous, and the politically reasonable. As Vattimo recognizes, "Atheism appears in this light as another catastrophic Tower of Babel" (Vattimo 1988, p. 31). Because we disagree as to when it is obligatory, licit, or forbidden to reproduce, have sex, transfer property, and to take human life, we are left in post-modernity with interminable disagreements about the content of bioethics. Without an objective standard, without a God's-eye perspective, platitudes about a common ground and/or a common good are either self-delusions or the recruitment of moral language for political rhetorical purposes. All of this is to say that secular claims with regard to a canonical morality cannot continue as before. Hegel saw this and was at peace with this state of affairs (Engelhardt 2010b).

This state of affairs already recognized by Hegel has in the 20th and 21st centuries been further explored by others such as Richard Rorty and Gianni Vattimo. The appreciation of the quite different character of morality "after foundations," that is, after God, allows a better understanding of the radical demoralization and deflation not just of any secular reconstruction of traditional Christian morality and bioethics, but of any secular morality and bioethics. All secular moralities are *Sittlichkeiten* in the sense that Hegel recognized: they are particular fabrics of moral understandings, commitments, and intuitions each shaped by its own socio-historical context and supported by one among a plurality of possible and in the end freestanding moral narratives. A concrete morality is always the discourse of a particular moral community with its particular moral narrative sustaining its own particular moral intuitions, hence its ethnocentric character. As such, a concrete secular morality without a unique anchor in reality cannot aspire to providing canonical norms for persons as such or, for that matter, for humans as such. Hence, Rorty's warning that the significance and force of secular morality must be rethought: "We can keep the notion of 'morality' just insofar as we can cease to think of morality as the voice of the divine part of ourselves and instead think of it as the voice of ourselves as members of a community, speakers of a common language" (Rorty 1989, p. 59). But which community? What common language? There is obviously a plurality of competing communities and competing languages of moral discourse. After foundations, not only the sense but also the force of secular morality and bioethics turns out to be quite different from what had for the most part been expected in Western moral philosophy, given philosophical commitments from Thomas Aquinas through Immanuel Kant.

Rorty wanted at least to keep the morality-prudence distinction. But matters are worse than Rorty acknowledged. The difficulty is that the traditional priority of a moral point of view over the perspective that affirms the good of a particular person or group can itself only be secured as long as the moral point of view is anchored in a God Who affirms it and enforces it. One needs a God's-eye perspective with teeth to anoint a particular point of view as the moral point of view. On behalf of the moral point of view, Rorty states:

> We can keep the morality-prudence distinction if we think of it not as the difference between an appeal to the unconditioned and an appeal to the conditioned but as the difference between an appeal to the interests of our community and the appeal to our own, possibly conflicting, private interests (Rorty 1989, p. 59).

The problem is that Rorty has no canonical community with which his "we" must identify. His "we", as he knows, is ethnocentric even if it is an anti-ethnocentric ethnocentrism. One simply has a plurality of normative points of view. Because any large society will always compass a plurality of communities, a plurality of "we's," a multiplicity of moral discourses, there is no canonical "we" to allow Rorty to maintain the morality-prudence distinction in favor of morality.

As Kant recognized, the priority of the moral point of view requires God, Who enforces, not just defines, His moral point of view. The "we" for Kant is the "we" that is in concert with God and enforced by God. The difficulty is that Rorty fails to add that any community (as Kant insisted) that hopes to draw the morality-prudence distinction, as it had traditionally been drawn, can do so only so long as the members of that community still hold at least as a practical moral postulate that the morality of their community is anchored in and enforced by God. But, of course, Rorty would not affirm this. A core difficulty, which Rorty does recognize, is that one cannot establish by sound rational argument which secular morality or bioethics is canonical, if any. One always needs the prior concession of basic premises and/or rules of evidence. Rorty does not as clearly concede that this same difficulty besets establishing the priority of the moral point of view. To establish the priority of the moral point of view, one needs foundational premises and rules of evidence to establish what morality is, as well as God Who enforces the morality. Without a God to define a canonical moral point of view and then to enforce it, one cannot even recognize which normative point of view with its bioethics is the point of view that a person should affirm and why. But one would not expect Rorty always to be clear in these matters, in that for him morality is in the end politics, a political agenda he hopes will be established at law and in public policy.

This is why we face the deflation of secular morality. If all is ultimately meaningless, why should I not act to advantage my family, even if this undermines the greatest good for the greatest number, or even when this violates important right-making conditions? Perhaps the moralist will quote John Rawls and say, "we are so constituted that we have in our nature sufficient motives to lead us to act as we ought without the need of external sanctions, at least in the form of rewards and punishments imposed by God or the state" (Rawls 1993, p. xxvii). But Rawls's considerations will not be sufficient. They would not have been sufficient for Alexander the Great or Julius Caesar, who pursued glory rather than morality. The immoralist can simply respond to the moralist, "So what?! I will act to advantage my family or pursue glory, and, if I am careful, there will likely be no price to pay, only advantage." The normativity of the moral point of view cannot be established without begging the question, arguing in a circle, or engaging in an infinite regress. For a community to regard the moral point of view as always trumping prudence, one must already have conceded particular basic premises or rules of evidence, as well as at least Kant's practical postulates of God and immortality.

One is left with a troubling conclusion that one cannot in general secular terms establish the priority of a community of anonymous persons (i.e., the so-called moral point of view) over the claims of the particular community of those for whom one is most concerned and with whom one is most intimately socio-historically bound: the community of one's family, friends, and close associates. There is no canonical secular perspective that can rule out the priority of the perspective that affirms the good of those for whom one is most concerned as *the* appropriate and guiding normative point of view. Consider, for example, a person who is confronted with the alternative of either killing an innocent person with whom he has no relationship and no interest, for which homicide he would be amply and securely rewarded (and let us also grant, with little chance of ever being discovered as the murderer), or refusing to do so, in which case he, his family, friends, and close associates would be brutally and expertly tortured for a year and then subjected to a degrading, painful, and slow death by those making the offer. Again, if one held the universe to be ultimately meaningless, why would it be irrational to reject the anonymous moral point of view and instead embrace a family- and associates-focused view? In that within the dominant secular culture one cannot invoke a God's-eye perspective, there is no final standpoint from which in principle to show that one should not embrace a normative perspective that affirms that one should advance the flourishing of those with whom one is most intimately bound and connected (i.e., family, friends, and associates), rather than the good of persons generally, anonymously considered.

Without begging the question, arguing in a circle, or engaging in infinite regress, no special priority can be given to a Kantian or utilitarian moral point of view with its bioethics versus a quasi-Confucian, normative perspective with its morality that places family members centrally, then friends, etc., along with affirming family over individual patient consent. In the absence of being able to speak from the God's-eye perspective (and of course the question then is *which God?* the Norse god, Odin?), neither the perspective of the anonymous community of all persons nor the perspective of the community to whom one is bound in love and ultimate loyalty can in general secular terms be shown conclusively to have a compelling rational priority, a more compelling claim to be *the* normative point of view that one *should* affirm. The attempt to preserve at least something of morality's traditional priority over prudence fails.[41] One is left with a plurality of secular moralities and normative fabrics, some even rejecting the traditional moral point of view itself and instead affirming the pursuit of the flourishing and advancement of those for whom one is most concerned and most intimately bound in love and affection (e.g., family, close friends, etc.), or indeed the pursuit of glory or even mere naked personal advantage. The claimed priority of the traditional view of morality's canonicity is unsecured, once one no longer affirms Kant's practical postulates of God and immortality.

Talk of a religion without God will not help (Dworkin 2013), because such discourse does not identify any non-socio-historically-conditioned point of reference. It is organ music with nothing happening. After God, there is no one, or no perspective, from which to give a final judgment that can endure. There is no one enduring perspective to give content to the good, the right, and the virtuous so that it can persist in its significance. Some may say with Ronald Dworkin (1931–2013) that "religion is deeper than God. Religion is a deep, distinct, and comprehensive worldview: it holds that inherent, objective value permeates everything, that the universe and its creatures are awe-inspiring, that human life has purpose and the universe order" (Dworkin 2013, p. 1). Without a God to anchor them, those are simply pious and inspiring words without substance. Without a final and eternal self-conscious point of view to give a final judgment regarding any reward for right, good, and virtuous behavior, all is lost without any enduring point of reference. The result is that after God all is changed.

To summarize, there is demoralization and deflation of morality and bioethics that involve a radical recasting of a domain that had once compassed moral matters. Choices regarding one's engagement in sexuality, reproduction, and self-killing within the dominant secular culture have become mere life-style or death-style choices. Again, decisions whether or not to fornicate, to engage in homosexual acts or bestiality, to define one's life as a heterosexual, homosexual, or shoe fetishist, or to have one's children within or outside of marriage have become non-moral life-style choices. Choices in these matters are no longer experienced as, or considered to be, moral choices about which one can be blameworthy or praiseworthy. This shift in the understanding of morality and bioethics constitutes a watershed change. Consider again how outrageous it has become in the dominant secular culture to state that it is immoral to live a homosexual life-style. So, too, the choice whether or not to use abortion has within the dominant secular culture become a personal reproductive choice, a personal life-style choice, not a moral matter. In addition, within the dominant secular culture the choice whether or not to use physician-assisted suicide or euthanasia has become a death-style choice, not a matter that should be held to be good or bad, praiseworthy or blameworthy. Such choices within the dominant secular culture have ceased to be characterized as choices bearing on one's moral character or virtue. An important domain of human choices is no longer appreciated as having a moral valence. As we will see, the demoralization and deflation of morality affect morality as a whole.

VI. Morality and Bioethics as Macro Life-style Choices

As the demoralization of traditional morality was occurring, it was initially hoped by most secular moralists that the emerging post-Christian secular morality and bioethics would at least be able to maintain the full moral force of the cardinal slogans of the Enlightenment and the French Revolution regarding liberty, equality, human dignity, tolerance, social justice, and human rights. After all, when making life-style and death-style choices, the social-democratic moral perspective demanded that persons be recognized as free, equal, and without moral reproof in their legitimate, peaceful, life- and death-style choices, while all along asserting a canonical moral significance for liberty and equality. The expectation had generally remained that life- and death-style choices would still necessarily need to be placed within moral constraints that would require affirming others as possessing equal human dignity. However, this cannot be established as more than a particular macro life-style choice. Given the implications of the failure to provide foundations, human rights claims as well as the traditional Western heterosexist mores as secular claims equally come into question, because as secular moral claims they remain at best assertions supported by particular moral intuitions set within a freestanding moral-political view, all of which exists floating within the horizon of the socio-historically conditioned. Claims of human rights, human dignity, human equality, and social justice can at best derive their significance from one among a plurality of diverse ethnocentric fabrics of moral intuitions supported by one among a plurality of diverse moral narratives, the canonical force of which is undermined, when all is approached after God, that is, as if all were in the end without any ultimate meaning.

Within the dominant secular culture, and in the field of bioethics in particular, it is still largely unrecognized that the demoralization that renders traditional moral choices into choices among life-styles also transforms the status of the central moral tenets of the dominant secular culture itself. That is, the demoralization and deflation of morality bear as well on the force of such liberal moral norms as human equality, human dignity, human rights, and even tolerance. These moral claims, and for the same reasons, are best appreciated as elements of a particular life-style choice, albeit a macro life-style choice. This is the case because such general moral claims are no more embedded in a canonical moral rationality than are particular choices such as whether to embrace a homosexual life-style. The result is that the affirmation of a social-democratic moral vision, along with the bioethics of individual informed consent and truthtelling, is nothing more than a macro life-style choice, a more comprehensive life-style choice. In contrast, Alexander the Great, Julius Caesar, and Napoleon pursued glory over morality. The possible content of morality and bioethics is plural. For example, Chinese bioethicists affirm a family-oriented bioethics over an individually-oriented bioethics (Fan et al. 2012; Fan 2007). Choices in this area are at best claims sustained within a particular freestanding moral or political narrative, a point that Joseph Raz admits in his affirmation of individual consent. "The puzzle is how one can give consent a viable role, without saying that only principles already agreed to by all can be relied upon" (Raz 1990, p. 46). Raz proceeds to invoke an intuition, because otherwise he cannot justify the political theory he wishes to embrace. Because neither secular morality nor secular political authority are embedded in the will of God, a cosmic order, metaphysics, or canonical moral rationality, one is left with particular moral and political visions as a plurality of accounts, each supported by simply one among a plurality of intuitions sustained by one among a plurality of freestanding moral and/or political accounts or narratives, floating within the horizon of the finite and the immanent. Because by sound rational argument none among these positions can be established as canonical, they lack a conclusive rational necessity.

For example, what can the assertion that "all men are created equal" mean after God and after metaphysics? If God does not in some sense make all persons equal, and if there is no socio-historically unconditioned perspective that in some way requires all humans, if not all persons, to be recognized as equal, then in what way and on what canonical grounds can humans be equal? What can the canonical moral force of claims of human equality be in the face of the actual stark disparities and inequalities in terms of virtue, intelligence, and talents that distinguish humans, as well as in the face of an intractable moral pluralism that undermines the possibility of a single canonical standard by which to compare humans and still speak of equality? If one attempts to ground equality in an equal capacity to give permission, the minimal capacity necessary to acquiesce in the minimal state, this is not enough to account for more complex human institutions. One is confronted with a wide variation in the rational self-conscious appreciation of what it means to give one's permission. Why should all consent or permission carry the same weight? How does one compare the consent of an eleven-year-old with a thirty-five-year-old, a person with an IQ of 85 with that of a person with an IQ of 140? Analogous puzzles arise regarding reason-giving in rational discourse. And for that matter, why should reasons be confined to immanently apprehensible reasons (whatever that may mean), rather than include transcendent considerations such as the will of God, if one holds that one knows the will of God? The result is that not even social-democratic affirmations of liberty, equality, and solidarity can be established as morally canonical outside of a particular ethnocentric context or framework. Again, after God, and therefore after a canonical metaphysics and after canonical foundations, any particular affirmation of human rights, human equality, and human dignity is at best grounded in one among a plurality of local or particular moralities, each with its own web of intuitions supported by its own moral narrative.

The implications are wide-ranging and dramatic. Any particular affirmation of human rights, human dignity, human equality, social justice, and tolerance can at most be regarded as integral to the affirmation of a particular macro lifestyle choice. Nor can any particular macro life-style choice be shown by sound rational argument to be necessarily integral to the proper, that is, canonical, secular appreciation of the good, the right, or the virtuous. For example, in the absence of a non-socio-historically-conditioned God's-eye view, it cannot be demonstrated that the affirmation of a social-democratic ethos replete with the liberal West's list of human rights and liberal bioethical commitments is more integral to a rightly-ordered secular morality or view of the secular politically reasonable than the mores and political vision of elitist capitalist oligarchies such as Singapore. Nor can the view that one should appeal to individual consent rather than family-based consent (Fan 2007; Fan & Li 2004) be shown to be canonically rationally warranted. Nor will a Western liberal approach to the bioethics of health care allocation be able to be rationally established in preference to one warranted by a Chinese moral vision (Fan et al. 2012). No particular secular morality or account of moral rationality or of the politically reasonable has a canonical status that can be established by sound rational argument. Secular views of morality as well as of the politically reasonable remain plural.

The result is not a nihilism, but it comes close. It is not merely that the claims of traditional Christian morality cannot be maintained within the dominant secular culture through being recast into a secular morality, as Kant attempted.[42] More radically, moral claims in general within the dominant secular culture are demoralized into individual macro life-style choices, which exist as freestanding viewpoints sustained by diverse narratives (e.g., the moral vision of Cambridge, Massachusetts, versus that of Singapore or Beijing). As Judd Owen observes,

> The growing consensus among intellectuals today is that liberalism itself, like everything else human, is the product of a "cultural bias." Rorty agrees. We are "without a skyhook with which to escape from the ethnocentrism produced by acculturation" (1991, 2). Liberal democracy does not transcend ethnocentrism; it is a form of ethnocentrism (Owen 2001, p. 16).

The demoralization and deflation of traditional morality recast the significance and force of the social-democratic moral project itself into a macro life-style choice. All moral discourse within the horizon of the finite and the immanent, including the social-democratic political project itself, is left without foundations and therefore without ultimate significance. Traditional secular morality, indeed bioethics, that had once claimed a universal validity and a necessary rational priority for its moral point of view in putatively being anchored in reality or reason itself is cut loose from any secure mooring. Is this nihilism?

Well, not quite. Within the horizon of the finite and the immanent, there is still surely meaning. There are projects that can capture human interest and fill one's life with purpose. There are limited, finite goals that can *de facto* move

individual humans and unite human communities. One can pursue fully immanent projects and ideals. One can show love and courage. There is meaning, but
this meaning must be recognized as narrative- or account-dependent, such that
the narratives live and die with the narrators, or at least with the narratives and
the communities that sustain those narratives. Each moral narrative or vision is
under these circumstances contingent, socio-historically conditioned, existing
as one among a plurality of competing visions of human meaning sustained by
some but not other communities. All meaning *qua* secular is as a consequence
ultimately transient. Any particular moral community can be and will be dis-
rupted, indeed eventually obliterated. Nothing endures forever within the horizon of the finite and the immanent. Moral communities can remember virtuous
men and their accomplishments only as long as those communities exist.

The memory and perspective of any particular moral community is a meager
substitute for the memory and perspective of God. Communities die and their
records are lost, with the result that the memory of the virtuous and the vicious
is equally in the end, in the long run, lost. Absent the personal Creator God,
Who is the Genesis of all, the ground of all morality, the certain motivator for
rightly-ordered conduct, and the One Who forever remembers and appropriately rewards and punishes the virtuous and the vicious, all is ultimately meaningless. The Western culture that created a synthesis of Christian, Platonic, and
Stoic concerns and that lived in the recognition of an ultimate and enduring
reality has been replaced by a culture in which nothing has ultimate meaning
and in which no meaning is anchored in reality as it is in itself. This side of the
rupture from the possibility of ultimate orientation, reality and secular morality
are not just intractably plural, but in the end fundamentally meaningless. The
meaning of secular morality and bioethics needs to be radically reconsidered.

VII. From Kant to Hegel: The State and Politics as a Substitute for God and Morality

After metaphysics and after God, the secular fundamentalist state becomes a surrogate for God because, once reality, morality, and bioethics are severed from an
unconditioned ground in being, and once moral reason is recognized as plural
in content, one is not just left with a plurality of moralities and bioethics, but also

the closest thing to a common morality and a common bioethics becomes that morality and bioethics that are established at law and in public policy, a matter to which we will turn in greater detail in chapter six. This morality and bioethics are radically different from, and deflated in their force in comparison with, the traditional morality and bioethics of Christianity, which are anchored in the commands of God. Secular morality and bioethics are even pale in comparison with the morality of Kant, which thought itself to have an anchor in rationality. The strongest general normativity and authority that secular morality and bioethics can enjoy are simply that they are imposed through law and within a particular state. Given moral pluralism, the dominant moral and bioethical understanding is not that about which there is good reason to claim a moral consensus, a secular equivalent of a *consensus fidei.* The dominant morality and bioethics are at best the morality and bioethics that, given a sufficient political consensus, have been established at a particular time in a particular polity by an effective ruling political coalition. The result is that the dominant secular morality and bioethics are the secular equivalent of an established religion, now presented as the secular state's established secular ideology. Again, the current dominant secular morality and bioethics, along with its claims regarding liberty, equality, human dignity, and social justice, can at best be recognized as a cluster of intuitions embedded within a free-standing narrative of a particular community that has succeeded in having this morality and bioethics temporarily established at law and in public policy. The moral becomes the political.

Secular morality and secular bioethics (as we will also see in chapter six with regard to clinical ethics) are sustainable only as a secular political agenda, a point to which we will return at greater length in the next chapter. Here, however, it is important to note what impels post-modernity's political turn. The need to reassess the meaning of a secular morality and bioethics became more apparent as Western morality became post-metaphysical following the death of God in Western culture. As already emphasized, G. W. F. Hegel's announcement of God's cultural death in his 1802 paper "Glauben und Wissen" ("Faith and Knowledge") reflected a realization that after God morality cannot be anchored in an unconditioned moral perspective, and as a consequence morality is always socio-historically conditioned (Engelhardt 2010a and 2010b). Hegel recognized that for secular morality there can be no vantage point beyond the socially and historically conditioned perspectives of particular moral narratives and their narrators.[43] That is, secular morality involves a shift from a metaphysical to a post-metaphysical discourse, which invites all to act guided not by a theistic methodological postulate affirming God's existence and immortality, but by an atheistic methodological postulate. Again, Kant tried to avoid this radical recasting of morality. Kant implicitly recognized that, in the absence of the theistic methodological postulates, the moral-philosophical assumptions supporting the traditional strong understanding of Western morality would be unmasked as unfounded, leading to the radical demoralization and deflation of what had been traditional secular Western morality.[44] It is for these reasons that Kant affirmed as practical postulates the existence of God and of immortality.[45] Kant, however, had not anticipated the political restatement of morality that after God and after foundations would reground morality as ideology.

Hegel marks the end of modernity and the threshold of post-modernity. Crucial elements of the theistic moral vision had been abandoned by the dominant secular culture of the nineteenth century. In Hegel's case, an atheistic postulate was embraced, albeit camouflaged by a discourse rich in theological terms and images. Nevertheless, Habermas correctly appreciates the dramatic implications of these developments. "[A] renewal [in the dominant secular culture] of a philosophical theology [is impossible] in the aftermath of Hegel" (Habermas & Ratzinger 2006, p. 41), because "the *methodical* atheism of Hegelian philosophy and of all philosophical appropriation of essentially religious contents" defines the secular culture (Habermas 2002, p. 68). Apart from God, Hegel realized that philosophers by default become gods, or at least the standpoint of philosophy becomes the standpoint of God as far as this is possible within the horizon of the finite and the immanent.[46]

One should note as well a peculiarity of the particularity of all-encompassing immanence. By default, persons become the ultimate origin of, focus for, and judge of their own moral concerns. In the absence of canonical moral standards, and in the absence of an authoritarian or non-individually directed ethos, the now-dominant secular culture of the West endorses each person's freedom in peaceable secular interaction to be equally the determinant of the character of moral propriety. The result is that, given such a cultural context, autonomous decisions and agreements among consenting adults serve as the lynchpin of the contemporary secular moral fabric (Engelhardt 1986, 1996). Because there is no final unconditioned moral perspective, within this culture each individual by default comes to regard himself as having a moral right to tell, authenticate, and peaceably realize his own moral narrative, as long as this narrative and the actions it warrants are tolerant in being in conformity with the now-emerging criterion of not morally disapproving of the peaceable, secularly accepted life-style and death-style choices of others. Apart from God and metaphysics, persons find themselves left to frame their own moral and bioethical narrative without any canonical normative guidance. Each person becomes a quasi-God's-eye perspective.

If God is not recognized as existing, as well as establishing and enforcing rewards for acting rightly and punishments for acting wrongly, then the state is by default the best available enforcer of morality within the horizon of the finite and the immanent in being able, as far as possible, to provide a positive correlation between happiness and worthiness of happiness.[47] It is for this reason, *inter alia*, that Hegel understands the state to be "the march of God in the world [*Es ist der Gang Gottes in der Welt, dass der Staat ist*]." The state under these circumstances is the "actual God [*der wirkliche Gott*]" (Hegel 1991, p. 279, §258 Zusatz). In summary, in the absence of a canonical morality to define the culture, and deaf to the commandments of God, if one aspires to a general morality, then the best one can have is the establishment of a morality at law and in enforceable public policy. The force of law then substitutes for what had been the supposed universal rational force of moral norms, which since the time of the Western medieval moral-philosophical synthesis had been held to be grounded in moral-philosophical rationality, and whose putative rational force had in Western modernity already replaced the commands of God.

In the face of intractable secular moral and bioethical pluralism, that is, in the absence of a non-socio-historically conditioned foundation or perspective from which one can identify one morality as *the* canonical morality and bioethics, the final force of secular morality and bioethics becomes the sanctions within a particular secular state for acting contrary to that morality established at law and in public policy. One is left with legal sanctions understood in terms of the punishments imposed by law and considered in light of the probability of one's actually being punished.[48] The political becomes the higher truth and full force of morality. Medical law and established health care policy become the higher truth of bioethics. In summary, absent God and immortality, and absent a canonical reason that can substitute for God, it is the state that in lieu of God and of a canonical moral rationality gives secular morality its standing and force. Hegel accepted and affirmed all of this. Hegel embraced what Kant had sought to avoid. Hegel recognized that in a secular culture one could not escape a substantive revision of the content and force of Western Europe's dominant morality that was becoming after God and after metaphysics, nor do without its political realization. Hegel also appreciated that morality could only be fully understood in terms of its political realization, a matter to which we will return in chapter three. Hegel recognized and embraced a culture fully beyond that of traditional Christianity.

VIII. The Demoralization and Deflation of Morality and Bioethics: A Summary

Once secular morality and bioethics are recognized as incapable of appealing to a God's-eye perspective to secure a non-socio-historically-conditioned, "objective" grounding and to a God's-eye perspective that can enforce morality, that is, once one recognizes that sound rational argument cannot establish a particular canonical secular morality, then the various secular moralities must be recognized as multiple alternative clusters of moral intuitions supported by diverse narratives, floating as freestanding accounts within the horizon of the finite and the immanent, all without a final reliable enforcer other than the state. As a consequence,

(1) secular morality and bioethics are intractably plural. Given a plurality of basic moral premises and of rules of evidence, and in the absence of access to an unconditioned ahistorical standpoint equivalent to a God's-eye perspective by which to define the content of *the* canonical morality, any attempt to identify a canonical secular morality and bioethics will beg the question, argue in a circle, and/or engage in infinite regress.

(2) This intractable secular moral and bioethical pluralism has wide-ranging implications. One is confronted with the circumstance that there

are insufficient grounds for holding that persons who act contrary to the norms of the dominant secular morality and/or bioethics must necessarily be held to be immoral or blameworthy in the eyes of rational persons in general. This is the case because there are no universal secular canonical grounds to establish any particular secular moral claims as necessarily rationally binding, for there will always be alternative orderings of goods, rights, and preferences, none of which can be shown to be canonical. Because there is no one canonical view of the right, the good, and the virtuous that can be established as canonical through sound rational argument, there is therefore no unbiased basis on secular moral grounds to hold that those who violate one particular deontological, utilitarian, or virtue-based account must in universal terms be held to have acted wrongly, badly, or viciously, because, given a different view of what should be the guiding right-making conditions, the proper ordering of goods or preferences, or the correct view of virtue, a different rule for action could have been affirmed as the governing norm. In short, there is no universal or canonical secular moral perspective or account. Thus, a utilitarian hunter can plausibly respond to a utilitarian animal-rights advocate that the self-reflective culture of the hunt produces enough intense pleasure for a sufficient number of hunters so as to outweigh the pain of the animals involved. The animal may suffer, but the hunters can extend and deepen their pleasure from the kill in their reflections on, and stories about, the hunt. The same could be said with regard to an audience in the Colosseum watching gladiators. As a consequence, the meaning of morality is demoralized into conflicting and incompatible life-style choices.

(3) Secular morality and bioethics are demoralized into life-style and death-style choices. If all is approached as if there were no God, that is, if all is approached as if there were no final God's-eye perspective, secular morality and bioethics are not just plural in significance and force, but radically demoralized into various life-style choices. This demoralization is not just manifest in choices regarding third-party-assisted reproduction, abortion, physician-assisted suicide, euthanasia, and consensual

sexual activity outside of the marriage of a man and a woman, which are regarded as non-moral life-style and death-style choices, but this same demoralization discloses the true status of the social-democratic ethos and its affirmations of liberty, fair equality of opportunity, and human rights as simply a particular, ethnocentric, macro life-style choice. Alternative moral and bioethical perspectives such as the Singaporean pursuit of security and familial prosperity within an effectively one-party oligarchical capitalist state become at best alternative macro life-style choices (Li & Wang 2012; Lim 2004 and 2012; Fan et al. 2012). Each morality is a macro life-style choice.

(4) Morality is deflated in its claims of having priority over against the claims of prudence. After God and after metaphysics, the moral point of view can no longer be regarded as necessarily trumping the pursuit of the good of those for whom one is most concerned, such as oneself, one's family, friends, and close associates, even when this undermines the good of persons generally and violates the rights of individual persons. If one does not recognize a God's-eye perspective so as to establish a particular morality and bioethics, along with the God Who enforces that morality and bioethics, it is impossible without begging the question, arguing in a circle, or engaging in infinite regress to hold that it will always be irrational or improper to reject the moral point of view, the anonymous and unbiased regard of persons, including patients as persons, along with an anonymous regard of the good and of right-making conditions, and instead to affirm a normative account focused on achieving the good of a particular group, even if this involves diminishing the good of the greatest number and/or violating right-making conditions. Morality itself becomes a macro life-style choice.

(5) Morality and bioethics are further deflated in their force and significance in the absence of any ultimate meaning. That is, the force of secular morality and bioethics is radically deflated if one regards everything as coming from nowhere, going nowhere, and for no ultimate purpose, because acting morally or alternatively immorally is itself without ultimate significance. Thus, the significance of having acted immorally or

against the established ethics of the medical profession will in the long run in the absence of a God's-eye perspective be lost in the surdity of an ultimately meaningless reality. In a fully ultimately meaningless and surd universe, it will not have mattered whether one has acted morally or immorally, professionally or unprofessionally. The result is that, after God, the meaning and force of morality and bioethics are foundationally changed. Indeed, as Friedrich Nietzsche (1844–1900) recognized in *On the Genealogy of Morals* (1887), after God, morality is at best a fiction in the sense that morality possesses neither canonical status nor enduring meaning. As Anscombe underscored, after God the whole meaning of morality must be radically reconsidered (Anscombe 1958).

(6) In the end, everything crucially turns on whether one can veridically encounter the God's-eye perspective. Does God exist, and has He revealed Himself to us? This crucial issue will be the focus of section eight of chapter seven, "Encountering God."

In short, the intractable pluralism, demoralization, deflation, and ultimate meaninglessness characterizing secular morality and bioethics have dramatic implications with respect to the force of the normative claims advanced by the contemporary dominant secular culture regarding matters such as the moral significance of autonomy, equality, fair equality of opportunity, as well as human rights, patient rights, the rights of research subjects, social justice, and human dignity. The morality and bioethics of secular culture is radically different from, and deflated in its force in comparison with, the traditional morality and bioethics of Christianity, which is anchored in the commands of God and which is enforced by God, or for that matter in contrast with moralities such as that of Kant, which were supposed to be anchored in rationality itself, not that mere rationality could substitute for God. Without God, the meaning of morality and bioethics is substantively altered. After God, all is changed.

IX. Looking into the Abyss

In a culture after God, moralities along with their bioethics are nothing more than freestanding fabrics of intuitions sustained by narratives that float without foundations within the horizon of the finite and the immanent. They are macro life-styles. They have no necessary grounding in a canonical rationality or in reality as it is in itself. They are not secured by a normative vision that has any necessity beyond its affirmation by its partisans who endorse a particular cluster of intuitions and their narrative. Insofar as one can speak of a justification for a particular secular morality and its bioethics, it is only to be found internally, that is, within a particular freestanding fabric of intuitions. Within a narrative, one can find reasons, grounds, considerations, and arguments that can be engaged and advanced, given the assumptions and commitments of that narrative's particular morality and its bioethics. Each alternative morality and bioethics enjoys its own internal justifications, with each alternative morality and bioethics having its own basic premises and its own rules of moral evidence. But there is no common canonical morality because there is no common moral ground, no common basic set of moral premises and rules of inference. Absent a God's-eye perspective, a common canonical morality cannot exist. Secular morality is intractably plural and deflated. One is adrift in a meaningless, contingent cosmos.

The demoralization and deflation of morality have dramatic implications for how one regards one's life. One is placed within a life-world after sin. People within the dominant secular culture can no longer recognize that certain actions alienate them from the Ground of everything, that is, from God. Of course, those within this secular life-world will be pleased to be beyond guilt and shame when they make their peaceable life-style choices to fornicate, commit adultery, engage in homosexual acts, use donor gametes for reproduction, and use physician-assisted suicide or euthanasia. Within the dominant culture, these decisions have become acceptable life-style choices. Within this life-world after God, they are after sin and after morality. They can do things their way. They can live on their own terms. There is no more fear of God. When one is very sure one will never be caught, one will seek one's own good, and the good of those one loves, even against established law and public policy. This re-orientation from God to love of one's self has had an all-pervasive impact on how one understands who one is. All that had been once recognized as sins remain sins, albeit now sins in ignorance. Such sins will still turn one to oneself and away from God, but without the opportunity for repentance and re-orientation. Having rendered oneself blind to what one ought to be, one has eliminated a whole dimension of moral striving. In a world without ultimate meaning, one is left ultimately adrift. The everyday fabric of life has changed dramatically.

We live in a life-world radically apart from what I encountered in 1954. All appears, and is experienced, quite differently, although only a little over a half century has passed. Traditional Western morality had regarded itself as having a supporting rationality grounded in, and in accord with, a rationality anchored in being as such, indeed in accord with the will of God. In 1954, traditional morality was still salient in much of everyday life, even if its norms were often violated. In contrast, the now-dominant morality, the now-public morality, is articulated without God. It is now clear that this public morality lacks the basis for securing any point of final orientation or canonical moral view beyond being one among a plurality of immanent moralities. The now-dominant public morality along with its bioethics is a particular artifact of a particular culture. In contrast, the traditional morality and its bioethics were not understood to be contingent. They were regarded as rationally and metaphysically necessary. Now, however, it is ever clearer that the dominant contemporary secular morality has no necessity. It is one from among a plurality of possibilities. Last but not least, for both traditional Western Christian morality and the morality of modernity as illustrated by Kant, the grounds for acting morally, the motivation and justification to be moral, could only be secured through the God Who commands, punishes, and rewards. The morality of the now-dominant secular culture has publicly separated itself from any anchor in reality as it is in itself and/or canonical rationality.

Now when I walk the streets of Italy, I pass through the ruins of not only what had been a pagan empire, but what had once been Western Christendom. The pope is still there.[49] However, Western Christianity is fragmented and in rapid decline. There are ancient and beautiful, largely empty churches. The priests at the altars now look *ad occidentem*, often straight into my eyes as I enter. The priests are as old as I am. They are tired. They are men from a world that exists no more, or that, insofar as it exists, has survived crippled and in decline. The congregation is generally meager and also old. My grandchildren ask me, "What could possibly have happened? How could Western Christianity have died out?" They see the grandeur reflected in the buildings of Rome. Yet from our conversations with Romans, it is clear to them that traditional Christianity has died in Rome. They can understand the victory of the barbarians. Their puzzle is about what made Rome and Western Christianity fail.

When I sit with Roman Catholic clerics to drink in the evening and to discuss theology, morality, and bioethics, even with the young priests of the Legionaries of Christ[50] there is an appreciation that Christianity has become a scandal. Roman Catholicism and its celibate priesthood have become an embarrassment for Christianity as a whole. After I gave a lecture at Regina Apostolorum Pontifical University in Rome in March of 2010, young Legionaries of Christ reflected with me about the difficulty of seemingly unending pleas by prelates for forgiveness, given the continuing disclosures of sexual indiscretions. The continued disclosure of sexual liaisons, homosexual and heterosexual, with adults and with children by a supposedly celibate clergy[51] have now become a public stumbling block to taking Christianity seriously (Engel 2006). In 1954, such things happened, but they remained a private shame. Now much more is public. Even the sense of shame has changed, because everything concerning sexuality, reproduction, the family, and the authority of the state is now embedded in a life-world radically different from that which I entered as I first set foot in Italy in 1954. Given political correctness, there now is liberty only to speak of the abuse of children, but not to underscore homosexual seductions. It is a different culture.

Yet in the midst of the cultural rubble of what had once been Christendom, even in Italy, there are still believers. Belief has far from disappeared. Many believers are fundamentalist Protestants cut off from the history of Christianity as a whole and without a coherent understanding of church, but they do recognize that God lives and that Jesus is the Messiah, the Son of the living God. They have been given the grace to know the right answer to the question: Who do you say I am? (Mt 16:16). There are still Roman Catholics fervently loyal to what remains of their traditions. There is as well the ever-increasing presence of Orthodox Christians in the very heart of Rome. All of these, along with Orthodox Jews and traditional Muslims, collide with the aspirations of the now-dominant secular culture and the claims of the secular fundamentalist state. It is the children of those who take God seriously who are increasingly in the streets of Italy. Their places of worship are full.

Notes

[1]This chapter developed from ancestral papers presented at the Centro Evangelico di Cultura "Arturo Pascal" and Consulta di Bioetica Onlus, Turin, Italy, January 31, 2012 ("Bioethics after Foundations: Feeling the Full Force of Secularization"), at the University of Salento in Lecce, Italy, on February 1 ("The Deflation of Morality: Rethinking the Secularization of the West"), at the Instituto Banco di Napoli, Naples, February 3 ("How can an Autonomy-based Morality Get along with a Quasi-Religious Profession like Medicine?"), and at the University of Naples Frederick II on February 3 ("Autonomy, Medical Professionalism, and the Culture Wars").

[2]The term *dominant secular culture* identifies the established ideology of contemporary secular fundamentalist states (Engelhardt 2010c, 2010d). In a society shaped by a secular fundamentalist state, a state in which one secular moral perspective is established and enforced by law and public policy, there nevertheless remain particular communities with their own quite different cultures (e.g., Orthodox Christian and Orthodox Jewish).

[3]The Frankfurt School identifies a cluster of neo-Marxist critical social theorists, which took shape around the Institute for Social Research and included persons such as Max Horkheimer, who returned to be director of the re-opened Institute in 1950. The Institute significantly influenced neo-Marxist philosophy and social theory in the 1960s. For an overview of the Frankfurt School, see Arato & Gebhardt 1987.

[4]The fall of Rome in A.D. 410 was for many Romans unimaginable. It had not been pillaged since it fell to the Celts in 386 B.C. Jerome, who was living in Palestine at the time, was overwhelmed by the news that the city had fallen.

> Whilst these things were happening in Jebus a dreadful rumour came from the West. Rome had been besieged and its citizens had been forced to buy their lives with gold. Then thus despoiled they had been besieged again so as to lose not their substance only but their lives. My voice sticks in my throat; and, as I dictate, sobs choke my utterance. The City which had taken the whole world was itself taken; nay more famine was beforehand with the sword and but few citizens were left to be made captives. In their frenzy the starving people had recourse to hideous food; and tore each other limb from limb that they might have flesh to eat. Even the mother did not spare the babe at her breast (Jerome 1994, Letter CXXVII.12, p. 257).

> [B]ut alas! Intelligence was suddenly brought me of . . . the siege of Rome, and the falling asleep of many of my brethren and sisters. I was so stupefied and dismayed that day and night I could think of nothing but the welfare of the community . . . But when the bright light of all the world was put out, or, rather, when the Roman Empire was decapitated, and, to speak more correctly, the whole world perished in one city. . . . Who would believe that Rome, built up by the conquest of the whole world, had collapsed, that the mother of nations had become also their tomb; that the shores of the whole East, of Egypt, of Africa, which once belonged to the imperial city, were filled with the hosts of her men-servants and maid-servants, that we should

every day be receiving in this holy Bethlehem men and women who once were noble and abounding in every kind of wealth, but are now reduced to poverty? We cannot relieve these sufferers: all we can do is to sympathise with them, and unite our tears with theirs (Jerome 1994, "Preface to Ezekiel," p. 500).

Shortly after my first visit to Italy, a final destruction of the remnants of Western Christendom would begin. In 1954 I could not have imagined how different Italy would be in a mere fifteen years.

[5]The meaning of post-modernity will be further explored in the course of this volume. Here it is enough, as has already been underscored in chapter one, to identify a culture as post-modern if it has recognized that all secular accounts of morality, bioethics, and reality are intractably plural and without ultimate meaning.

[6]One might think of Richard Rorty's reflection on the detheologized Christian theology of Paul Tillich (1886–1965). "He would say, in effect, that it was precisely the job of a Christian theologian these days to find a way of making it possible for Christians to continue using the term 'Christ' even after they had given up supernaturalism (as he hoped they eventually would)" (Rorty 1991, p. 70).

[7]There is a considerable dispute about the force of the Enlightenment on modernity, ranging from Karl Löwith's secularization thesis (Löwith 1949) to the quite different position of Hans Blumenberg that the idea of progress is not a secularization of Christian eschatology, but a dynamic process from within human history itself (Blumenberg 1983).

[8]Peter Gay correctly perceives that, although there were many Enlightenments, they were still joined together in one general project.

> There were many philosophes in the eighteenth century, but there was only one Enlightenment. A loose, informal, wholly unorganized coalition of cultural clerics, religious skeptics, and political reformers from Edinburg to Naples, Paris to Berlin, Boston to Philadelphia.... The men of the Enlightenment united on a vastly ambitious program, a program of secularism, humanity, cosmopolitanism, and freedom, above all, freedom in its many forms—freedom from arbitrary power, freedom of speech, freedom of trade, freedom to realize one's talents, freedom of aesthetic response, freedom, in a word, of moral man to make his own way in the world (Gay 1966, p. 3).

[9]Even deism involves a recognition of a God's-eye perspective. One should note the difference between theism and deism. Immanuel Kant crafts a helpful distinction.

> Those who accept only a transcendental theology are called *deists*; those who also admit a natural theology are called *theists*. The former grant that we can know the existence of an original being solely through reason, but maintain that our concept of it is transcendental only, namely, the concept of a being which possesses all reality, but which we are unable to determine in any more specific fashion. The latter assert that reason is capable of determining its object more precisely through analogy with nature, namely, as a being which, through understanding and freedom, contains in itself the ultimate ground of everything else. Thus the deist represents this being

merely as a *cause of the world* (whether by the necessity of its nature or through freedom, remains undecided), the theist as the *Author of the world* (Kant 1964a, p. 525, A631–632=B659–660).

Kant in his account of empirical knowledge is a deist in invoking the idea of God as a regulative idea (A670–671=B700–701). In this regard, Kant is a defender of Intelligent Design in arguing that one must view the world as if it were created and designed by God. However, in his moral theology, Kant embraces a theism.

> . . . if we consider from the point of view of moral unity, as a necessary law of the world, what the cause must be that can alone give to this law its appropriate effect, and so for us obligatory force, we conclude that there must be one sole supreme will, which comprehends all these laws in itself. For how, under different wills, should we find complete unity of ends? This Divine Being must be omnipotent, in order that the whole of nature and its relation to morality in the world may be subject to his will; omniscient, that He may know our innermost sentiments and their moral worth; omnipresent, that He may be immediately at hand for the satisfying of every need which the highest good demands; eternal, that this harmony of nature and freedom may never fail, etc. (Kant 1964a, pp. 641–642, A815=B843).

Hear, O Kantians, your god is two: one deist and one theist!

[10]In the United States, secularization is reflected in movements to remove public acknowledgements of God through, *inter alia*, removing the phrase "one nation under God" from the Pledge of Allegiance (*Elk Grove Unified School District v. Newdow*, 542 U.S. 1 [2004]). There has also been opposition to the American motto "in God we trust" (*Aronow v. United States*, 432 F.2d 242 [9th Cir. 1970]; *O'Hair v. Blumenthal*, 462 F. Supp. 19 [W.D. Texas 1978]), as well as suits to remove displays of the Ten Commandments from public buildings (*McCreary County v. ACLU of Kentucky*, 545 U.S. 844 [2005]; *Van Orden v. Perry*, 545 U.S. 677 [2005]; and *Glassroth v. Moore*, 335 F.3d 1282 [11th Cir. 2002]).

[11]Traditional Christians will consider what John Rawls regarded as a "reasonable pluralism," as "a disaster," albeit given the fallen human condition unavoidable (Rawls 1993, p. xivf). Traditional Christians are in this sense fundamentalists.

[12]The so-called autumn of the Middle Ages showed a society coming apart in decadence and extremes. See, for example, Huizinga 1996.

[13]The idea of the Middle Ages as a period spanning from either the Council of Nicea (A.D. 325), the sack of Rome (A.D. 410), or the resignation of the last Augustus in the West (Romulus Augustulus, A.D. 476), was influenced by Flavio Biondi's (1392–1463) *Historiarum ab inclinatione Romanorum imperii decades*, a work in 32 volumes, written between 1439 and 1453, which spanned the history of Europe from 410 to the fall of Constantinople in 1453 (Masius 1879).

[14]European culture came to regard its new science, technology, and literature as superior to that of the ancients. "As early as the eighteenth century, the word 'modern' acquired something of the ring of a war cry, but then only as an antithesis of 'ancient'—implying contrast with classical antiquity" (Schorske 1985, p. xvii). The assertion of modernity's superiority over

against the ancients was captured in the term "the *querelle*." The *querelle* or quarrel focused on whether the culture of the moderns had surpassed that of classical Greece and Rome. The result was the emergence of the notion of cultural and scientific progress with its face to the future contrasted with the first period of the modern age, the Renaissance, with its face still turned to the past. See Baron 1959 and Lorimer 1956.

[15]One should recall the importance of episcopal principalities in the Western empire. For example, with the Golden Bull of Emperor Karl IV in 1351, three of the seven electors who determined who would be emperor were ruling bishops (Cologne, Mainz, and Trier).

[16]An immense transfer of church properties to the state had already occurred in the Austro-Hungarian empire under Emperor Joseph II (ruled 1763–1790), who in 1790 closed seven hundred religious houses.

[17]For a critical assessment of the Secularization of 1803, see Joseph Freiherr von Eichendorff (1788–1857): Eichendorff 1958, vol. 4, pp. 1133–1184.

[18]Into the early 20th century, courts in the United States affirmed Christianity. In 1892 the Supreme Court even opined:

> American life, as expressed by its laws, its business, its customs, and its society, we find every where a clear recognition of the same truth [that the Christian religion is a part of the common law]. Among other matters, note the following: the form of oath universally prevailing, concluding with an appeal to the Almighty; the custom of opening sessions of all deliberative bodies and most conventions with prayer; the prefatory words of all wills, "In the name of God, amen;" the laws respecting the observance of the Sabbath, with the general cessation of all secular business, and the closing of courts, legislatures, and other similar public assemblies on that day; the churches and church organizations which abound in every city, town, and hamlet; the multitude of charitable organizations existing every where under Christian auspices; the gigantic missionary associations, with general support, and aiming to establish Christian missions in every quarter of the globe. These, and many other matters which might be noticed, add a volume of unofficial declarations to the mass of organic utterances that this is a Christian nation (*Church of the Holy Trinity v. United States* 143 U.S. 457 [1892]).

Indeed, Christianity (generally Protestant Christianity) constituted an essential component of American common law (*United States v. Macintosh*, 283 U.S. 605 [1931]).

This continued cardinal moral role of Christian mores was accepted because this was in full harmony with the constitutional prohibition against the establishment of religion in the First Amendment to the compact styled the Constitution of the United States. This is the case because as written the amendment prohibits only a *federal* establishment of a religion. "Congress shall make no law respecting an establishment of religion, or prohibiting the free exercise thereof. . . . " The First Amendment originally meant in practice that ministers of one particular denomination could not be federally supported to the exclusion of other denominations. The prohibition against the establishment of a religion was not taken to require a separation of the state from religion in the sense of purging Christian moral norms from law and public policy (consider the legal prohibition of the marriage of adult sterile siblings). The American legal framework was accepted as "self-evidently" shaped by, and receiving guidance from, Christianity. As a consequence, until the last part of the 20th century, Christianity was in different states in different ways *de facto* and generally *de jure* the established religion. For a history of the continued establishment of Christianity in particular American states in the early 19th century, see McConnell 2003.

This establishment of Christianity in the United States was only brought into question in the mid-20th century as the Supreme Court through a set of rulings secularized American law and public policy by imposing the First Amendment on the states and public institutions generally. See, e.g., *Zorach v. Clauson,* 343 U.S. 306 (1951); *Torcaso v. Watkins,* 367 U.S. 488 (1961); and *Abington School District v. Schempp,* 374 U.S. 203 (1963). One should note that the Supreme Court itself has remained divided about how to regard the remnants of Christianity in public spaces.

> From 1947, when the U.S. Supreme Court first applied the non-establishment norms to the states, to the present, the justices of the Court have been sharply divided about what it means to say that government may not establish religion. They have been divided both about what the nonestablishment norm means as a general matter and, especially, about what the norm means, about what its implications are, for government aid to religiously affiliated schools. The division among the present justices is as great as it has ever been: The four most relevant recent cases decided by the Court (in 1995, 1997, 2000, and 2002) were decided by votes of five to four or six to three (Perry 2003, p. 6).

Despite this ambivalence, confessional Christianity has in general been removed from the public forum.

[19]The general cultural and legal acceptance of religious belief lay behind the United States Congress's adopting on April 22, 1864, the motto "In God we trust" for American coinage (The Congressional Globe, p. 144), which appeared for the first time on the two-cent coin that year. The Coinage Act of February 12, 1873, requires that "the Director of the Mint, with the approval of the Secretary of the Treasury, may cause the motto 'In God we trust' to be inscribed upon such coins as shall admit of such motto. . . . " Appendix to the Congressional Globe, February 12, 1873, §CXXXI, Sec. 18, p. 237. As late as July 30, 1956, the 84th Congress approved legislation by which "The national motto of the United States is declared to be In God We Trust" (P.L. 84–140), Law 36 U.S.C. 186.

[20]Until the mid-20th century, Christianity, and in most parts of the United States Protestant Christianity (save for anomalies such as southern Louisiana), constituted the civil religion of the United States. "Evidence that Protestant Christianity [was] the functional common religion of [American] society would overwhelm us if we sought it out" (Wilson 1986, p. 113). Until then, the American ethos was that of Protestant Christianity; see Huntington 2004. This general establishment of Protestantism allowed the American federal government to persecute Orthodox Christians in Alaska. See Oleksa 1992, pp. 171–186. For an account of

the weakening and transformation of mainline Christianity, see Hutchinson 1989; Roof & McKinney 1987; and Turner 1985.

[21]*Lautsi v. Italy*, no. 30814/06, §55, 3 November 2009 (referred to the Grand Chamber on 1 March 2010). For a discussion of this ruling, see Andreescu & Andreescu 2010 and European Court of Human Rights 2011.

[22]Hegel's "Glauben und Wissen" originally appeared in *Kritisches Journal der Philosophie*, vol. 2, number 1 (Tübingen: Cotta, 1802).

[23]One might note that the term social justice arose in the first half of the 19th century, coined by Luigi Taparelli, S.J.

[24]Paul Gottfried perceptively recognized that the move to values discourse transformed the German political party, the Christian Democratic Union (CDU).

> German political historian Karlheinz Weissmann presents an argument about "value conservatism" similar to mine in explaining the "leftward lurch" of the Christian Democrats on social and natural questions under Helmut Kohl and even more under Angela Merkel. According to Weissmann, in the 1970s the center-right CDU decided to exchange the defense of "structural conservatism," identified with the family, church, army, and nation, for a less confrontational "Wertekonservatismus," a position that signified a "dwindling of its conservative content." Instead of rising to the defense of German refugees from Eastern Europe, upholding the honor of its nation and the traditional concept of marriage, Christian Democratic leaders could leave behind divisive issues, which were likely to draw charges of flirting with fascism from the left, and to focus on inoffensive electoral slogans. In Germany, Weissmann insists that this substitution was deliberate and took place for opportunistic reasons (Gottfried 2007, p. 163).

[25]Contemporary Europe's embarrassment about its Christian past is grounded not just in its secularization, but also in its radical embrace of the supposedly universal, non-particularist commitment of the Enlightenment that produced a view of human equality, human dignity, and human rights built around a vision of humans as bare individuals.

[26]*Fundamentalism* is not a univocal term; it identifies both religious and secular fundamentalisms. The term originally arose in American fundamentalism when the American Bible League in 1907 produced twelve pamphlets entitled "The Fundamentals" defending traditional elements of Christian doctrines (e.g., the Virgin Birth, the atonement, the physical resurrection of Christ, and the Second Coming of Christ) under critical assault by liberal theologians. In this volume, a fundamentalist position is one that holds that the commands of God or of one's morality trump the requirements of the state, including what the secular state and the dominant secular culture hold to be the secularly politically reasonable. *Fundamentalist* has come to identify anyone with the view that his particular religious, moral, or metaphysical understandings, whether secular or religious, trump contrary claims in all matters addressed by that account. As Rawls puts it,

> Many persons — call them "fundamentalists" of various religious or secular doctrines which have been historically dominant — could not be reconciled to a social world

such as I have described. For them the social world envisaged by political liberalism is a nightmare of social fragmentation and false doctrines, if not positively evil. To be reconciled to a social world, one must be able to see it as both reasonable and rational. Reconciliation requires acknowledging the fact of reasonable pluralism both within liberal and decent societies and in their relations with one another. Moreover, one must also recognize this pluralism as consistent with reasonable comprehensive doctrines, both religious and secular. Yet this last idea is precisely what fundamentalism denies and political liberalism asserts (Rawls 1999, pp. 126–127).

Those who recognize revealed religious truth as traditionally understood within the Abrahamic religions (e.g., Orthodox Jews, Orthodox Christians, traditional Protestants, conservative Roman Catholics, and traditional Muslims) are fundamentalists in this sense. They have grounds to find the fragmentation of society into communities organized around false, not to mention sinful, moral and metaphysical viewpoints as a default position that is for the time being to be tolerated in the face of intractable and not-to-be-celebrated moral and metaphysical diversity. It is not a state of affairs to be celebrated.

[27]Of course, many philosophers constructed their accounts without God. See, for example, Antony 2010.

[28]The differences separating Confucian versus Rawlsian approaches to justice may involve not just different rankings of cardinal goods, but also different goods, as well as the role of different categories of basic approaches through which morality, law, and public policy concerns are addressed, as for instance the role of *li* or ritual. See Solomon et al. 2014.

[29]Rawls's acknowledgement of the family as the enemy of fair equality of opportunity leads him to be troubled about the proper place of the family within a society organized in terms of liberal social-democratic principles.

> The consistent application of the principle of fair opportunity requires us to view persons independently from the influences of their social position. But how far should this tendency be carried? It seems that even when fair opportunity (as it has been defined) is satisfied, the family will lead to unequal chances between individuals (§46). Is the family to be abolished then? Taken by itself and given a certain primacy, the idea of equal opportunity inclines in this direction. But within the context of the theory of justice as a whole, there is much less urgency to take this course (Rawls 1971, §77, p. 511).

[30]Agrippa, who lived towards the end of the first century or during the second century, showed why philosophical controversies such as moral controversies cannot be resolved by sound rational argument. His views are summarized by Diogenes Laertius, *Lives of Eminent Philosophers*, Pyrrho 9, 88–89, as well as by Sextus Empiricus, "Outlines of Pyrrhonism" I.15.164–169. To resolve a moral dispute by sound rational argument, the disputants must already embrace common and true basic premises, as well as common and correct rules of evidence.

[31]In his biography of Kant, Kuehn concludes that "Kant did not really believe in God" (Kuehn 2001, pp. 3, 391–2). Kuehn came to this conclusion on the basis of reports by persons

such as Johann Brahl, who stated that Kant did not "believe in God, even though he postulated him" (Kuehn 2001, p. 392). Nevertheless, God or at least the idea of God, along with the postulate of God's existence, played cardinal roles for Kant (Insole 2013). But none of these roles justified for Kant traditional recognition of man's relationship to God. As J. H. W. Stuckenberg noted, "reason did not postulate the existence of God for the purpose of prayer; therefore the idea of His existence does not justify prayer" [for Kant] (Stuckenberg 1990 [1882], p. 355). For Kant, the only proper role for prayer was a rhetorical one when it was engaged to encourage moral action. As for himself, Kant had nothing to do with religious ritual or personal prayer. "Thinking it contemptible for any one to become devout in the weakness of old age, he declared that this should never be the case with him; and he kept his promise, for during his greatest weakness and with death staring him in the face, there was a remarkable absence of all religious expressions" (Stuckenberg 1990, p. 355). Given the Enlightenment spirit of the time, "Kant was lauded as the saviour of religion and morality, and some regarded him as the improver and perfecter of the Christian religion" (Stuckenberg 1990, p. 374). The result was that "Creeds and the cultus, as well as the Scriptures, were now to be conformed to the Critical Philosophy and its religion and morality. A Reformed minister declared that the Kantian morality surpasses that of Christianity" (Stuckenberg 1990, pp. 374–5). The Kantian moral reduction of Christianity allowed a post-Christian culture still to call itself Christian, although it had with malice aforethought turned to set God as existing aside.

[32]Through his reference to God's holy will, Kant implicitly recognizes God as providing a canonical unity for the kingdom of ends. As the uniquely complete and canonical moral perspective, God secures for Kant a single, canonical morality. See Kant, *The Foundations of the Metaphysics of Morals*, AK IV.414.

[33]In the *Opus Postumum*, God is for Kant the foundation for a single and coherent moral law.

> There exists a God, that is, one principle which, as substance, is morally law-giving. For morally law-giving reason gives expression through the categorical imperative to duties, which, as being at the same time substance, are law-giving over nature and law-abiding. It is not a *substance* outside myself, whose existence I postulate as a hypothetical being for the explanation of certain phenomena in the world; but the concept of duty (of a universal practical principle) is contained identically in the concept of a divine being as an ideal of human reason for the sake of the latter's law-giving [*breaks off*] (Kant 1993, 204, AK XXII, 122–123).

Pace Kant, God gave different laws to different people, seven laws to the sons of Noah and then 613 laws to the Jews. Even in this case, the unity of both sets of laws is in God.

[34]Hegel was a somewhat high-church Lutheran atheist. Walter Kaufmann gives Heinrich Heine's (1797–1850) account of an evening with Hegel as an indication of Hegel's atheism.

> I, a young man of twenty-two who had just eaten well and had good coffee, enthused about the stars and called them the abode of the blessed. But the master grumbled to himself: "The stars, hum! Hum! The stars are only a gleaming leprosy in the sky!" For God's sake, I shouted, then there is no happy locality up there to reward virtue

after death? But he, staring at me with his pale eyes, said cuttingly: "So you want to get a tip for having nursed your sick mother and for not having poisoned your dear brother?"—Saying that, he looked around anxiously, but he immediately seemed reassured when he saw that it was only Heinrich Beer, who had approached to invite him to play whist. . . .

I was young and proud, and it pleased my vanity when I learned from Hegel that it was not the dear God who lived in heaven that was God, as my grandmother supposed, but I myself here on earth (Kaufmann 1966, p. 367).

For a slightly different translation of Heine's remarks, see Heine 1910, p. 114.

Hegel did not consider himself obliged to explain to others that, although he was a Lutheran, he was an atheist in the sense of denying the existence of the transcendent God. After all, he believed in God insofar as God existed, as incarnate in the community of philosophers. Terry Pinkard sees a further example of Hegel's views in Hegel's ambiguous answer to his wife as to whether he credited immortality: "when she asked him what he thought of [personal immortality], he simply without speaking pointed to the Bible, which she of course interpreted in her own way" (Pinkard 2000, p. 577).

[35]There is much disagreement about what Hegel understood his undertaking to be. My account of Hegel is indebted to Klaus Hartmann (1925–1991), who recognized that Hegel's mature project was not grounded in a metaphysics, but was instead post-metaphysical, or, as Hartmann puts it in his best-known article in English, "non-metaphysical" (Hartmann 1972). A presentation of Hartmann's understanding of Hegel's project can be found in Hartmann 1999, 1988, 1981, 1976, 1970, 1966. For an assessment of Hartmann's account of Hegel, see Engelhardt & Pinkard 1994. Hegel is best interpreted as setting aside the metaphysics that had reigned from the High Middle Ages into the 18th century.

As will be noted in chapter eight, Kreines describes Hegel's non-metaphysical account of reality in terms generally in accord with Hartmann's interpretation of Hegel. For example, Kreines states:

> Hegel seeks to advance yet farther Kant's revolution *against* pre-critical metaphysics . . . Hegel denies all need to even conceive of Kant's things in themselves, leaving no contrast relative to which our own knowledge could be said to be merely limited or restricted. That is, Hegel aims not to *surpass* Kant's restriction so much as to *eliminate* that restriction from the inside (Kreines 2007, p. 307, emphasis is in the original).

In all these accounts, it is recognized that for Hegel thought and being are one.

[36]The sophists and physicians of Greece played major roles in undermining the traditional character of Greek culture, in particular its recognition of traditional, religiously based norms. See Versenyi 1963.

[37]In his attempt to provide a rational ground for morality, Kant in *The Critique of Practical Reason* (1788) retreated to the assertion that morality is a fact of reason, holding that "The consciousness of this fundamental law may be called a fact of reason, since one cannot ferret it out from antecedent data of reason, such as the consciousness of freedom" (Kant 1956, AK V.31, p. 31).

[38]For Hegel, God was dead in the sense that the vanguard culture of Hegel's time no longer acknowledged God as a personal God or a transcendent noumenal entity. The result was a change in the character of the culture from one that experienced the centrality of at least a God's-eye perspective to a culture marked by "the feeling that 'God Himself is dead'" (Hegel 1977, p. 190; Hegel 1968, p. 414). This death of God for Hegel included the death of metaphysics in the sense that it had become clear that philosophy could not establish claims about the deep nature of reality as it is in itself apart from its being socio-historically conditioned. This Hegelian turning point, the lodging of transcendence within immanence, was crucial, a point that will be emphasized at a number of steps along the way of developing the arguments in this volume.

[39]By "after metaphysics" I identify a culture's loss of a sense that morality is anchored in reality, in being-as-it-is-in-itself.

[40]G. W. F. Hegel in the section "Die Moralität" of Grundlinien der Philosophie des Rechts (1821) criticizes Kant and similar moral-philosophical attempts to establish by rational argument alone a canonical, content-full morality. Such is not possible without covertly importing a particular content. Instead, as Hegel recognizes, all content comes from a particular socio-historically-conditioned circumstance, a particular ethical community (Gemeinwesen, or to use a later term, Gemeinschaft). "In an ethical community, it is easy to say what someone must do and what the duties are which he has to fulfil in order to be virtuous. He must simply do what is prescribed, expressly stated, and known to him within his situation. Rectitude is the universal quality which may be required of him, partly by right and partly by ethics" (Hegel 1991, §150, p. 193). "Was der Mensch tun müsse, welches die Pflichten sind, die er zu erfüllen hat, um tugendhaft zu sein, ist in einem sittlichen Gemeinwesen leicht zu sagen.—es ist nichts anderes von ihm zu tun, als was ihm in seinen Verhältnissen vorgezeichnet, ausgesprochen und bekannt ist. Die Rechtschaffenheit ist das Allgemeine, was an ihn teils rechtlich, teils sittlich gefordert werden kann" (Hegel 1986, §150, p. 298).

[41]Richard Rorty understood that once one recognized the absence of foundations for secular morality, the significance of morality and human life is radically recast. "The German idealists, the French revolutionaries, and the Romantic poets had in common a dim sense that human beings whose language changed so that they no longer spoke of themselves as responsible to nonhuman powers would thereby become a new kind of human beings [sic]" (Rorty 1989, p. 7). Rorty failed to sufficiently appreciate the scope of the unintended adverse consequences for society defined by a secular morality without foundations, lacking a God's-eye perspective with teeth: a God Who imposes sanctions and rewards. In contrast with Rorty, Dostoyevsky foresaw with foreboding what it would mean to live after God, the consequences of which were displayed by Hitler's National Socialism and the international socialisms of Lenin, Stalin, Mao Zedong, and Pol Pot. One might consider, for example, the brutal policies of Mao Zedong and his regime (Dikötter 2010 & 2013).

[42]Kant attempted a secular reconstruction of most of Western Christian morality. For example, he argued with regard to masturbation that it involved a use of oneself as a means in a way equivalent to self-murder. "The ground of proof surely lies in the fact that a man gives up his personality (throws it away) when he uses himself merely as a means for the gratification of

an animal drive. But this does not make evident the high degree of violation of the humanity in one's own person by the unnaturalness of such a vice, which seems in its very form (disposition) to transcend even the vice of self-murder" (Kant 1964b, p. 86, AK V.425).

[43]In the 5th century before Christ, Protagoras recognized that the death of God, that is, the denial of God's existence, entailed the death of metaphysics and of objectivity in ethics, such that humans became the only criterion of truth, with the consequence that secular moral pluralism is intractable.

[44]Kant recognized the necessity of God for morality and immortality. As Kant puts it already in the first edition of *The Critique of Pure Reason* (1781),

> . . . if we consider from the point of view of moral unity, as a necessary law of the world, what the cause must be that can alone give to this law its appropriate effect, and so for us obligatory force, we conclude that there must be one sole supreme will, which comprehends all these laws in itself. For how, under different wills, should we find complete unity of ends. This Divine Being must be omnipotent, in order that the whole of nature and its relation to morality in the world may be subject to his will; omniscient, that He may know our innermost sentiments and their moral worth; omnipresent, that He may be immediately at hand for the satisfying of every need which the highest good demands; eternal, that this harmony of nature and freedom may never fail, etc. (Kant 1964a, pp. 641–642, A815=B843).

Here Kant anticipates his articulation of his moral postulates of God and immortality in the *Critique of Practical Reason* (1788).

[45]Kant requires for the coherent engagement in moral action that we act as if there were ultimate enduring meaning. Otherwise, the rationality of morality would be brought into question. As Kant puts it in the *Critique of Pure Reason*: "These postulates are those of immortality, of freedom affirmatively regarded (as the causality of a being so far as he belongs to the intelligible world), and of the existence of God" (Kant 1956, p. 137, AK V.133). He rejects embracing the atheistic methodological postulate.

[46]For Hegel, it is philosophers and intellectuals generally who within the horizon of the finite and the immanent constitute the only equivalent of a God's-eye perspective, although the content of that perspective is socio-historically conditioned. For Hegel, it is philosophers who give the only available final rational answers to rational questions about morality and rationality. Philosophers as such are Absolute Spirit. They are the secular equivalent of God (Engelhardt 2010a). This will be examined in further detail in chapter eight.

[47]For Hegel, a morality becomes fully actual only when it is realized through becoming law and public policy. Hegel, *Elements of the Philosophy of Right*, 279, §258 Zusatz. The state provides a morality with an objectivity through rendering that morality into law and public policy. Hegel, *The Philosophy of Right*, §§244, 247.

[48]Christians understand that one is required by God to recognize the authority of the state so as to maintain the rule of law, one of the seven laws given to Noah. The state in this sense acts with Divine authority. "Let every person be subject to the governing authorities; for there is no authority except from God, and those authorities that exist have been instituted

by God. Therefore whoever resists authority resists what God has appointed, and those who resist will incur judgment. For rulers are not a terror to good conduct, but to bad. Do you wish to have no fear of the authority? Then do what is good, and you will receive its approval" (Rom 13:1–3).

[49]If one credits the arguments of some traditional Roman Catholic thinkers, Pope John Paul II significantly changed what the Roman Catholic church teaches (Ferrara & Woods 2002). The view that the papacy has adopted a fundamentally different view regarding Christianity appears fully vindicated by the interview on October 1, 2013, of Pope Francis in *La Repubblica* (Scalfari 2013). This issue will be further examined in chapter seven.

[50]At the end of the 20th century, the Legionaries of Christ had become a financially very well-endowed, "conservative," and successful order with over 800 priests. All I met were devout and committed to Roman Catholicism. The Legionaries were founded by Fr. Marcial Maciel (1920–2008) in 1941. By the late 1990s, allegations were surfacing that Fr. Maciel had had homosexual relationships with seminarians and other priests. In addition, there were indications of his having two families with two different women. It is interesting to note that, "following the 1997 charges made against Fr. Maciel, the Holy Father [John Paul II] went out of his way to demonstrate his confidence in and support for the priest [Maciel], who as the head of a religious congregation reports to and is directly responsible to the pope. On December 31, 2001, Angelo Cardinal Sodano, Vatican Secretary of State, second in command at the Vatican, blessed and inaugurated the new headquarters of the Pontifical Athenaeum Regina Apostolorum, the Legion's University in Rome" (Engel 2006, p. 973). John Paul II's support of Fr. Marcial Maciel once constituted a stumbling block to his canonization. Benedict XVI banished Fr. Maciel from ministry to a "life of prayer and penitence" in 2006; Fr. Maciel died in disgrace in 2008.

[51]As to my views of the Roman Catholic general requirement that clergy be celibate, I note with joy that the father of seven of my grandchildren is an Orthodox priest who was ordained after the birth of his first child.

References

Alora, Angeles Tan & Josephine M. Lumitao (eds.). 2001. *Beyond a Western Bioethics: Voices from the Developing World*. Washington, DC: Georgetown University Press.

Andreescu, Gabriel & Liviu Andreescu. 2010. The European Court of Human Rights's *Lautsi* decision: Context, contents, consequences, *Journal for the Study of Religions and Ideologies* 9.26 (Summer): 47–74.

Anscombe, G.E.M. 1958. Modern moral philosophy, *Philosophy* 33.1 (January): 1–19.

Antony, Louise M. (ed.). 2010. *Philosophers without Gods*. New York: Oxford University Press.

Arato, Andrew & Eike Gebhardt (eds.). 1987. *The Essential Frankfurt School Reader*. New York: Continuum.

Baron, Hans. 1959. The *querelle* of the ancients and the moderns as a problem for Renaissance scholarship, *Journal of the History of Ideas* 20 (January): 3–22.

Bernstein, Richard. 2003. Continent wrings its hands over proclaiming its faith, *New York Times*, November 12.

Blumenberg, Hans. 1983. *The Legitimacy of the Modern Age*, trans. Robert M. Wallace. Cambridge, MA: MIT Press. Translation of *Die Legitimität der Neuzeit*, 2nd rev. ed. 1976.

Brunner, Otto, Werner Conze, & Reinhart Koselleck (eds.). 1978. *Geschichtliche Grundbegriffe*. Stuttgart: Klett-Cotta.

Clement of Alexandria. 1994. *The Stromata*, in *Ante-Nicene Fathers*, vol. 2, eds. Alexander Roberts & James Donaldson. Peabody, MA: Hendrickson Publishers.

Copernicus, Nikolaus. 1543. *De Revolutionibus orbium coelestium*, 6 vols. Norimbergae: Johannes Petrium.

Cumper, Peter & Tom Lewis (eds.). 2012. *Religion, Rights and Secular Society: European Perspectives*. Cheltenham, UK: Edward Elgar.

Cvijic, Srdjan & Lorenzo Zucca. 2004. Does the European constitution need Christian values? *Oxford Journal of Legal Studies* 24.4: 739-748.

Dann, G. Elijah. 2011. Philosophy, religion, and religious belief after Rorty, in *An Ethics for Today*, Richard Rorty (pp. 27–76). New York: Columbia University Press.

Dikötter, Frank. 2013. *The Tragedy of Liberation: A History of the Chinese Revolution 1945–1957*. New York: Bloomsbury.

Dikötter, Frank. 2010. *Mao's Great Famine: The History of China's Most Devastating Catastrophe 1958–1962*. New York: Walker & Company.

Diogenes Laertius. 2000. Protagoras, in *Lives of Ancient Philosophers*, vol. 2 (pp. 321–367), trans. R. D. Hicks. Cambridge, MA: Harvard University Press.

Dworkin, Ronald. 2013. *Religion Without God*. Cambridge, MA: Harvard University Press.

Edelman, Nathan. 1939. Other early uses of *moyen âge* and *moyen temps*, *The Romanic Review* 30 (December): 327–330.

Eichendorff, Joseph Freiherr von. 1958. *Werke und Schriften*. Stuttgart: Cotta'sche.

Engel, Randy. 2006. *The Rite of Sodomy*. Export, PA: New Engel Publishing.

Engelhardt, H. T., Jr. 2010a. Moral obligation after the death of God: Critical reflections on concerns from Immanuel Kant, G.W.F. Hegel, and Elizabeth Anscombe, *Social Philosophy & Policy* 27.2: 317–340.

Engelhardt, H. T., Jr. 2010b. Kant, Hegel, and Habermas: Reflections on 'Glauben und Wissen', *The Review of Metaphysics* 63.4: 871–903.

Engelhardt, H. T., Jr. 2010c. Religion, bioethics, and the secular state: Beyond religious and secular fundamentalism, *Notizie di Politeia* 26.97: 59–79.

Engelhardt, H. T., Jr. 2010d. Political authority in the face of moral pluralism: Further reflections on the non-fundamentalist state, *Notizie di Politeia* 26.97: 91–99.

Engelhardt, H. T., Jr. 2000. *The Foundations of Christian Bioethics*. Salem, MA: Scrivener Publishing.

Engelhardt, H. T., Jr. 1973. *Mind-Body: A Categorial Relation*. The Hague: Martinus Nijhoff.

Engelhardt, H. T., Jr., & Terry Pinkard (eds.). 1994. *Hegel Reconsidered*. Dordrecht: Kluwer.

European Court of Human Rights. 2009. *Lautsi v. Italy, Second Section*, November 3.

European Court of Human Rights. 2011. *Lautsi v. Italy, Grand Chamber*, March 18.

Fan, Ruiping (ed.). 2011. *The Renaissance of Confucianism in Contemporary China*. Dordrecht: Springer.

Fan, Ruiping. 2010. *Reconstructionist Confucianism*. Dordrecht: Springer.

Fan, Ruiping. 2007. Which care? Whose responsibility? And why family? A Confucian account of long-term care for the elderly, *Journal of Medicine & Philosophy* 37.5 (October): 495–517.

Fan, Ruiping, Xiaoyang Chen, & Yongfu Cao. 2012. Family-oriented health savings accounts: Facing the challenges of health care allocation, *Journal of Medicine and Philosophy* 37.6: 507–512.

Fan, Ruiping & B. Li. 2004. Truth telling in medicine: The Confucian view, *Journal of Medicine & Philosophy* 29.2 (April): 179–94.

Ferrara, Christopher A. & Thomas E. Woods, Jr. 2002. *The Great Façade: Vatican II and the Regime of Novelty in the Roman Catholic Church*. Wyoming, MN: Remnant Press.

Gay, Peter. 1966. *The Enlightenment: An Interpretation*. New York: W. W. Norton.

Gildea, Robert. 2008. *Children of the Revolution: The French, 1799–1914*. Cambridge, MA: Harvard University Press.

Gottfried, Paul E. 2007. *Conservatism in America: Making Sense of the American Right*. New York: Palgrave Macmillan.

Habermas, Jürgen. 2002. *Religion and Rationality*, ed. Eduardo Mendieta. Cambridge, MA: MIT Press.

Habermas, Jürgen & Joseph Ratzinger. 2006. *The Dialectics of Secularization*. San Francisco: Ignatius Press.

Hartmann, Klaus. 1999. *Hegels Logik*, ed. Olaf Müller. Berlin: Walter de Gruyter.

Hartmann, Klaus. 1988. *Studies in Foundational Philosophy*. Amsterdam: Rodopi.

Hartmann, Klaus. 1981. *Politische Philosophie*. Munich: Alber.

Hartmann, Klaus. 1976. *Die ontologische Option*. Berlin: Walter de Gruyter.

Hartmann, Klaus. 1972. Hegel: A non-metaphysical view. In *Hegel*, ed. Alasdair MacIntyre (pp. 101–124). Garden City, NY: Anchor Books.

Hartmann, Klaus. 1970. *Die Marxsche Theorie*. Berlin: Walter de Gruyter.

Hartmann, Klaus. 1966. On taking the transcendental turn, *Review of Metaphysics* 20.2: 223–249.

Hegel, G.W.F. 1991. *Elements of the Philosophy of Right*, ed. Allen W. Wood, trans. H. B. Nisbet. Cambridge: Cambridge University Press.

Hegel, G.W.F. 1986. *Grundlinien der Philosophie des Rechts*. Frankfurt/M.: Suhrkamp.

Hegel, G.W.F. 1977. *Faith and Knowledge*, trans. Walter Cerf and H. S. Harris. Albany: State University of New York Press.

Hegel, G.W.F. 1968. *Jenaer kritische Schriften*, in *Gesammelte Werke*, vol. 4. Hamburg: Meiner.

Heine, Heinrich. 1910. *Heinrich Heine's Memoirs from his Works, Letters and Conversations*, ed. Gustav Karpeles, trans. Gilbert Cannan. London: Heinemann.

Hofmann, H.H. (ed.). 1976. *Quellen zum Verfassungsorganismus des heiligen römisches Reiches deutscher Nation*. Darmstadt: Wissenschaftliche Buchgesellschaft.

Huizinga, Johan. 1996. *The Autumn of the Middle Ages*, trans. Rodney J. Payton & Ulrich Mammitzsch. Chicago: University of Chicago Press.

Huntington, Samuel P. 2004. *Who Are We: The Challenges to America's National Identity*. New York: Simon & Schuster.

Hutchinson, William R. (ed.). 1989. *Between the Times: The Travail of the Protestant Establishment in America, 1900–1960*. New York: Cambridge University Press.

Insole, Christopher J. 2013. *Kant and the Creation of Freedom*. Oxford: Oxford University Press.

Jerome. 1994. *Letters and Select Works*, in *Nicene and Post-Nicene Fathers*, Second Series (vol. 6), ed. Philip Schaff and Henry Wace. Peabody, MA: Hendrickson Publishers.

Kallscheuer, Otto. 1996. *Das Europa der Religionen*. Frankfurt am Main: Fischer.

Kant, Immanuel. 1993. *Opus Postumum*, ed. Eckart Förster, trans. Eckart Förster & Michael Rosen. Cambridge: Cambridge University Press.

Kant, Immanuel. 1964a. *Immanuel Kant's Critique of Pure Reason*, trans. Norman Kemp Smith. New York: Macmillan.

Kant, Immanuel. 1964b. *The Metaphysical Principles of Virtue*, trans. James Ellington. Indianapolis: Bobbs-Merrill.

Kant, Immanuel. 1959. *Foundations of the Metaphysics of Morals*, trans. Lewis White Beck. Indianapolis: Bobbs-Merrill.

Kant, Immanuel. 1956. *Critique of Practical Reason*, trans. Lewis White Beck. Indianapolis: Bobbs-Merrill.

Kaufmann, Walter. 1966. *Hegel: A Reinterpretation*. New York: Doubleday Anchor.

Kreines, James. 2007. Between the bounds of experience and divine intuition: Kant's epistemic limits and Hegel's ambitions, *Inquiry* 50: 306–334.

Kuehn, Manfred. 2001. *Kant: A Biography*. Cambridge: Cambridge University Press.

Kuhn, Thomas. 1962. *The Structure of Scientific Revolutions*. Chicago: University of Chicago Press; 2nd ed., enlarged, 1970.

Laforgue, Jules. 1958. The impossible, trans. William Jay Smith, in *An Anthology of French Poetry from Nerval to Valéry in English Translation*, ed. Angel Flores. Garden City, NY: Doubleday.

Latreille, André. 1948. *L'Église catholique et la révolution française*, 2 vols. Paris: Hachette.

Leigh, Edward & Alex Haydon (eds.). 2009. *The Nation that Forgot God*. London: Social Affairs Unit.

Li, Jun & Jue Wang. 2012. Individuals are inadequate: Recognizing the family-centeredness of Chinese bioethics and Chinese health system, *Journal of Medicine and Philosophy* 37.6: 568–582.

Lim, Meng-Kin. 2012. Values and health care: The Confucian dimension in health care reform, *Journal of Medicine & Philosophy* 37.6: 545–555.

Lim, Meng-Kin. 2004. Shifting the burden of health care finance: A case study of public-private partnership in Singapore, *Health Policy* 69: 83–92.

Lorimer, J. W. 1956. A neglected aspect of the 'querelle des anciens et des modernes', *The Modern Language Review* 51 (April): 179–185.

Löwith, Karl. 1949. *Meaning in History: The Theological Presuppositions of the Philosophy of History*. Chicago: University of Chicago Press.

Lyotard, Jean-François. 1984. *The Postmodern Condition*, trans. G. Bennington and B. Massumi. Manchester: Manchester University Press.

Marauhn, Thilo. 2004. Die Bewältigung interreligiöser Konflikte in multireligiösen Gesellschaften, in *Koexistenz und Konflikt von Religionen im vereinten Europa*, ed. Hartmut Lehmann (pp. 12–29). Göttingen: Wallstein.

Masius, Alfred. 1879. *Flavio Biondo, sein Leben und seine Werke*. Leipzig: B. G. Teubner.

Masterman, Margaret. 1970. The nature of a paradigm, in *Criticism and the Growth of Knowledge* (pp. 59–89), eds. Imre Lakatos & Alan Musgrave. London: Cambridge University Press.

Mathiez, Albert. 1977. *Les Origines des cultes révolutionnaires*. Geneva: Slatkine. 1st ed. 1904.

McConnell, Michael W. 2003. Establishment and disestablishment at the founding, Part I: Establishment of religion, *William & Mary Law Review* 44.5: 2105–2208.

Oleksa, Michael. 1992. *Orthodox Alaska*. Crestwood, NY: St. Vladimir's Seminary Press.

Owen, J. Judd. 2001. *Religion and the Demise of Liberal Rationalism*. Chicago: University of Chicago Press.

Paz, Octavio. 1974. *Children of the Mire*, trans. Rachel Phillips. Cambridge, MA: Harvard University Press.

Pera, Marcello. 2011. *Why We Should Call Ourselves Christians: The Religious Roots of Free Societies*, trans. L. B. Lappin. Jackson, TN: Encounter.

Perry, Michael J. 2003. *Under God? Religious Faith and Liberal Democracy*. New York: Cambridge University Press.

Pinkard, Terry. 2000. *Hegel: A Biography*. New York: Cambridge University Press.

Puppinck, Grégor. 2012. The case of Lautsi v. Italy: A synthesis, *Brigham Young University Law Review* 873, issue 3. Available at: http://digitalcommons.law.byu.edu/lawreview/vol2012/iss3/7

Puppinck, Grégor & Kris J. Wenberg. 2010. Legal memorandum, ECHR—Lautsi v. Italy, *European Centre for Law and Justice*. Available at: eclj.org/pdf/ECLJ-MEMO-LAUTSI-ITALY-ECHR-PUPPINCK.pdf

Rawls, John. 1999. *The Law of Peoples*. Cambridge, MA: Harvard University Press.

Rawls, John. 1993. *Political Liberalism*. New York: Columbia University Press.

Rawls, John. 1971. *A Theory of Justice*. Cambridge, MA: Belknap Press.

Raz, Joseph. 1990. Facing diversity: The case of epistemic abstinence, *Philosophy & Public Affairs* 19.1 (Winter): 3–46.

Reclus, Maurice. 1947. *Jules Ferry*. Paris: Flammarion.

Rendtorff, Trutz. 1975. Die Beziehung von Kirche und Staat—zur Wirklichkeit der Volkskirche, in *Trennung von Kirche und Staat?* ed. Klaus Wegenast et al. (pp. 50–60). Hamburg-Bergstedt: Herbert Reich Evangelischer Verlag.

Roof, Wade Clark & William McKinney. 1987. *American Mainline Religion: Its Changing Shape and Future*. New Brunswick, NJ: Rutgers University Press.

Rorty, Richard. 1991. *Objectivity, Relativism, and Truth*. New York: Cambridge University Press.

Rorty, Richard. 1989. *Contingency, Irony, and Solidarity*. New York: Cambridge University Press.

Sajó, András. 2008. Preliminaries to a concept of constitutional secularism, *International Journal of Constitutional Law* 6.3-4: 605–629..

Scalfari, Eugenio. 2013. The pope: how the church will change, *La Repubblica* (October 1) http://www.repubblica.it/cultura/2013/10/01/news/pope_s_conversation_with_scalfari_english-67643118/ [accessed October 3, 2015]

Schorske, Carl E. 1985. *Fin-de-Siècle Vienna*. New York: Alfred Knopf.

Schreiber, Monica. 2012. *Kirche und Europa*. Berlin: De Gruyter.

Schutz, Alfred & Thomas Luckmann. 1973. *The Structures of the Life-World*, trans. Richard M. Zaner and H. T. Engelhardt. Evanston, IL: Northwestern University Press.

Secher, Reynald. 2003. *A French Genocide: The Vendée*, trans. George Holoch. Notre Dame, IN: University of Notre Dame Press.

Sigfusson, Saemund. 1906. The high one's lay, in *The Eddas*, ed. Rasmus Anderson, trans. Benjamin Thorpe. London: Norroena Society.

Smith, Steven D. 1995. *Foreordained Failure: The Quest for a Constitutional Principle of Religious Freedom*. New York: Oxford University Press.

Solomon, David, Ping-Cheung Lo, & Ruiping Fan (eds.). 2014. *The Common Good: Chinese and American Perspectives*. Dordrecht: Springer.

Stuckenberg, J. H. W. 1990 [1882]. *The Life of Immanuel Kant*. Bristol: Thoemmes.

Turner, James. 1985. *Without God, without Creed: The Origins of Unbelief in America*. Baltimore, MD: Johns Hopkins University Press.

Uitz, Renata. 2012. The pendulum of church-state relations in Hungary, in *Religion, Rights and Secular Society: European Perspectives*, eds. Peter Cumper & Tom Lewis (pp. 189–214). Cheltenham, UK: Edward Elgar.

Vattimo, Gianni. 1988. *The End of Modernity*, trans. Jon R. Snyder. Baltimore: Johns Hopkins University Press.

Versenyi, Laszlo. 1963. *Socratic Humanism*. New Haven, NJ: Yale University Press.

Vesalius, Andreas. 1543. *De humani corporis fabrica*. Basel: A Operinus.

Vovelle, Michel. 1991. *The Revolution Against the Church*, trans. Alan José. Columbus: Ohio State University Press.

Weiler, Joseph H. H. 2003. *Un Europa Cristiana. Un saggio esplorativo*. Bologna: Biblioteca Univ. Rizzoli.

Weiler, Joseph H. H. 1999. *The Constitution of Europe: 'Do the New Clothes Have an Emperor?' and Other Essays on European Integration*. Cambridge: Cambridge University Press.

Wiedemann, Richard. 2012. *Der Streit um das Schulkreuz in Deutschland und Italien*. Berlin: Duncker & Humblot.

Wilson, A. N. 1999. *God's Funeral*. New York: W. W. Norton.

Wilson, John. 1986. Common religion in American society, in *Civil Religion and Political Theology* (pp. 111–124), ed. Leroy S. Rouner. Notre Dame, IN: University of Notre Dame Press.

Zucca, Lorenzo. 2012. *A Secular Europe*. Oxford, UK: Oxford University Press.

Zucca, Lorenzo. 2009. The crisis of the secular state—A reply to Professor Sajó, *International Journal of Constitutional Law* 7.3: 494–514.

CHAPTER THREE

More on Secularization, Thoughts on Sex, and the Authority of the State[1]

I. Varieties of Secularization Reconsidered

God is no longer worshipped publicly. Even sex has changed. Sex no longer has moral significance. Having sex has become like playing tennis: one just needs a consenting partner if one is not playing solitaire. A whole domain of human life has been deflated in its significance. How is one to understand these vast recent transformations of Western culture? How is one to understand secularization and its consequences, especially given the demoralization and deflation of morality? The removal of God from the public square by taking away any point of ultimate orientation has brought across the radical force and meaning of secularization. The place in which we find morality and bioethics is new. So, too, is the meaning of health care policy. Secularization not only changes sex, and therefore the bioethics of such issues as the artificial insemination of unmarried women, as well as of abortion, but also the legitimacy of the state is brought into question, along with the standing of health care policy.

At the outset, one must acknowledge that secularity, secularism, and secularization are multivalent and ambiguous. For example, the secularity of the minimal state outlined in *The Foundations of Bioethics* (Engelhardt 1986, 1996) is not the secularity of contemporary secular fundamentalist states. The English term "secular" derives from the Latin *saeculum*, which itself has a range of meanings. Lewis and Short give the following definitions of the Latin:

1. the body of individuals born at a particular time, a generation; a generation within a single family; (pl.) the succession of generations; 2. a breed, race;

3. the present time, the contemporary generation, the age; 4. the period of a time corresponding to the lifetime of a particular person or persons, age; 5. a human lifetime, generation; 6. 1 period of one hundred years, a century; 7. one of the imaginary divisions or ages (golden, silver, etc.) of human history; 8. (pl.) future ages, posterity; 9. (pl.) through the ages, for ever; the course of human affairs; 10. human life, the world (Lewis & Short 1879, pp. 1613–1614).

The word *saeculum* is rich in meaning. For example, *saeculare* also refers to a hymn, the *carmen saeculare*, which Horace composed at the command of Augustus Caesar and was first sung in A.U.C. 737 (i.e., 17 B.C.). A *saeculum* marked a period of about 100 to 120 years and had a sense of *sacramentum* and *sacerdotum* (Mommsen 1858, esp. pp. 168–189). The word was once heard in Roman Catholic churches throughout the world in the refrain, "per omnia saecula saeculorum", "through ages of ages".

The English terms *secular* and *secularization* also compass a complex variety of meanings. These include (1) the religiously neutral context of ordinary life that a monk renounces so as through asceticism to pursue the Kingdom of Heaven (*saeculo renunciare*),[2] (2) a cleric or the property of a cleric who has not taken special "religious" vows (e.g., poverty, chastity, and obedience), (3) the process of rendering a religious cleric and/or his property into being secular (e.g., freeing the cleric from those vows), (4) the process that renders a cleric or church property into a layman or a layman's property, (5) the attempt to annul or limit the powers, immunities, and influence of the church, (6) secularism as a movement or ideology aimed at removing religious discourse and presence from the public forum and/or the public space, and (7) secularization as the process by which the dominant culture is cleansed of any reference to God and religion. The minimal state, as for example in the account of Robert Nozick (1938–2002), is secular in the first sense (Nozick 1971). However, there is on the face of the earth no minimal state. The sixth sense is exemplified in the movement, secularism, founded by George Holyoake (1817–1906) (Goss 1908; Holyoake 1896, 1871). The laicism that structures current secular fundamentalist states draws on both the sixth and the seventh senses (Engelhardt 1991, pp. 22–23; 2010a, 2010d).

These senses of *secular* and *secularism* in the end led to a laicism that gained salience after the French Revolution but especially after 11 December 1905 with the Separation Law and the repudiation of the 1801 Concordat and that now frames the dominant secular culture. Here, following James K. A. Smith's reflections on the meaning of secular in the thought of Charles Taylor, there is secular$_2$. According to this account of secularism,

> Political spaces (and the constitutions that create them) should carve out a realm purified of the contingency, particularity, and irrationality of religious belief and instead be governed by universal, neutral rationality. Secularism is always secularism$_2$. And secularization theory is usually a confident expectation that societies will become secular$_2$—that is, characterized by decreasing religious belief and participation. People who self-identify as "secular" are usually identifying as areligious (Smith 2014, p. 21).

There is also a secular$_3$. "A society is secular$_3$ insofar as religious belief or belief in God is understood to be one option among others, and thus contestable (and contested)" (Smith 2014, pp. 21–22). Secularism$_3$ is equivalent to the seventh sense of the secular mentioned above in which a cultural space exists that gives no decisive place for God and His claims.

One must note that *laïcité* has become a complex French Republican concept. As Cécile Laborde defines it,

> *Laïcité* is often translated as "secularism," but I argue that it in fact encompasses a comprehensive theory of republican citizenship, articulated around three ideals: equality (religious neutrality of the public sphere or secularism *stricto sensu*), liberty (individual autonomy and emancipation from religious oppression), and fraternity (civic loyalty to the community of citizens) (Laborde 2008, pp. 7–8).

Laïcité and secularism are thus often associated with a particular secular constitutional project.

The secular character of the culture now dominant in Western Europe and the Americas is more radical than Charles Taylor appreciates (Taylor 2007). First, contemporary secularity is nested within a robust and aggressive laicism. It is not just that, in the now-dominant culture, belief in God has become optional,[3] which involves secularity in the first sense, or that concern for God and the transcendent have weakened, but that reference to God and the transcendent have with prejudice been removed from public spaces,[4] involving secularization in the sixth and seventh senses. It is rather that this secularization is occurring in a very aggressive fashion, such that the now-dominant culture has made public confession of belief in God highly politically incorrect. As David Hollinger observes, in America by the 1960s "Religion was increasingly private, and public discussion was increasingly secular" (Hollinger 1996, p. 28). Among other things, in America's elite colleges and universities, "the open profession of Christian belief in the course of one's professional work is uniquely discouraged" (Hollinger 1996, p. 28). As Michael McConnell puts it, "in most of academia, and in many walks of life dominated by the secular elite, the news of the death of God has been taken to heart and the voice of religion is all but silenced" (McConnell 1993, p. 166). This provides a strong instance of the sixth and the seventh senses of secularization. Religious faith is something one should not have, or at least have only privately and then only with embarrassment, and about which one should not speak in public. The contemporary dominant secular culture creates a pervasive sentiment against any speech or behavior that suggests belief in God and against believers who confess their belief in the public space. Belief in God is something about which one should even feel ashamed. The secularization of the public forum and public space, as well as of the dominant culture, excludes not just religious acknowledgements of God and of the importance of worshipping God, but it even excludes public philosophical, non-religious reflections on whether one needs to acknowledge God in order to make sense of morality and reality. Secularization is many-faceted and multi-dimensional (Connolly 1999; Dreyfus & Kelly 2011; Gregory 2012; Warner et al. 2010). In the face of this secularization, one is not even to ask whether the idea of God is essential to traditional notions of morality and bioethics.

There is a resolute animus against any public consideration of God or of the transcendent, because many now regard even a philosophical consideration of God as a prelude to religious violence, in particular the violence of believers against non-believers. As Santiago Zabala puts it, "Thought must abandon all objective, universal, and apodictic foundational claims in order to prevent Christianity, allied with metaphysics in the search for first principles, from making room for violence" (Zabala 2005, p. 13). Such secularists hold themselves justified in mounting a pre-emptive strike against what they perceive to be the dangers of even the most abstract theological reflection, though in the 20th century more were killed by atheist governments than have ever been killed by religious fanaticism. These secularists have embraced a strong sense of *laïcité* so that religious beliefs or even natural theological reflections have come to be regarded as superstitions that constitute threats to civic peace, which threats must be contained if they cannot be eradicated. Laborde understands such defenders of a secular space (a view that Laborde does not affirm) as seeking to remove even personal religious symbols (e.g., yarmulkes) from the public space. Energies have in particular been directed against the wearing of the hijab, which can be seen as

(i) an ostentatious religious sign, which infringes the neutrality of the public sphere, in itself a guarantee of equality between all citizens,

(ii) a symbol of sexist oppression, which denies the liberty and autonomy of the girls wearing it,

(iii) a demand of recognition of cultural difference, which undermines national identity and trans-ethnic solidarity (Laborde 2008, p. 8).

This animus against the presence of religious faith has even produced a proselytizing atheist movement (Dawkins 2006; Harris 2005). Religion, in particular Christianity, threatens the re-moralization of morality and bioethics.

It is not simply, as Max Weber (1864–1920) puts it, that there has been a disenchantment (*Entzauberung*) of reality so that mysticism and the presence of spirits are neither acknowledged nor appreciated.[5] Most particularly, the cosmic struggle between good and evil as spiritual and personal is not to be mentioned in public even by those who still recognize it. An *Entzauberung* has surely occurred. One might consider Duffy's description of the life of Christianity in England before the Reformation to appreciate a non-disenchanted life-world.

Mass began with an elaborate procession round the church, at the commencement of which salt and water were solemnly exorcised, blessed, and mixed. In the course of the procession the altars of the church, and the congregation, were sprinkled with holy water, which would later be taken to the households of the parish, where it was used to banish devils and ensure blessing (Duffy 1992, p. 124).

With a few emendations, this picture of pre-Reformation England is still true of the life of an Orthodox church in 21st-century America, where holy water is blessed to be taken home, where oil is sanctified for anointing at home,[6] where the priest is invited at least yearly to bless each home, and where the Our Father concludes with "and deliver us from the evil one." Fully "enchanted" Christian life-worlds still exist, alive with the recognition of devils and angels and their attachment to things, persons, and places. It is not just that the dominant culture has lost an appreciation of the cosmic dimension of the struggle between good and evil, but that any hint of a recognition in the public space by believers of this struggle is actively to be suppressed. The cultural space in which morality is articulated is now fully after God.

Harvey Cox (1929–) in *The Secular City* regards secularization as integral to "the liberation of man from religious and metaphysical tutelage, the turning of his attention away from other worlds and toward this one" (Cox 1966, p. 15). The rupture has been so radical that the Roman Catholic dissident theologian Edward Schillebeeckx (1914–2009) stated:

> The Christian revelation, in the form in which it has been handed down to us, clearly no longer provides any valid answer to the questions about God asked by the majority of people today. Neither would it appear to make any contribution to modern man's meaningful understanding of himself in this world and in human history. It is at once evident that more and more of these people are becoming increasingly displeased and dissatisfied with the traditional Christian answers to their questions (Schillebeeckx 1969, p. 156).

Although he revised his earlier views in important ways, Peter Berger in 1969, in the midst of the cultural and sexual revolution that produced the contemporary dominant secular culture, observed:

> Probably for the first time in history, the religious legitimations of the world have lost their plausibility not only for a few intellectuals and other marginal individuals, but for broad masses of entire societies. This opened up an acute

crisis not only for the nomization of the large social institutions but for that of individual biographies. In other words, there has arisen a problem of "meaningfulness" not only for such institutions as the state or the economy but for the ordinary routines of everyday life (Berger 1969, p. 130).

However, Islam appears as a counter-example to Cox's assertion that "urbanization means a structure of common life in which the diversity and the disintegration of tradition are paramount" (Cox 1966, p. 4). Within Muslim countries, desecularization, not secularization, has occurred despite urbanization, a phenomenon to which we will turn in the next chapter. In addition, many such as the Hasidic Jews have learned how to live in the secular city without themselves being secularized (Fader 2009).

Berger's characterization identifies a radical change in the possibilities for meaning in the once-Christian West, whose dominant culture is now secular. This change was quite apparent after the First World War, as the commitments of the dominant intellectual class became increasingly post-Christian. As a result, there was a subtle but significant shift that secularized the mainline Christianities themselves and the character of the public culture, so that a secular view was favored over a religious. In 1939, on the brink of the Second World War and the armed conflict among the secularized polities of Germany, the Soviet Union, and the United States, T. S. Eliot wrote:

> We must remember also that the choice between Christianity and secularism is not simply presented to the innocent mind, *anima semplicetta*, as to an impartial judge capable of choosing the best when the causes have both been fully pleaded. The whole tendency of education (in the widest sense—the influences playing on the common mind in the forms of "enlightenment") has been for a very long time to form minds more and more adapted to secularism, less and less equipped to apprehend the doctrine of revelation and its consequences. Even in works of Christian apologetic, the assumption is sometimes that of the secular mind (Eliot 1982, p. 190).

By the late 1960s and 1970s, the secular transformation of the public culture had become pervasive (Bloom 1992; Cox 1966; Hutchison 1989). Given America's dominantly Protestant character, as Harold Bloom observes, "the American

Religion, which is so prevalent among us, masks itself as Protestant Christianity yet has ceased to be Christian" (Bloom 1992, p. 32). This secularization has been wide-ranging because it was tied to the demoralization and deflation of morality that would bring bioethics into question and to the delegitimization of the state that would also bring the force of health care policy into question.

The agenda of the dominant secular culture has been in particular to deprive religion of any political significance. Religion is not to be a political project. Only secular, democratic constitutionalism is to have legitimacy. In many cases, the secular and anti-religious project goes beyond that of Rawls' notion of public reason in which public discourse is to be sustained independently of "comprehensive doctrines of any kind" (Rawls 1999, p. 143). In the case of András Sajó, as Lorenzo Zucca points out, Sajó "genuinely believes that secular public reason is our common comprehensive doctrine at the foundation of Western political systems" (Zucca 2009, p. 507). This aspiration to an official secular discourse for the public forum and the public space surely begs the question as to which discourse should be normative.

> The trouble is that secular reason, as a comprehensive doctrine, is not shared by everyone in our societies, as there are other competing comprehensive doctrines, mainly religious ones. How does one find a compromise between religious and nonreligious comprehensive views without appealing to secular reason? That is the question that preoccupies Rawls, though it does not seem to preoccupy Sajó in the least. This explains why Sajó does not hesitate to call religious arguments a burden on secular people. But the problem is that our societies impose secular burdens on religious people without paying the slightest attention to religious arguments. Hence, Sajó's suggestion to exclude religious arguments totally has an authoritarian ring (Zucca 2009, p. 507).

Nevertheless, the secular agenda is to mount a project of cleansing religion from the public space.

This cleansing of religion from the public space is to be undertaken in part by directly forbidding as far as possible religiously grounded public speech, especially that with a political focus. This is also to be undertaken indirectly through undermining the religious significance and identity of religious institutions in the public space. As András Sajó has put it, "Secularism in constitutional law means that social functions of 'churches' are taken over by the state or are privatized. This is the result, at least partly, of the changed self-perception of mainstream churches" (Sajó 2008, p. 609). This occurs, for example, by removing Roman Catholicism from involvement in adoption by requiring the placing of adoptees with homosexual couples. The agenda of removing any strong presence of religion from public services is shaped by the secular requirement of keeping "religion out of the public sphere. . . . Religion cannot be a political project" (Sajó 2008, p. 621). This secularizing project requires progressively limiting religious freedom and strong religious expressions in the public square when they have political implications.

This goal is often pursued by constraining religious institutions so that they can no longer publicly proclaim the presence of God but are instead left affirming "values," in that "values" are cut loose from any transcendent anchor and are thus more compatible with the secular social-democratic project. Although a values discourse is already prominent with Friedrich Nietzsche (1844–1900), Max Weber (1864–1920), and Carl Schmitt (1888–1985), values discourse becomes salient in Germany only in 1975 with Erhard Eppler (Eppler 1975) and in the United Kingdom in 1983 with Margaret Thatcher (1925–2013). Gertrude Himmelfarb observed that "the discussion of 'values' . . . started in England in the election campaign of 1983, when an interviewer of Margaret Thatcher observed, rather derisively, that she seemed to be approving of 'Victorian values'" (Himmelfarb 1995, p. 3). This shift in discourse away from God, Christ, or virtues had already occurred with Eppler. What occurred in German public discourse was an abandonment of a direct support of structural conservatism focused on issues of church, family, and nation.[7]

The goal is as well to transform the character of private religious education so as to encourage if not require instruction in private religious schools that (1) brings traditional religious views into question and (2) requires the translation of religious requirements into secular terms. As Ian MacMullen puts it, this would involve a

> commitment to secular reason-giving inside and outside the classroom, balance religious instruction with critical perspectives on the faith, insulate

significant parts of the academic curriculum from the religious ethos of the
school, teach about other ethical doctrines in a way that makes children
aware of viable alternatives to their family's faith, and demonstrate a sincere
willingness to open the school to teachers and students outside the community of faith (MacMullen 2007, p. 175).

Religious schools would be allowed to maintain their religious identity, even if
they "run mandatory classes of instruction in a particular religious doctrine, so
long as these classes include some secular, critical perspectives by way of balance" (MacMullen 2007, p. 175). Religious commitment is to be recast in terms
of the demands of secularity.

This volume explores these vast changes in the dominant culture of the West
that have driven and are driving its further secularization, recasting the context
for understanding contemporary morality and bioethics. These changes are tied
to the end of Christendom, as well as to the marginalization of Christianity. In
addition, many of the mainline Christianities of the West have rendered themselves post-traditional. These changes are complex and have many intertwining
sources. Procrusteanly, they can be gathered under eight headings.

1) The Enlightenment's pursuit of emancipation has been associated with an
antipathy not just to the clergy, but to Christianity generally. In its turn
away from the past, the Enlightenment supported a search for emancipation from Christendom and a liberation from the constraining hand
of tradition. This search for emancipation was expressed in the Enlightenment's fascination with autonomy, which gained further salience in
the 20th century (Schneewind 1998). Being a Christian became suspect
because of Christianity's particular non-philosophical, non-universalist
core acknowledgement of a Messiah Who is God, Who was born in a
particular place with a particular genealogy. This particularity collides
with the Enlightenment's claims regarding universal rights, such as those
around which the European Union has sought to articulate its identity,
its morality, and its bioethics.

2) The Enlightenment viewed persons as first and foremost members of a
universal moral community. This account encourages regarding moral

agents as individuals apart from their sex, race, family, history, nationality, and particular community. The universal moral community is to bind persons simply as naked moral agents. This leads not just to discounting the significance of intermediate institutions, so that there is nothing separating the individual and the state, but also to considering persons as bare individuals making fully plausible, *inter alia*, the self-assignment of sexual identity. Individuals are to find their primary moral orientation in terms of universal allegiances as humans *qua* persons, not as Christians or Jews, or members of families, citizens of nations, or as men and women. They are to be citizens of the world apart from any particularity.

3) The Enlightenment's endorsement of equality has led to the pursuit of fair equality of opportunity, for all persons are to be fully interchangeable, thus bringing both the family and religious communities into question as stumbling blocks to fair equality of opportunity. There is a particular animus against the family because families invest their energies primarily in raising and giving advantages to their own children, rather than the children of others. So, too, religious communities as particular communities give psychological support and identity first and foremost to their own members.

4) The Enlightenment's endorsement of the pursuit of happiness has become informally construed as the pure pursuit of pleasure or bare preference satisfaction, so that happiness has been shorn of any particular normative content. Moved by a universalist and morally vacuous solidarity, persons are not just to be guaranteed that amount of food, clothing, and shelter needed for survival, but to be given the opportunity for that amount of food, clothing, shelter, and resources needed to feel satisfied. This commitment to satisfaction has led to the emergence of the hook-up culture, as well as to an affirmation of soft if not hard pornography. Traditional Christian culture is thus undermined by a culture of seduction.

5) The Enlightenment rejected a traditional theistic view of the transcendent in part because it divides. Traditional Christianity is regarded as a

particular threat to the possibility of a full identification with a universal moral communality. The current dominant culture requires all normative concerns to be articulated and understood within the horizon of the finite and the immanent, so that a concern for a transcendent orientation will not fragment the secular community.

6) In order to pursue emancipation, respect the bare individual, achieve fair equality of opportunity, pursue happiness as pleasure, and locate all meaning within the horizon of the finite and the immanent, the now-dominant culture requires that religion, especially Christianity, be tolerated in the public space only if its meaning is subject to a full secular translation so that it is given an immanent meaning as a mere element of culture. Once translated into secular terms, religion can be allowed to serve as a moral heuristic, following Jürgen Habermas, or can be recognized as an enrichment of culture, as a *Kulturgut*, becoming a detheologized ritual, among other things. Differences are to be set aside through a homogenizing interreligious and intercultural dialogue. The goal is to banish attempts to convert the other through a characterization of proselytizing as violence against the other.

7) These immense cultural challenges to traditional Christianity have had numerous impacts on society and culture. Salient among these has been the disestablishment of Chrisatianity in Christian universities, a matter to be addressed in chapter seven. The rapidity of these changes in Western Europe and the Americas during the 1960s was driven by the significant chaos engendered in Western Christianity during and following Vatican II, which changes accelerated the decline of the mainline Christianities of the West. The moral vacuum that resulted enabled the European Union to embrace an ethos of transformative secularization, with aggressively post-Christian characteristics. A similar process is taking place in the Americas and elsewhere. These changes recast the background assumptions or paradigm framing morality and bioethics, a point to which we will turn in greater detail in chapter seven.

8) Morality and bioethics, as a consequence, have been subjected to a demoralization and deflation because of their full severance from a God's-eye perspective. This robust secularization is more forceful and transformative than most have acknowledged.

This volume explores these intertwining roots of the contemporary, dominant, secular culture and its character of being after God, which determines the situation within which contemporary morality and bioethics must be understood.

II. A New Sense of Toleration: Toleration as Acceptance

With wide-ranging implications, as the previous chapter shows, secular morality is increasingly recognized to be without foundations. Because of the acknowledgement of the absence of metaphysical roots, of foundations, all morality and bioethics, which have been regarded as justified through moral-philosophical argument, are demoralized and deflated. The bioethics of the artificial insemination of unmarried women, abortion, physician-assisted suicide, and euthanasia becomes a bioethics of life- and death-style choices. When all is approached as if everything ultimately came from nowhere, went to nowhere, and for no ultimate purpose, Protagoras is vindicated: there is no vantage point beyond the sphere of the socio-historically conditioned. Each person becomes the measure and standard of all things.[8] As has already been shown, morality becomes a macro life-style choice. As Santiago Zabala in his essay, "A Religion Without Theists or Atheists," recognizes, these changes in how reality and morality are appreciated are tied to the character of contemporary secularization.

It is indeed secularization that teaches us that questions about the nature of God are useless because of the weakness of our reason. We are not told that God does not exist, only that it is not clear what it actually means to affirm or deny his existence. Postmodern man, who has lived out the end of the great unifying syntheses produced by traditional metaphysical thought, manages to live without neurosis in a world where God is no longer present, therefore in a world where there are no longer stable and guaranteed structures capable of supplying a unique, ultimate, and normative foundation for our knowledge and for our ethics (Zabala 2005, p. 11).

All is rendered contingent and therefore in the end unstable and without ultimate meaning. "All that is solid melts into air" (Berman 1982). The loss of ultimate meaning is to be accepted with equanimity.

Given the loss of moral objectivity, given the demoralization and deflation
of morality and bioethics, the secular culture forbids a condemnatory moral
attitude regarding peaceable life-style and death-style choices (e.g., engaging in
homosexual acts, reproducing outside of marriage, or using physician-assisted
suicide). In addition, the central importance within the dominant secular culture of respect of persons is taken to require that one respect persons in their
life- and death-style choices, however perverse and misguided these choices
may be. That is, it is judged to be immoral to judge peaceable life- and death-
style choices to be immoral, because one is required to respect persons in the
choices that they are free to make within secular polities. Although in the face
of intractable moral pluralism one can no longer discern the immorality of particular life- and death-style choices, the hope is still to recognize the canonical
character of the higher-level moral obligation to be non-judgmental. Of course,
this is impossible, for morality and bioethics themselves have become a macro
life-style choice.

The prohibition of being judgmental has thus become core to the new secular ethos and its life-world. One is not to speak judgmentally about what secular
bioethics allows (e.g., one is not to say "abortion is immoral and a sin"). Charles
Murray notes in his account of the increase of out-of-wedlock births in the
United States primarily among lower socio-economic classes that the upper
socio-economic whites who have far fewer illegitimate births are nevertheless
disinclined to make adverse moral judgments regarding the life-style choices
that lead to births outside of marriage, even if such births are associated with
generally negative social outcomes for both the women and their children.

> Nonjudgmentalism is one of the more baffling features of the new-upper-
> class culture. The members of the new upper class are industrious to the
> point of obsession, but there are no derogatory labels for those who are
> not industrious. The young women of the new upper class hardly ever have
> babies out of wedlock, but it is impermissible to use a derogatory label for
> non-marital births. You will probably raise a few eyebrows even if you use a

derogatory label for criminals. When you get down to it, it is not acceptable in the new upper class to use derogatory labels for anyone, with three exceptions: people with differing political views, fundamentalist Christians, and rural working-class whites (Murray 2012, pp. 289–290).

This non-judgmentalism is less puzzling when set against the demoralization and deflation of morality.

The dominant secular culture's demoralization of major dimensions of traditional morality is accompanied by a commitment not to tolerate the intolerant, not to tolerate those who fail to be non-judgmental with regard to legal life- and death-style choices. Herbert Marcuse (1898–1979) finally triumphs (Wolff et al. 1965). The phrase "no tolerance for the intolerant" serves as a rallying cry for secularists in the culture wars against any who would remoralize what in the dominant culture have become life-style and death-style choices. Christian bakers, for example, who refuse to make wedding cakes for homosexuals are visited with opprobria such as "bigot." A powerful wall of aversive emotions is recruited against "fundamentalists" who seek to re-anchor morality in the will of God. Tolerance has become a code word for the culturally required demoralization of a wide range of sexual, reproductive, and end-of-life choices. The new secular, demoralized, and deflated culture requires that one be adversely judgmental regarding those who are judgmental.[9] The result has been a foundational recasting of the meaning of toleration.

The English word "toleration" has roots in the Latin *tolerans*, which like the original English indicates enduring, suffering, or putting up with something about which one disapproves. One finds this meaning of *tolerance* in the English Act of Toleration (24 May 1689), which under certain conditions allowed freedom of worship to particular non-conformists, but not to Roman Catholics and Unitarians. Moreover, despite the Act of Toleration, only Anglicans could sit in Parliament, although specified non-conformists were free to have their own churches for their own worship. It was clear that those who were tolerated had not through this toleration received approval of their religion or of their form of worship. They were members of communities often publicly despised. They were members of religious communities holding dogmas that were recognized by the state as wrongheaded and heretical, but nevertheless as "tolerable."

Again, traditionally one tolerates only that of which one does not approve. In this sense, certain heretical religious bodies and their members were tolerated, and coercive force was not used against them, although they and their members were still subject to social opprobrium and pressure because they were understood as worshipping and believing wrongly (Sowerby 2013). Even John Locke's *Letter Concerning Toleration* (1689), which is generally regarded as a defense of the English Act of Toleration, excludes atheists from toleration. "Those are not at all to be tolerated who deny the Being of a God" (Locke 1983, p. 51). Thus, as Lorenzo Zucca observed, there emerged a trichotomy between right beliefs, proscribed wrong beliefs, and tolerable wrong beliefs (Zucca 2009, p. 21). Toleration grew in its scope, as the state attempted to come to terms with intractable religious pluralism. As Hegel appreciated, this created a space for the emergence of the open space of contemporary civil society, along with the eventual secularization of that society and the state.[10]

The recently recast meaning of toleration requires not just that one forbear from using force against those whom one tolerates, but that one in addition indirectly affirm the views that are tolerated. This transformed meaning of toleration socially prohibits one from stating publicly that, although one has taken the position that persons holding particular disapproved-of views and/or engaging in particular disapproved-of actions (e.g., fornication, adultery, homosexual acts, false worship, particular doctrines) should be free of state coercion, they nevertheless act immorally. That is, one is to be prohibited from saying, "you should be free to practice your religion, but it is an evil heresy"; "you should not be jailed for your life-style; however, it is perverse and immoral"; "physicians who are willing should not be legally forbidden to inseminate unmarried women artificially, but it is sinful." Persons with wrongheaded views or those who engage in perverse or immoral actions are not to experience the discomfort of publicly-voiced adverse moral judgments. Instead, the dominant secular culture requires an indirect affirmation of the life-style choices of others through phrases such as: "Different people have different life-styles; your life-style is simply not right for me, although it is good for you." The result is that the dominant secular culture affirmatively requires that public morality and bioethics make space for a wide range of life-style and death-style choices, of which sexual and reproductive choices (e.g., the artificial insemination of lesbians) are among the most salient about which no moral or bioethical criticism is to be allowed. Such tolerance is integral to a particular macro life-style choice, a "morality" that requires an at least weak acceptance of that which is tolerated.

III. Sex Matters

The emergence of post-modern, secular societies with their radical recasting of the meaning of toleration requires that one move from toleration *sensu stricto* to tolerance now understood as soft acceptance of the life-style and peaceable moral commitments of the other without a public hint of moral rejection.[11] This change is tied to profound changes in ordinary expectations. Among them is the demoralization and deflation of traditional sexual and reproductive norms with the consequent dramatic alteration of the very texture of everyday life. The tolerance of difference in sexual activity (e.g., choosing one's sexual partner as a member of a different sex, the same sex, or an animal) involves more than abandoning the implicit negative moralization involved in toleration and requires not only acceptance of what had once been able to be recognized as sinful, but what is now according to the secular culture to be accepted as a life-style choice. The category of sin in general and of sexual sin in particular is now forbidden by the dominant secular culture. The results are widespread and dramatic. After all, sex is a major motive force. How one regards sex and engages in sexual relations as well as how men and women bond sexually significantly shapes the life-world. Sex is powerful. Sex matters. Sex is one of the major framing forces that shape a society. The dominant secular culture seeks to render consensual sexual acts beyond sin and beyond moral judgment, thus transforming and further secularizing society. How we regard ourselves, our bodies, and carnal relations structures large areas of life. These are complex matters about which quite different accounts can be and are given.[12]

We now live in a life-world in which concubinage has become ubiquitous and is as acceptable as marriage. It is now taken for granted that men and women may live together, hook up, and be sexual partners, all without benefit of clergy. Mothers now without hesitation or shame speak of their daughters having moved in with their boyfriends (Fernandez-Villaverde et al. 2012; Finer 2007; Greenwood & Guner 2010). It is no longer an embarrassment, at least in many social circles, to have one's daughter reproduce outside of marriage (Murray 2012). Given the norms of the dominant secular culture, one is not publicly to evince one's embarrassment. Public advertisements and discussions have come to substitute "partner" for "spouse", as in "Your partner wants the spartan purity of uncarpeted hardwoods" (Anonymous 2013, p. D1). There has been the emergence of a dominant culture in which sexual relations and reproducing outside of marriage are no longer recognized as shameful or marked by guilt. As Vattimo has observed, "Belief in the importance of sexuality in human life is gradually waning" (Vattimo 2011, p. 56). Sex has become a civil right (Wheeler 2012). The taken-for-granted character and moral significance of sexual activity, pair bonding, and reproduction have changed radically from what they had been in the 1950s. Moreover, the new ethos of toleration requires that one not speak publicly in condemnation of these immense changes in sexual mores, or even publicly seriously consider their adverse consequences.

To repeat the above with a slightly different emphasis: sexual activity and reproduction have been demoralized into life-style choices as the West has become fully post-Christian, indeed after God. With the loss of the language of sin, it is no longer a subject of guilt and/or shame to have sex or to live together outside of wedlock. Moreover, it is no longer a subject of guilt and/or shame to have children outside of wedlock (Murray 2012, chapter 3). This is not to claim that in the past fornication or adultery was infrequent, or that many did not give illegitimate issue. Popes of the 15th and 16th centuries were well known for advancing the interests of their bastard children. What is different is that in the past, vice through hypocrisy regularly paid tribute to virtue. Sexual and reproductive indiscretions *ceteris paribus* brought official social disapproval and established social costs, which the rich and/or powerful such as Pope Alexander VI (1431–1503, elected 1492) could avoid. However much honored in the breach, there were publicly established sexual mores that reflected traditional Christian commitments and views of the body. This is no longer the case. Western public sexual and reproductive mores have changed fundamentally. In the process, the meaning of the body in Western culture has changed as well. Although the recent changes were long in coming, and although they have deep roots in Western culture, the changes over the last half-century have been rapid and dramatic.

To give an example from Germany as it was before the recent cultural transformations: on the 6th of March, 1970, I took my wife to the university hospital in Bonn, Germany, so that she could be delivered of our second child. I was there as a Fulbright post-graduate fellow studying Kant and Hegel. On entering the hospital, the admitting clerks asked for proof of marriage in order to determine whether to record our child as legitimate or as a bastard. Not having traveled to Germany with a copy of our marriage license, I explained to the hospital officials that we were citizens of Texas and that a common-law marriage was sufficient to ensure legitimacy. Then I elaborated that the necessary and jointly sufficient conditions for a common-law marriage were that the couple be male and female, that they hold themselves openly and notoriously to be husband and wife, and that they have had intercourse. We manifestly met the conditions. The next morning after the birth of our daughter, I was visited in my wife's room by a hospital official who joyfully informed me that he had called the American Embassy in Bad Godesberg, which had confirmed that my account of common-law marriage in Texas was correct; my daughter would be registered as legitimate.

In stark contrast, the Evangelische Kirche Deutschlands (EKD) in June of 2013 took an important step towards the erasure from the public consciousness of the dominant German culture of distinctions such as between legitimate and illegitimate unions with reference to a marriage of a man and a woman (Kirchenamt of EKD 2013). In the statement, the EKD sought to forge a view of the family that encompassed not just a husband and a wife with children (in the past, widows and widowers with children constituted a deficient case of a family), but families of single women, along with homosexual unions. Absent was the traditional Christian recognition that sexual activity or reproduction outside of the marriage of a man and a woman was deeply misdirected. The body was assumed to be open to peaceable consensual use in sexual activity and reproduction. The body *qua* body had become at least implicitly regarded as a neutral instrument available for peaceable sexual and reproductive uses by consenting persons. The body is no longer recognized as bringing with it constraining norms.

The view advanced by the EKD regarding sexual acts and reproduction is, to say the least, very distant from the position taken by St. Paul in his first letter to the Corinthians.

Now the body is not for fornication, but for the Lord; and the Lord for the body. And God both raised up the Lord, and will raise up us by His own power. Ye know that your bodies are members of Christ, do ye not? Having taken up then the members of Christ, shall I make them members of a harlot? May it not be! Or know ye not that he that is joined to the harlot is one body? For, "The two," saith He, "shall be into one flesh." But he who is joined to the Lord is one spirit. Keep on fleeing fornication. Every sin whatsoever a man might do is outside the body, but he who committeth fornication sinneth against his own body. Or know ye not that your body is a temple of the Holy Spirit Who is in you, Whom ye have from God, and ye are not your own? For ye were bought with a price; glorify then God in your body and in your spirit, which are God's (I Cor 6:13–20).

Unlike the EKD's statement, St. Paul gives special attention to the evil of fornication. In our dominant culture, opposing fornication is by itself astonishing enough. The reason for St. Paul's condemnation of fornication is now even more culturally alien: the special evil of illicit sexual unions lies in uniting one's body with the body of another person who is not one's spouse. More precisely, the evil of fornication is best understood in terms of its being a use of one's body that is improper in being incompatible with the sanctification of one's body. Sexual intercourse for traditional Christians is a serious matter because of the union effected between two bodies. As Christ puts it with regard to marriage, "the two shall become one flesh" (Mt 19:5). The body is central and so, too, is the sanctification of sexual acts. While the marriage bed is undefiled, that of fornicators and adulterers is defiled. "Let marriage be held in honor by all, and let the marriage bed be kept undefiled; for God will judge fornicators and adulterers" (Heb 13:4). This view has remained integral to traditional Christianity.

St. Paul's statements should not be taken to deny that before Christ patriarchs and kings were at liberty without wrong-doing to take concubines, a point attested to in Genesis (25:6) and elsewhere, and about which Moses Maimonides reflects in the *Mishneh Torah*.[13] The issue of concubinage is important and complex, but it is irrelevant to Christians for whom concubinage and fornication are now materially equivalent. With the Resurrection, the normative monogamy of Adam and Eve is restored. Within traditional Christianity, unabsolved fornicators who have not been re-admitted to the chalice are barred from receiving Communion,[14] which exclusion is a cardinal criterion for Christians. When before the distribution of the Holy Gifts the deacon says: "With fear of God and faith and love, draw near" (*Liturgikon* 1994, p. 307), this warning reminds congregants that one should only approach the chalice after prayer, fasting, and the approval of one's spiritual father. The Liturgy, in concert with the canons of the Church, takes account of what has happened to the body.

In the dominant secular culture, in contrast, the very notion of sexual immorality has become a puzzling, if not an inaccessible notion. Why the consensual use of donor gametes should be a problem for morality and bioethics is no longer apparent. A complex set of normative changes has altered a broad sweep of everyday life, changing the life-world and the experience of the body within the dominant culture. The widespread valorization of fornication, the broad acceptance of concubinage, and the increasing percentage of children born outside of marriage, all of which are grounded in the pursuit of self-fulfillment and a negative regard of tradition, made terms such as "bastard" politically incorrect but affirmed the acceptance of homosexual acts and homosexual liaisons. The widespread cultural acceptance of heterosexual sins undermined the plausibility of denouncing homosexual sins. The result is that the consensual use of the body in sexual activity and reproduction has been demoralized into the concerns of life-style choices, so that such use is no longer of direct moral concern. Consensual uses of the body in sexual activity and reproduction have come to involve choices that the dominant secular culture cannot find right or wrong, good or bad. Within the life-world of the dominant secular culture, sex and reproduction outside of marriage have become as unproblematic as having a meal on the run.

How did this watershed change in the public culture occur? Crucial was the loss of the traditional Christian understanding of the body. The dominant secular culture, given its commitments, ceased to endorse the traditional Christian project of sanctifying the body, of turning it into a holy relic. This change has roots in the Western moral-philosophical project of specifying and justifying through reason the appropriate character of the moral life. The good, the right, and the virtuous came to be understood without any necessary reference to the holy, much less to the sanctification of the body.[15] The inability of the dominant secular culture properly to appreciate the importance of the body in the human encounter with the transcendently holy is a function of contemporary Western thought having given central place to a view of agency within which the body becomes a means as instrument for the realization of merely immanent goals. In contrast, for traditional Christians, the sanctification of the body was and is understood in terms of a transforming encounter with the transcendently Holy. Instead, the body is now understood in terms of the narratives that persons tell about their own bodies.

Surely, a number of views can be advanced about how one ought to characterize the now-dominant secular culture and its appreciation of the body. Here, I underscore one dimension of these changes, one that has roots in a way of regarding the human condition that grew out of the Enlightenment through Kant, and that was then importantly transformed by cultural forces crucially appreciated and reinforced by, among other people, G. W. F. Hegel. The result is the contemporary post-modern view of the moral life in which each person is free peaceably with consensual others to have and pursue his own vision of sexual and reproductive flourishing. The meaning of the body is now nested within a narrative of the Spirit, Geist, Absolute Spirit (a notion to which more attention will be given in chapter eight). It is a view through which traditional Christian morality, including the sexual and reproductive morality that was still embraced by Kant, became demoralized and deflated. The result is that much of what had been understood as moral choices regarding sexuality and reproduction are transformed into personal life-style choices. Among the consequences is that heterosexual marriage and the traditional family have at the very least been culturally marginalized. As Hegel recognized, Kant's Christian morality, which Kant sets after Christ as Messiah and God, cannot be sustained. The morality of sexual acts, reproduction, and the family becomes a morality located within a Christianity, indeed a culture, after God.[16]

The body is central in the life of the Church. This is the case because, among other things, the bodies of true theologians, the bodies of holy fathers and mothers, have been sanctified so that to touch them is to make physical contact with the uncreated energies of God. It is for this reason that traditional Christians seek to touch relics and that relics are placed in the altars of churches, becoming central to the Liturgy. Indeed, Canon VII of the Seventh Ecumenical Council

(Nicea II, A.D. 787) affirms the tradition of having relics in the altar of a church. As Ecumenical Patriarch Bartholomew remarked regarding the culture of traditional Christianity and the centrality of the sanctification of the body:

> ... the change of man's essence, theosis by grace, is a fact that is tangible for all the Orthodox faithful. Grace is not only obtained through the transformed relics of the saints, which is totally inexplicable without acceptance of the divine. Grace also radiates from living Saints who are truly in the likeness of the Lord [Lk 8:46]. ... Grace can also be obtained by the presence of the Saints who have influenced and sanctified, and to a degree transformed, natural objects and places (Bartholomew 1997).

At stake is that sanctification of the body as recorded in Acts regarding the living body of St. Paul. "God did extraordinary miracles through Paul, so that when the handkerchiefs or aprons that had touched his skin were brought to the sick, their diseases left them, and the evil spirits came out of them" (Acts 19:12). St. Paul's body was sanctified. To touch his body was to make contact with God's uncreated energies.

Because of this early Christian appreciation of the sanctification of the body, there was from Christianity's beginning a concern to gather up the relics of the martyrs. Even after their deaths, it was recognized that their bodies remained sanctified. With regard to St. Ignatius of Antioch, it is recorded after his martyrdom: "For only the harder portions of his holy remains were left, which were conveyed to Antioch and wrapped in linen, as an inestimable treasure left to the holy Church by the grace which was in the martyr" (Roberts & Donaldson 1994, The martyrdom of Ignatius vi, vol. 1, p. 131). Again, for example, "The Martyrdom of Polycarp" records that after his death

> ... the jealous and envious evil one who resists the family of the righteous, when he saw the greatness of his martyrdom, and his blameless career from the beginning, and that he was crowned with the crown of immortality, and had carried off the unspeakable prize, took care that not even his poor body should be taken away by us, though many desired to do this, and to have fellowship with his holy flesh (Lake 1965, p. 335, XVII.1).

"The Martyrdom" reports that after St. Polycarp's body was burned by the Romans, "we, at last, took up his bones, more precious than precious stones, and finer than gold, and put them where it was meet" (Lake 1965, p. 337, XVIII.1). The Christians were interested in the relics of St. Ignatius and St. Polycarp because their bodies had been sanctified and provided contact with the uncreated energies of God. It was for this reason that Liturgies were (and are) celebrated on the relics of martyrs.[17]

This understanding is vividly alive in Orthodox Christianity, which recognizes the importance of sanctifying both body and soul. For example, due to the importance of sanctification of the body, the priest during the Liturgy in the "Prayer of the Thrice-Holy Hymn" (the Trisagion) asks, "Pardon us every transgression both voluntary and involuntary; sanctify our souls and bodies" (*Liturgikon* 1994, p. 263). The goal is not just that one's soul becomes holy, but that one's body becomes holy. Again, in the "Prayer before the Gospel" the priest says, "For thou art the Illumination of our souls and bodies, O Christ our God" (*Liturgikon* 1994, p. 267). There is no sense of seeking a spiritual transformation apart from the body. The body is no mere prison of the soul. The same point is underscored when, after the second "Litany of the Faithful" in the Liturgy of St. John Chrysostom, the priest asks God to "cleanse our souls and bodies from every defilement of flesh or spirit" (*Liturgikon* 1994, p. 272), as well as in the prayer before the Our Father in the Liturgy of St. Basil the Great. "Purify us from every defilement of flesh and spirit . . ." (*Liturgikon* 1994, p. 299). Finally, in the thanksgiving prayer after Communion in this same Liturgy, the priest prays, "We give thanks unto Thee, O Lord our God, for the participation in Thy holy, immaculate, immortal and heavenly mysteries, which Thou hast given unto us for the welfare and sanctification and healing of our souls and bodies" (*Liturgikon* 1994, p. 309). The project is to seek through grace, that is, through the uncreated energies of God, to transform not just the soul but also the body.

This approach of traditional Christianity is not the approach to the body found in the morality and bioethics that characterize the contemporary dominant secular culture. Given the thoroughgoing disenchantment of the world within the contemporary dominant secular culture, the holiness of relics and bodies is incomprehensible. That the power of God's energies can enter into physical reality cannot be admitted. In this contemporary culture, one finds instead a narrative cut off from any anchor in being beyond the being supported by particular narratives sustained within particular free-standing accounts, all articulated within the horizon of the finite and the immanent. How did we end up in this current state of affairs? Faced with the challenges posed by David Hume, Immanuel Kant attempted not only to vindicate the necessary character of claims made by Euclidean geometry and Newton's physics, but to preserve the content and binding force of Christian morality, however without Christ as God and surely without the energies of God entering into matter. Kant as the ultimate Protestant radically disenchants matter. Kant's grand project, grounded among other things in his solution to the Third Antinomy in the First *Critique* (i.e., the issue as to whether humans are causally determined or free), led Kant to conceive of moral agents *qua* moral (and therefore for him noumenal) agents as choosing apart from any causal nexus, including socio-historically conditioned forces. Kant's solution to the Third Antinomy imposed a cleft between humans as bodies and humans as free agents. This approach made impossible any appreciation of the sanctification of the body, the rejection of which had been underscored in the destruction of relics during the Protestant Reformation and the French Revolution. As already noted, Hegel realized that the emerging secular culture had taken things much farther. The dominant secular culture had radically recast traditional Western Christian views through averting the cultural gaze from everything that could claim to be in itself apart from its being for us. As we saw in chapter two, this is the force of Hegel's famous pronouncement in 1802 of God's death. In his essay "Glauben und Wissen" [Faith and Knowledge], Hegel recognized the cultural change ingredient in "the feeling that 'God Himself is dead,' upon which the religion of more recent times rests" (Hegel 1977, p. 190; Hegel 1968, pp. 413–4).

Not only was Hegel willing to face the death of God in the vanguard culture of his day, but he had also come to terms with the consequences Kant had hoped to avoid: without a God's-eye perspective, not only would the right not always trump the good, but morality would not always trump prudence (Engelhardt 2010a, 2010b). In the contemporary culture, being is only for us, and all categories, including all morality, are socio-historically conditioned. Hegel realized that the very sense of morality was transformed, once it was placed after God. As we will see more clearly by the end of this chapter, without a transcendent

God's-eye perspective, law and public policy by default become the higher truth of morality (Hegel, *Grundlinien der Philosophie des Rechts*, #211). Law and public policy are the reality of a secular society's effective norms. As a further consequence, the state becomes an immanent substitute for God (ibid., #258). This restatement of morality as the ethics incarnate in and reduced to law and public policy provided the basis for Richard Rorty and the later John Rawls to have politics substitute for morality. After all, no one canonical morality can be identified. But law can be established. In the absence of a God's-eye perspective to ground secular morality and bioethics, the state sustains the unity and specific meaning of a society's norms by establishing those norms at law and in public policy. Although many saw the earlier Rawls as vindicating the powers of moral philosophy, by 1985 Rawls had rejected the claim that his *Theory of Justice* provided a generally justifiable moral defense of justice as fairness. He was left with advancing a political rather than a moral proposal (Rawls 1985).

This state of affairs has vast implications for how one ought to understand the morality and bioethics of the body, sexual activity, and reproduction. Within the dominant secular perspective, there is nothing to be said about the sanctification of the body as a result of an encounter with the transcendentally Holy. There is nothing that one can say concerning acts that defile, that preclude sanctifying contact with the Holy. In liberal democracies, one has at best the requirement that one peaceably pursue the satisfaction of one's sexual and reproductive preferences (dare one say, one's desires), whatever they may be, with consenting others within perhaps the constraints of law. But what should those constraints be? In the absence of philosophy's being able to establish canonical moral constraints, that is, after the immanentization which Hegel recognized (Engelhardt 2010b), there is nothing that can be specifically affirmed to bind persons in general. One has at best a thin aesthetic to replace moral norms. One's body is whatever one makes of it peaceably within the horizon of the finite and the immanent. It is persons who weave a narrative about their bodies, not bodies that set nonnegotiable limits to these narratives.

Once there is no ultimate point of reference, the meaning of the body is to be fabricated, that is, constituted, through various life-style choices that nest the body within various and diverse free-floating narratives. Bodies, along with sexuality and reproduction, become what one peaceably makes of them with consenting others, and increasingly with the assistance of medicine as through technologically mediated reproductive means (e.g., *in vitro* fertilization and embryo transfer). That is, humans are recognized rather as rights and dignity bearers (whatever that might mean) who with other humans are at liberty peaceably to constitute within their own narratives the meaning of their bodies with consenting others. In the contemporary dominant culture, an appreciation of the body as it had been recognized in traditional Christianity is gone. The body has been relocated within a culture in which an agnostic if not an atheistic methodological postulate dominates. All is to be appreciated as if it were ultimately meaningless, receiving only provisional meaning from particular narratives. The body is no longer acknowledged, set within God-imposed norms, as central to the human encounter with a radically transcendent God Who conveys sanctification, and through Whom there is the resurrection of the body.

IV. Sexuality and Reproduction: A Life-world After Sin

The transformation of the public mores of sexuality and reproduction, as Francis Fukuyama correctly observes, was abetted by many factors, important among them the easy availability of effective, reliable, cheap contraception. Effective and cheap contraception allowed one fairly reliably to separate the reproductive dimension of sexuality from the social and recreational dimensions of sexuality (Fukuyama 1999). There was no longer the same fear that sexual activity before marriage might produce a child out of wedlock, a burden to the woman, as well as to her family, along with the duty on the part of the man to marry the woman or at least to provide child support. An important economic motivation for traditional sexual morality was weakened. However, the availability of cheap and effective contraception is not the sole factor that produced this radical change in sexual mores (Goldin & Katz 2000). At the same time effective contraception became available, it also became more acceptable for a woman to have a child without being married, leading to a comprehensive change in cultural expectations regarding sexual activity, child-bearing, and marriage. There has been a foundational change in sexual and reproductive mores. Among the major themes of conflict and contrast is that defining the gulf separating secular career-oriented women from traditional Christian and Orthodox Jewish women who hope to be housewives, have five or more children, and thus do the will of God. These housewives, contrary to liberal secular women, see true fulfillment for a woman to be realized through being the mother of many children and raising them for the Lord. They realize not just that she who rocks the cradle will shape the future of the world; they have a transcendent focus ("the woman shall be saved through childbearing" [I Tim 2:15]).

Within the dominant secular culture, the traditional Christian family is counter-cultural and sexist. Among other things, it is grounded in a gender-essentialism that affirms the authority of husbands. Genesis states that humans were created so as to be two different sexes ("Male and female he created them" [Gen 1:27]), a point that Christ Himself emphasizes: "But from the beginning of creation, 'God made them male and female'" (Mark 10:6; see also Matthew 19:4). Moreover, the resulting relationship of husband and wife goes against the grain of a socio-democratic culture. Eve, the proto-typical woman, is made for Adam to be his helpmate, not the man for the woman (Gen 2:18; I Tim 2:11-15; I Cor 11:9). This relationship requires that wives submit to their husbands (Eph 5:22) and show respect for their husbands as they would for Christ (Eph 5:33). The traditional Christian vision of the family as the domestic church united under the headship of the husband goes against contemporary egalitarian passions. As St. John Chrysostom summarizes, the family is "not to be a democracy, but a monarchy; and as in an army, this order one may see in every family. In the rank of monarch, for instance, there is the husband; but in the rank of lieutenant and general, the wife; and the children too are allotted a third station in command" (Chrysostom 1994, p. 204). This inequality in the authority of husbands and wives has broad implications and lies at the root of the impossibility of having Christian priestesses. The traditional Christian family finds itself grounded in a structure that is before and beyond the consent of its members.

Of course, men are instructed by the dominant secular culture that it is improper, indeed morally exploitative, of them to seek a wife who wishes to be a housewife and mother. Men are told that they are not to be obstacles to their wives' (partners') self-realization, self-fulfillment, and self-expression. The whole image of being a father and breadwinner has thus also been transformed. A complex realignment of social roles has occurred so that if women have children, they are placed in daycare centers and/or men are asked to take on their share of what traditionally had been "women's work". In contrast, within fundamentalist patriarchal Christianities, men are expected to find a virtuous woman who will be a suitable helper (Gen 2:20), bearing his children and tending to the home, while he keeps righteous order while supporting the family, raising sons and daughters for the Lord. As always, the roles of men and women dialectically influence each other. As the contraceptive and abortion revolution placed fewer costs on women for sexual activities outside of marriage, the roles of men changed as well, which then further changed the roles of women. That is, sexual freedom for women led to more sexual license for men. No longer concerned about siring children and living up to the role of prime breadwinner and authoritative father, the man is also freed from his responsibilities, so that pre-marital sex and extra-marital sex are merely life-style choices. Indeed, boys who do not bed a girl early in their teens are often told by Western culture that they are "gay"—creating more "gay" men. It is now expected by many that men will be unfaithful, and there are even "marriage therapists" who will encourage married partners to have open marriages, based on the view that it is better to have open marriages than to have husbands and wives who "cheat" on each other, where "cheat" does not mean committing adultery, but only having clandestine sexual affairs.

This re-evaluation or more precisely devaluation of choices regarding sexual behavior, reproduction, and abortion from moral issues into issues of life-style choices is a surrender before the power of the drive to have sex. Over the history of mankind, the avoidance of fornication, adultery, and homosexual acts has been notoriously difficult. Yet, the recognition of norms allowed the possibility of repentance and the struggle towards virtue. The positive side of sinning is that after sinning one can with full energies repent and know the mercy of God. The struggle with sin is also the struggle to salvation. Now that sexual choices have been placed beyond morality and sin, none of this can be appreciated. A central dimension of human moral struggle and spiritual experience has been radically altered, if not fully forgotten. Sexuality no longer offers an opportunity to re-orient human concerns to God, but provides only an opportunity for acquiescence in the pursuit of the plurality of human desires.

These changes in the sexual mores of the dominant culture were strongly promoted by feminism and by the women's liberation movements,[18] along with movements that forthrightly endorsed personal sexual fulfillment on the part of women. Women were informed that they are now in control of their own sexual lives and that this among other things means that they are free on a par with men to make sexual choices and to enjoy sex without marriage.[19] An example is the emergence of a "hook-up" culture, particularly on college campuses, within which women in the pursuit of success eschew emotional involvement but have "hook-up buddies" to provide some level of sexual satisfaction without emotional or other encumbrances.[20] These changes in sexual mores are not simply the consequence of cheap and effective contraception, but are part of a major cultural change connected to the secularization and de-Christianization of the dominant culture of the West, which demoralized traditional morality. It was driven in part by what Bernice Martin terms the expressive revolution.

> In the last few decades the Western world has experienced a transformation in the assumptions and habitual practices which form the cultural bedrock of the daily lives of ordinary people. . . . The shift began as a sort of cultural revolution among a small minority of crusading radicals, and finished by altering some of our deepest—and therefore most customary and common-place—habits and assumptions (Martin 1981, p. 1).

The focus is both hedonic and reproductive, on both pleasure and the possibility of new social structures framing reproduction (e.g., a single woman reproducing contrary to traditional norms and outside of traditional social structures), combined with a discounting of personal responsibility, especially regarding the negative effects of raising children outside of marriage.[21]

Traditional sexual norms, including traditional views of marriage, were brought into question by being regarded as obstacles to self-fulfillment, self-realization, and self-expression. Traditional sexual mores became surd constraints from the past that were to be removed. The result was a cultural revolution aimed against the traditional Christian ethos of sex, reproduction, and marriage.[22]

> The counter-culture of the 1960s was an attempt to make all life into an evening of freedom when the 'thou' had full sway. It wanted to dispense with the masks too, to integrate the self below the mask with the freedom which the mask alone had hitherto conferred (Martin 1981, p. 15).

An epiphanic assertion of the new sexual mores was the Woodstock gathering (August 15–18, 1969).[23] Norms that had for centuries directed sexual behavior (hypocrisy and non-compliance notwithstanding) were weakening, if not collapsing. Not only was the character of sexual choices changed through the advent of cheap and effective contraception, but a new, post-Christian, countercultural ethos emerged. Woodstock constituted the secular equivalent of the Great Awakening of Protestantism at Cane Ridge, Kentucky, 6 August 1801. Rather than involving spasmodic responses to whatever spirits ruled that day (the 1801 revival was characterized by strange spasmodic dancing marked by uncontrollable jerky movements), the Woodstock gathering focused on setting Christian sexual norms aside. The transformation of the sexual and reproductive ethos was in the end so thoroughgoing as to render what had been a counter-culture into the social norm, or at least into choices that, given the transformation of the meaning and norms of toleration, no longer produced a public, adverse, moral judgment.[24] Sexual life-style choices were no longer matters about which physicians should in chastisement talk with their patients.

The established public morality bearing on sexual relations, pair bonding, reproduction, and the meaning of marriage was thus altered, with implications far beyond sexual relations. The geography of moral authority changed. In particular, the traditional authority of fathers and husbands was brought into question. How men and women tended to relate to each other changed as well. Within the dominant secular culture, sexual choices that had been recognized as involving important right-making conditions, goods, and virtues were rendered into life-style choices directed only by vague, quasi-aesthetic, but surely not by traditional moral and bioethical norms. The moral and bioethical norms that did become salient reflected liberal concerns regarding autonomy, equality, human dignity, and notions of human rights born of the Enlightenment and the French Revolution, which carried with them no prohibition against consensual sexual activities. These norms and the ethos they valorized envisaged persons as bare self-determining individuals without religion, race, history, family, or sex. As long as general Enlightenment norms were not violated, sexual and reproductive choices were taken to fall within the domain of the morally and bioethically acceptable.

These changes in mores were associated with various societal changes through which, *inter alia*, young women came to live apart from their parents, absent parental supervision and in the absence of social structures that placed their activities within a communally shared vision of traditional mores. This occurred in part because of more young women entering college, combined with the abolishment of often strictly overseen single-sex college housing for women in favor of common housing for both male and female students. Away from parental oversight, under the pressure of college life, confronted with a post-traditional sexual ethos, and beset by their own strong sexual urges, many women forgot their mothers' warning that if men have easy access to sex, men will not be as motivated to marry, much less remain bonded to one woman. The ethos of sexual liberation instructed and encouraged young women to adopt a different attitude to sexual intercourse, changing the strategies that once encouraged stable monogamy. Casual sexual relations were valorized as authentic expressions of a young woman's freedom from arbitrary parental authority and outworn cultural norms. With the advent of cheap and effective contraception, along with the availability of abortion, combined with a cultural endorsement of sexual self-fulfillment and self-realization, and in the face of the sexual passions of youth, college sexual life-styles, indeed sexual life-styles in general, were transformed.

The transformation of the dominant sexual mores was also associated with the influence of the Frankfurt School, which grew out of the Institute for Social Research, founded in the University of Frankfurt in 1923, and influenced by Georg Lukacs (1885–1971). Lukacs was an early defender of free love and a critic of the mores of the bourgeois family, as were others associated with the Frankfurt School. Herbert Marcuse in his very popular *Eros and Civilization* (1955) spoke of "the fulfillment of man and nature, not through domination and exploitation, but through release of inherent libidinal forces" (Marcuse 1955, p. 176). Here, too, Wilhelm Reich (1897–1957) should be included with his book *The Sexual Revolution* (1963). These intellectuals, as well as others, provided the justification for the sexual revolution of the 1960s and following.

The result has been a continuing, indeed accelerating transformation of the ethos and ethics of sexuality, reproduction, and marriage within the dominant culture. There has been a dramatic change in what is socially acceptable, as well as a change in the moral norms by which behavior is to be judged. This has been connected with a weakening of guidance from the Western Christianities. In a retreat from the language of sin and an embrace instead of the attitude "Who am I to judge?" (Christians should condemn the sin but not judge the sinner), "[t]he preaching of premarital chastity, which used to feature so prominently in the education of Catholic youth down to the 1960s and even beyond, has faded from view" (Vattimo 2004, p. 61). Having sex has become as morally significant as having a drink of water when thirsty. Sociologically, Vattimo has it right: "Belief in the importance of sexuality in human life is gradually waning" (Vattimo 2011, p. 56). This radical deflation of the significance of sexuality is tied to the centrality given to the pursuit of happiness understood as the pursuit of pleasure. On this point, Rorty summarizes the issue succinctly in claiming that we "have no moral obligations except helping one another satisfy our desires, thus achieving the greatest possible amount of happiness" (Rorty 2011, p. 8). Sexual satisfaction has become recognized as integral to the pursuit of happiness.

A culture emerged in which the erotic has become omnipresent, while at the same time being stripped of moral significance. In addition, the moral significance of the bond between marriage and reproduction has been abolished. There is not only more open casual sex and more open cohabitation, but there are fewer children born per woman with a greater percentage of those children entering the world from outside of a traditional marriage. In 1960 there were 18.1 children born for every thousand Italian women; by 2012 there were only 9.06. Also in 1960 only 2.4% of Italians were born outside of a traditional marriage; by 2012 this had risen to 24.9%.[25] The changes in the United States were as dramatic (Martin et al. 2012). In the United States, 23.7 children were born for every thousand women in 1960 and 13.66 children in 2013. As to illegitimacy, 5.3% of all children were born outside of marriage in 1960; this had risen to 40.7% in 2011.[26]

As just observed, these profound changes are the result of many factors, including not just the availability of effective contraception that made sexual intercourse seem more risk-free, but also the influence of various movements that placed an enhanced positive accent on individual autonomy as well as on individual self-realization, self-fulfillment, self-satisfaction, and self-expression. In addition and crucially, there was an expansion of a state-supported welfare system for unmarried women that made it economically easier, and at times even attractive, to reproduce outside of marriage. Welfare programs encouraged extramarital reproduction. The goal of such welfare programs was to liberate women from a dependence on men so as to allow women "greater freedom" to choose as they wished. In the United States, these welfare programs *de facto* targeted blacks and their impact was disproportionately greater on blacks (Moynihan 1965). In 1965 only 24% of black children were born outside of marriage (Akerlof et al. 1996). By 2011 this had risen to 72.3% (Hamilton et al. 2012). Such significant adverse consequences effected the large-scale destruction of the black family, leading to the loss of significant moral and social capital.

This all happened as there was at the same time the emergence of a suspicion of authority figures, especially the authority of husbands and fathers. The result has been that an increasing proportion of children now grow up without the coherent presence of a father, especially of a biological father who is the husband of their mother. The phenomenon of one-parent families has been shown to be strongly associated with poverty and other significant social costs (Mayer 1998; Pearlstein 2011). The authority of religion and the authority of God were discounted as well during this period. Those who in the past would have strongly restrained such sexual license (e.g., the Roman Catholic clergy) did so less often, while some of these authority figures did the very opposite and affirmed sexual and reproductive license, while also engaging in the sexual abuse of children. A culture emerged that marginalized the disciplinary, authoritative father who preserved the virginity of his daughters. Sexual urges that have always been notoriously difficult to discipline and contain found an affirmation in this newly dominant secular ethos of sexual self-realization, self-satisfaction, self-fulfillment, and self-expression.

A new sexual and reproductive ethos had taken shape and was established as a dimension of the now-dominant secular culture forming a basis for contemporary secular bioethics. The erotic had been re-valorized, while giving birth to children became regarded with some suspicion. After all, raising children interferes with the wholehearted pursuit of self-satisfaction; children are a burden. This devaluation of reproduction in the 1960s was supported by various apocalyptic views of a population explosion in the face of limited resources. It became plausible to many that the decoupling of sexual pleasure from reproduction was not only to be affirmed for various self-directed reasons, but it was also to be affirmed on altruistic grounds in order to avoid supposed threatening ecological disasters.[27] As a consequence, the erotic became more salient just as the number of children produced dropped. This sexual and reproductive ethos was tied to a new normative understanding of how women should live their lives. Among other things, the new ethos was built around an affirmation of women entering and succeeding in the workplace on an equal footing with men. Women were to find as much fulfillment as men in having a job and, if possible, a profession. Any interest that might exist in having children was to be relocated within the commitment to placing women fully and equally alongside men in the workplace. At the same time, women are to seek sexual pleasure and fulfillment on a basis equal to men, as described by Helen Gurley Brown, who valorized the role of sexual activity in career advancement (1962, 1965). But the difficulty remains: women, not men, get pregnant. In order to ensure the equality of women in sexual activity and in their entrance into the workplace on a par with men, there has to be robust protection against unplanned motherhood.

There was, of course, the possibility that the traditional culture would have been able to maintain itself along with traditional structures and boundaries. As Martin also notes, "If structure and boundary maintenance become strong enough, then expressive pleasure—food, sex—can *only* occur at unspontaneous, programmed times" (Martin 1981, p. 15). However, as a matter of fact, the traditional culture failed to respond effectively to the emerging post-traditional culture. The dominant culture did not encourage but rather undermined restraint. The dominant culture was transformed by a counter-culture. "At the heart of the counter-culture was a single-minded, often fanatical onslaught on boundaries and structures, a crusade to release Ariel, the infinite, expressive chaos into the everyday world" (Martin 1981, p. 15). Sexual pleasure and satisfaction, which had been traditionally affirmed only in marriage, became valorized in their own right through the Kinsey Reports (1948, 1953), the work of Masters and Johnson (1966, 1970, 1974, 1979, 1994), and such erotic best-sellers as *The Hite Report* (2003), leading to the emergence of genteel soft pornography and the contemporary cultural phenomena associated with an "easy" sexuality portrayed in the *Fifty Shades* trilogy (James 2012). All of this happened after the restraints of Western Christianity were foundationally weakened in the wake of the theological, cultural, and personal chaos that followed Vatican II (1962–1965), during which many Roman Catholic clerics left their calling in order to marry or otherwise "find themselves" (Roman Catholicism's contribution to the chaos in, and the transformation of, the dominant culture is addressed in chapter seven). Rather than defend traditional sexual norms, many priests and nuns often embraced the new spiritual and sexual *aggornamiento*, thus supporting the massive cultural changes that were under way. The changes in Roman Catholicism were reflected in similar transformations of mainline Christianity and liberal Judaism. Many religious institutions that could have effected restraint were themselves caught up with and in fact abetted the turmoil and moral chaos.[28] One thus finds the Evangelische Kirche Deutschlands (EKD), which compasses Lutheran, Reformed, and United churches, endorsing a post-modern vision of the family that identifies as families sexual reproductive units of any sort, including traditional families, families from divorce and re-marriage, single-parent households, and same-sex couples (Root 2013; Kirchenamt der EKD 2013).

Martin notes how this counter-culture, along with its new sexual mores, was tied as well to the ethos associated with the culture of rock music, which at the same time was gaining cultural salience.

> Rock music from its beginnings in the early 1950s was *par excellence* the cultural medium through which young people explored and expressed the symbolism of liminality (p. 154). Of all the features of social order which rock organizes, mediates and reflects, sexuality is probably the most important single element (Martin 1981, p. 183).

These profound alterations that occurred in the mores of the dominant culture of the West were the result of a complex constellation of factors, as Martin underscores.

> The sexual revolution of the late twentieth century also has hard social foundations in the chemical technology of contraception, the medical provision for safe early abortion, and the control of venereal diseases. All these have radically altered the social and personal meanings of sexual behaviour. They make it possible for sexuality to be *reduced* to the expressive dimension, denuded of all attendant physiological, social, and moral consequences, and

thus *of all risk.* Since the advent of the contraceptive pill and the medical capability of safe termination of pregnancy, human beings (significantly the female half of that plural) can separate sexuality from reproduction, and both from marriage, with greater ease than has ever before been the case (Martin 1981, p. 242).

The bottom line is that there were wide-ranging changes in norms bearing on sexuality, reproduction, and marriage, as well as in the general normative character of roles for men and women, fathers and mothers, husbands and wives. Because it is women who get pregnant, not men, much of this depended on changes regarding when women should agree to sexual intercourse, leading to an increase in the frequency of cohabitation and child-bearing outside of marriage, and to a change in the significance of marriage that has been reflected in rising divorce rates and births outside of marriage (Allen & Atkins 2012).

This dramatic recasting of sexual life-styles within the dominant secular culture has created numerous important points of significant conflict between the now-dominant secular culture and the normative sexual and reproductive life-styles of traditional Christians. Because traditional Christians live, experience, and know sexuality as properly nested within heterosexual marriage and tied to bringing children into the world, sexual activity and sexual self-fulfillment are affirmed, but only within marriage. This state of affairs not only underscores the traditional Christian moral affirmation of heterosexual marriage, but also condemns homosexual liaisons, along with heterosexual liaisons and reproduction outside of marriage. As a consequence, the traditional Christian ethos and ethics of sexuality and reproduction are saliently politically incorrect and against the grain of the contemporary age. In traditional Christian communities, sexual mores are as a result radically different from what occurs in the dominant secular culture. God-oriented language of sin remains robust. In traditional Christian communities, men tend to be schooled in sexual responsibility by women who explain to men that they can get access to sexual satisfaction only through marriage. Traditional Christian women defend cultural constraints that focus men on remaining faithful to one woman and on committing men to earning enough to support a wife and children, because among other things it is in their self-interest.

In traditional cultures, both men and women are schooled in moral habits that look beyond the affluence of a consumerist society and that instead focus on a commitment to each other and to God that supports heterosexual marital unions. The traditional focus is on men and women's intertwining obligations, but not on equality. Again, the traditional Christian moral vision, rather than underscoring the liberation of women, regards women as the protectresses of the morality of a culture in controlling access to sexual satisfaction. In a traditional Christian culture, it is recognized that if women provide sex before marriage, women diminish the incentives of men to marry, thus undermining the likelihood of women finding an acceptable partner willing to marry (again, as the traditional adage puts the matter, "if you give the milk away free, why should he buy the cow?"). Mothers will tell their sons to act like a man, embracing the special virtues of self-possession, courage, self-sacrifice, self-denial, self-control, and responsibility required in order to be a good husband, a good father, and the breadwinner for a large family with a stay-at-home wife. Traditional Christians will regard the sexual liberation movement for women as in fact having become a means for the sexual exploitation of women by men. The governing ideals of traditional Christian men and women are not contained within the horizon of the finite and the immanent. Hence, the importance of the language of sin.

Within the new life-world of sexuality and reproduction sustained by the dominant secular culture, the deportment of traditional Christian physicians will not only appear puzzling but highly immoral, given the dominant secular culture's demoralization of consensual sexual and reproductive choices. Imagine a traditional Christian physician who posts on his website and in his waiting room a statement (in addition personally to informing all new patients) that he will not provide contraception for unmarried women or refer for abortion. Secular bioethics can but recognize such ethics as unethical. Because sexual and reproductive choices are reduced to life-style choices set within a particular vision of human flourishing, it becomes a violation of secular bioethics for physicians, nurses, and other health care professionals to express adverse judgments regarding fornication, the insemination of lesbians, the use of donor gametes in reproduction within marriage, the use of transsexual surgery, and abortion. It becomes a violation of secular bioethics to fail to provide these services or even refer for them, a point to which we will turn in particular in chapter five.

In contrast, within the dominant secular culture the ethos of sexual and reproductive responsibility has been transformed so that men within a post-traditional culture can eschew marriage and reproduction. If they do find themselves the father of a child, the men, if they are in the lower socio-economic classes and judgment-proof, can easily avoid responsibility by never working sufficiently to be obliged to pay child support. Thus, a man can reproduce with more than one woman, usually finding some lonely woman to accept him. A new life-world of sexuality has taken shape in which women can be more easily exploited. Men are now at liberty to have sex with multiple women and not get married. They need only "respect" the women with whom they have sex by affirming the woman's personal self-fulfillment, all the while trying to avoid enduring commitments, especially any commitment to marriage (Edin & Nelson 2013). This strategy helps satisfy male sexual desires without reinforcing any notion of enduring responsibility on the part of men to the women with whom they have intercourse. The life-worlds of traditional Christianity and of the now-dominant culture collide. They involve incompatible views of the status and obligations of men and women regarding sexuality, reproduction, equality in the workplace, marriage, children, and the family.

For women who wish eventually to marry and have children, the playing field between men and women has become even more unequal. In the secular culture, women are encouraged to delay marriage and children in order to enter the workplace, while nevertheless being sexually active. Men can do the same, but they can outlast the women. A woman who delays marriage until after 35 will be neither as attractive as a marriage partner nor as fertile as she was in her twenties. On the other hand, a man in his late thirties or early forties when his career is established will look quite attractive to a woman in her twenties. As a consequence, the deferral of marriage by women in order to enter the workforce and to find sexual fulfillment equally with men appears to traditional cultures as a failure to appreciate two of the stark inequalities of men and women: women live longer than men, while their reproductive life is shorter than that of men. Men can marry and raise a large family, starting even in their sixties, while women cannot.[29] Men and women are not equal.[30] This, among other things, has increased the demand for third-party-assisted reproduction and shaped the character of contemporary secular morality and bioethics.

Against the background of these profound cultural changes, it is important to note not only how opaque the future is, but even how opaque the present is. It is difficult accurately to assess all that is even now taking place after the erosion of the traditional roles for men and women. Immense changes are occurring in how men and women engage the world within the contemporary secular culture. Post-industrial societies have a decreasing percentage of jobs for which the physical prowess that characterizes men is useful. It is a world in which verbal expression is becoming much more important than physical strength. The implications are significant and complex. They are associated, for example, with more women than men completing higher education (OECD 2011). Many men are having difficulty in adapting to the new environment. Some attribute the difficulty at least in part to a failure in male maturation (Hymowitz 2011).[31] As Hanna Rosin has observed in *The End of Men and the Rise of Women*: "Boys of every race and background have a much higher incidence of school disciplinary and behavior problems and suspensions, and they spend far fewer hours doing homework" (Rosin 2012, p. 163). These changes have also interestingly been associated with some decrease in sexual promiscuity. "In 1988, half of boys aged fifteen to seventeen reported having sex; by 2010 that number fell to just under a third. For teenage girls, the numbers dropped from 37.2 to 27 percent" (Rosin 2012, p. 19). What this all means is far from clear, and it surely does not mean the same thing for all communities within a society (Murray 2012). Hasidic Jews, for example, appear to be surviving relatively unscathed within a very secular New York City (Fader 2009). On the other hand, young Japanese appear to be losing interest in sex with others (Haworth 2013). Is a mass culture of solitary sex emerging?

Also at stake in all that has happened is a contrast between radically different understandings of the family. On the one hand, there remains a traditional, ontological, or metaphysical recognition of the family as a social possibility that should be realized by actual families, and that brings with it predetermined roles for husbands and wives, as well as for fathers, mothers, and children. This appreciation of the family encompasses previous generations and looks forward to the generations that are to come. Such families possess an integrity and autonomy of their own, amassing both social and financial capital, so as to give care and support to previous as well as following generations. Such families embrace a commitment to having children, as well as to caring morally and financially for them. Such views of the family are affirmed by traditional Christianity and Judaism (Fader 2009), as well as by Confucianism, with important implications for bioethics and health care policy (Fan 1997, 2010, 2011). In contrast, a libertarian/liberal view of the family construes the family as rising out of the agreement of its constituent members, as well as being shaped by commitments to the liberty, equality, and self-satisfaction of its members. Roles within the family are held to reflect no pre-existing reality, but are held instead to be grounded in choice and social forces. Such socio-sexual units have no necessary commitment to producing children. After all, children can be major impediments to self-satisfaction. Finally, reality appears to impose constraints: children in "families" other than those constituted from the marriage of their father and mother appear to be subject to significant risks.[32]

The changes we have reviewed in the dominant sexual ethos are intimately tied to more general cultural developments, which are associated with the emergence of a new post-traditional cultural elite. Reproduction outside of marriage, along with the increasing phenomenon of children being raised apart from their biological father, now characterizes the lower socio-economic class, while reproduction within marriage has remained salient in the upper socio-economic class. The upper socio-economic class has come to be characterized not only by more income and capital, but also by intact families and, with some important qualifications, the persistence of traditional religious belief and practice. In addition, society now falls into four classes: the unemployed (and radically under-employed), workers, service providers, and the creative intellectual class (Bishop 2009; Cherlin 2009; Florida 2011; Himmelfarb 2001; and Murray 2012). The last class has involved as a salient element the synthesis of bourgeois and bohemian characteristics (Brooks 2000). In the process, communities and cities have changed substantively (Ehrenhalt 1995), as well as being characterized by a large number of persons who live alone (Klinenberg 2013). Finally, it must be remembered that the upper socio-economic class is morally complex, including Hasidic Jews (Fader 2009).

V. The New Sexual Mores: The Cultural Importance of Abortion

Given the changes in sexual and reproductive mores, it is no accident that in the 1960s many of the states in the United States liberalized access to abortion, leading to the watershed cases of Roe v. Wade, 410 U.S. 113 (1973) and Doe v. Bolton, 410 U.S. 179 (1973). These 1973 holdings "normalized" elective abortion and further "empowered" women who now, *inter alia*, could have abortions without the permission of their husbands. Within the dominant secular culture abortion came to be regarded as an ordinary, accepted medical procedure, thus further securing the new sexual ethos of self-fulfillment and self-expression. The Supreme Court decisions constituted an important element of the profound secularization of the United States. A new post-Christian life-world of sexuality, work, and the family was entrenched in constitutional law, which became integral to the dominant secular morality. Similar changes have occurred in Europe. Abortion has been positively valorized by the dominant secular culture and its morality as integral to the new life-styles of women. Again, the affirmation of abortion was regarded as especially important, given more women attending college, the passage of laws opening the workplace to equal access by women, the affirmation of an ethos of sexual engagement by women on a par with men, and the loss of the assumption that one should have children.

A new life-world with its legal framework and bioethics has emerged for women in which sexuality, reproduction, and abortion have taken on new significance (Alvaré 2013). The way in which young women regard themselves has in the process radically changed and become integral to a new self-image tightly bound to economic engagement in the established consumerist society. Women, outside of religions that have maintained a traditional ethos,[33] are no longer encouraged to think of themselves primarily as future wives and mothers, but as women who should earn their own living on a par with men while also pursuing sexual fulfillment on a par with men, while perhaps also considering whether to marry and have a child.[34] The result has been a radical change in social ideals for women, which the availability of contraception and abortion made feasible. Women are no longer encouraged to look forward to finding a man capable of supporting them while they tend the home and care for the children. Instead, women are to pursue a life of their own, characteristically marked by their own search for sexual, personal, and workplace fulfillment, in which marriage and having a child (children) are optional, and for which abortion is crucial in maintaining this optional character. The actual compatibility of entering into the workplace and engaging actively in sex while still perhaps contemplating an eventual role as a mother is often explored through conflicts, for which abortion is frequently the "solution." All of these factors have led to the current form of the dominant secular bioethics of reproduction (Delkeskamp-Hayes 2013; Delkeskamp-Hayes & Imrényi 2013).

Central to being engaged in the pursuit of a career while being sexually active is the ability to avoid having children at the wrong time, or too many children, so as not to impede the pursuit of a complex interplay of secular educational, career, companionship, and marriage ideals, along with the various goods and goals of a consumer-oriented culture. Again, this state of affairs has given a powerful positive valence to abortion, in that access to abortion is an indispensable insurance against the disruptions that an unplanned pregnancy would impose on the pursuit of the full fabric of freedom in sexual, career, and consumer-oriented choices. In this light, one can understand the passion with which the dominant secular culture supports abortion "rights." Abortion allows women and men to live in this new, post-Christian life-world, unbound by the constraints of biology, traditional culture, and sin, especially without the fear of the personal, career, and economic disruptions attendant on an unwanted child. As a consequence, there have been books published that give a strong positive value to abortion with titles such as *Abortion is a Blessing* (Gaylor 1975), *Abortion is a Woman's Right* (Grogan 1985), *The Sacrament of Abortion* (Paris 1992), and *Sacred Choices* (Maguire 2001). Along with the postponement of marriage, there are fewer children, not just because of decreasing fertility with age as women marry later, but due to a greater accent on a perceived obligation of women to stay in the workforce in the pursuit of full participation in the economy, which is equated with self-fulfillment as a woman. The focus on maintaining one's job and advancing one's career, when combined with financial and opportunity costs associated with children, especially in a consumerist society, creates significant disincentives against having children, or at least any significant number of children. Again, because there will always be contraceptive failures, abortion is cardinal to sex roles in such secularized societies. It is for this reason as well that members of patriarchal fundamentalist religions, which are less influenced by these factors, out-reproduce liberals (Longman 2004). A new dominant ethos, morality, and bioethics of sexuality and reproduction have taken shape.

VI. Beyond Heterosexuality: The Secular Normativity of Bare Sexuality

There has been a watershed change in the established dominant sexual norms defining contemporary post-religious polities, a change that runs profoundly counter to the norms of traditional Christianity. Set within the horizon of the finite and the immanent, and given the contemporary dominant secular culture, peaceable sexual inclinations and passions are not to be disparaged. The now-dominant secular culture requires in addition to the acceptance of at-will heterosexual sexual liaisons, the acceptance of peaceable, consensual homosexual life-styles along with homosexual marriage. Withholding acceptance of homosexual acts has become a form of bigotry, if not hate-speech and hate-behavior. It is not just that the appreciation of fornication as a sin or as an act of immorality has been set aside, and the practice of concubinage generally accepted through the demoralization of morality into alternative life-styles. Sexuality in addition has been reduced to an all-purpose building block for pleasure and happiness as one conceives these, and the interpersonal relationships one wills to fashion with consenting others. This demoralization of the norms for sexual choices involves not only the dismissal but also the condemnation of both traditional Jewish and traditional Christian understandings of sexuality. These understandings support an essentialist appreciation of what it is to be a man and to be a woman, as well as a normatively heterosexualist appreciation of sexual pleasure as properly enjoyed only in the married union of a man and a woman. Both traditional Jews and Christians recognize that being a man or a woman reflects initial as well as enduringly essentially different ways of being human. "So God created man in His own image, in the image of God He created him; male and female He created them" (Genesis 1:27). Indeed, Christ says, "Haven't you read . . . that at the beginning the Creator 'made them male and female,' and said, 'For this reason a man will leave his father and mother and be united to his wife, and the two will become one flesh'?" (Matthew 19:4–5). To be a man or a woman is to be different in ways intrinsic to being human. Humans are foundationally dimorphic.

The sexual union of these dimorphic humans, the union of a man and a woman in marriage, is recognized as blessed of God. The Jewish marriage ceremony, which is preceded by a fast, is taken to forgive sins: "for the wedding day is by tradition a time when all their sins are washed clean and for Jews atonement is coupled with fasting" (Heilman 1992, p. 289). Further, marital intercourse is a mitzvah. For Jews as well as for Christians, marriage is in general an obligation.

> If any Bishop, or Presbyter, or Deacon, or anyone at all on the sacerdotal list, abstains from marriage, or meat, or wine, not as a matter of mortification, but out of an abhorrence thereof, forgetting that all things are exceedingly good, and that God made man male and female, and blasphemously misrepresenting God's work of creation, either let him mend his ways or let him be deposed from office and expelled from the Church. Let a layman be treated similarly (Sts. Nicodemus & Agapius 1983, "The 85 Canons of the Holy and Renowned Apostles," Canon LI, p. 91).

In addition, sexual pleasure in marriage is affirmed as blessed of God.

> And how become they one flesh? As if thou shouldest take away the purest part of gold, and mingle it with other gold; so in truth here also the woman as it were receiving the richest part fused by pleasure, nourisheth it and cherisheth it, and withal contributing her own share, restoreth it back a Man. And the child is a sort of bridge, so that the three become one flesh, the child connecting, on either side, each to other (Chrysostom 1994, Homily XII on Colossians iv.12, 13, vol. 13, p. 319).

Sexual contact and pleasure are known by Christians to exist properly only within the marriage of a man and a woman.

Traditional Christians also know, as St. Paul teaches, that, in contrast to heterosexual desires and contact, homosexual desires and sexual contact are in their very character not rightly related to God. Getting sexuality and sex right requires getting things with God right. Sexual perversion is rooted in a distorted relationship with God. It is for this reason that worshipping the creature rather than the Creator distorts human nature, including sexual orientation. As St. Paul puts it,

> They exchanged the truth of God for a lie, and worshiped and served created things rather than the Creator—who is forever praised. Amen. Because of this, God gave them over to shameful lusts. Even their women exchanged natural relations for unnatural ones. In the same way the men also abandoned natural relations with women and were inflamed with lust for one another. Men committed indecent acts with other men, and received in themselves the due penalty for their perversion (Romans 1:25–27).

Among the sequellae from the loss of a rightly-ordered relationship to God is that the normativity of heterosexuality is obscured, so that sexuality is mistakenly considered as merely a general building block for pleasure and happiness. Sexuality, outside of a rightly-oriented relationship to God, thus becomes merely a resource for building consensual human relationships unguided by a normative relationship to God.

The traditional Christian recognition of the normatively heterosexual character of marriage constitutes a major affront against a secular, post-modern vision of human dignity grounded in human freedom, all understood after God. Traditional Christianity denies the legitimacy of a canonical secular thin theory of the good, as for example that which Rawls presupposed for the fabric of justice within a secular, social-democratic state (Rawls 1971, #60, pp. 347–350), which understanding of the family brings the family into question as undercutting fair equality of opportunity (Rawls 1971, #77, p. 51). Rawls holds that the secular state presupposes an affirmation of that plurality of life-styles that can be nested in thick theories of the good that fit within the framework of a secular thin theory of the good that gives priority to liberty, then to equality, and then to social and economic advantages, as long as these redound to the advantage of the least-well-off class (Rawls 1971, #46, p. 303f). Second, traditional Christianity recognizes that even involuntary engagement in sinful acts, despite its involuntary character, reshapes the character of persons so that as a consequence of such sin one will tend not to aim perfectly at God (Engelhardt 2000, pp. 249, 278). One will fall short of the mark (*hamartia*), even if one cannot control one's engagement in certain acts, especially sexual acts, for sexual acts define our way of being human, as men and women. Such a recognition of involuntary sin is an offensive oxymoron for a moral vision that sets centrally free choice as *Wilkür* (free choice as setting one's own ends in terms of one's own wishes, not free choice as *Wille*, as will turned to God).[35]

The recognition of involuntary sin acknowledges proper ends for human volition beyond human choice. In the contemporary dominant culture and after the death of God, there is no perspective beyond that of individuals, in particular beyond individuals as the community of liberty-oriented moral agents deaf to God. Hence, the profound collision of the now-dominant secular morality with the norms of traditional Christianity. From the perspective of the contemporary dominant secular moral vision that is after God, the rejection of the legitimacy of homosexual marriage and other elements of consensual homosexual lifestyles offends deeply against the vision of human dignity grounded in one's willful self-constitution in accord with one's inclinations and passions. The pursuit of one's inclinations is not to be disparaged by a call to repentance, for no moral norm is recognized beyond oneself as a free peaceable agent collaborating with consenting others. *Wilkür* qua *Wilkür* has become *Wille*.

VII. Timeo Danaos et dona ferentes:[36]
Moral Philosophy as a Political Agenda

Any critique of equality is challenging to the dominant secular culture that wishes to regard persons qua persons and thereby not recognize them in important moral ways as differing due to history, circumstance, and/or sex. Rather, persons are approached as bare individuals fully interchangeable and not marked by defining roles as men and women, husbands and wives, fathers and mothers, grandfathers and grandmothers, teachers and students, etc. Morality along with bioethics is sought to be understood from a view from nowhere. In contrast, the viewpoint of the God of Christians is not a view from nowhere. The particularity of place, history, and even sex is not ignored. This goes against the Greek hope, especially salient among the Stoics, which developed further after the Western Middle Ages, that sought a viewpoint that treats all anonymously and equally.[37] As with all Greek thought, it had a cardinal impediment against appreciating the individual (Gorovitz & MacIntyre 1976). As the exploration of sexuality in the previous sections showed, the mores of the dominant secular culture wish to recast all persons in fully interchangeable terms. This follows from the Greek prejudice to see reality in universalist terms. Neither Judaism nor Christianity is grounded in universalist conceptual terms. Hence, in the perspective born of Greece and transformed by the Enlightenment, there is acceptance of homosexuality, bisexuality, fornication, and consensual adultery because persons are regarded as bare persons able to consent to their mutual interactions. In this barren conceptual geography, there are to be no fixed and normative sexual roles such as married and unmarried, husband and wife. All is to be open to all persons through free choice. This micro-level interchangeability of human roles has implications as well for the appreciation of the state: if the individual is the source of all authority, how can the state have any authority beyond that of the minimal state where all is grounded in consent and only in the consent of individuals?

The state of affairs at the micro-level and macro-level are thus closely interconnected. Among other things, the unraveling of the Western grand narrative regarding sexuality, reproduction, and marriage is closely associated with the unraveling of the Western grand narrative regarding state authority. The Greeks had supplied the basis for the emergence of the Western dream of a moral and political account that can bind all persons in a universal narrative supporting a web of universal rights. This universalist vision has its roots in the universalist character of most Greek moral philosophy, a vision that was reborn in the Western Middle Ages and is at odds with the Jewish and Christian experience of a personal God Who calls individual people to salvation, as He called Abraham (Gen 12:1–3), Who is merciful on a person-by-person basis (Ex 33:19), and Who has established a particular Church, at a particular place, and at a particular time in history, not to mention with particular and different obligations for men and women. For this universalist narrative, traditional Christianity remains scandalous in its particularist character and claims.

Again and most importantly for the Christianity of the first centuries, alive today in Orthodox Christianity, morality and bioethics are not third things between God and man that possess a rational foundation in moral philosophy, or even admit to a rational further development, as, for example, is fallaciously held by John Paul II in *Fides et ratio* (John Paul II 1998). Traditional Christianity, indeed Orthodox Christianity, embraces the theocentric horn of Plato's dilemma in the *Euthyphro*, that the good, the right, and the virtuous can only be rightly understood in terms of their leading to God, and not in terms of philosophical argument apart from God. In contrast, Western Christianity came to embrace the rationalistic horn, namely, that the good, the right, and the virtuous can be understood apart from God, in particular through a moral philosophy open in a universalist fashion to all men independent of right worship. Morality could also be rationally revised and developed. As a consequence, moral philosophy could reshape the dogmas of the mainline Christian denominations on such matters as the headship of the husband and the unacceptability of homosexual liaisons, rendering their dogmas along with their bioethics more compatible with the demands of the current secular view of the morally rational. Because rationalist Christian denominations affirmed norms of a universalist character, it was easy to act to erase ontological differences distinguishing men and women, homosexual acts and heterosexual acts.

The culture of modernity, which the contemporary, post-modern, dominant secular culture is replacing, grew out of this Western medieval Christian culture that had been shaped by a robust faith in reason and in particular in the capacity of philosophical reflection to determine the canonical content of morality. Moral philosophy as the ground of moral norms had been introduced in Greece of the 5th century B.C. to replace appeals to religious grounds for moral conduct as Greece was secularized and moved from being a traditional to a post-traditional culture; among other things, this led to the trial and execution of Socrates.[38] A post-religious faith in reason became the distinguishing mark of Athens. It was this faith in reason that Plato underscores in the *Euthyphro*, when Plato affirms that the good, the right, and the virtuous can be known apart from God. In the 5th century before Christ, moral rationality was developed in order to be substituted for the gods. In particular, moral rationality was to supply the ground for a canonical vision of the good, the right, and the virtuous. The rationalistic answer to the *Euthyphro* became central.

This cultural transformation of the very particular moral and ontological vision of Jews and Christians into a universalist account in which all persons are interchangeable was not only philosophically but politically plausible.[39] After the bloody religious wars of the 17th century, the Thirty Years' War on the

Continent (1618–1648), and the Civil War in England (1642–1651), the integrity of Christendom had been shattered, creating a moral and cultural vacuum.

> The Treaties of Westphalia finally sealed the relinquishment by statesmen of a noble and ancient concept, a concept which had dominated the Middle Ages: that there existed among the baptized people of Europe a bond stronger than all their motives for wrangling—a spiritual bond, the concept of Christendom. Since the fourteenth century, and especially during the fifteenth, this concept had been steadily disintegrating. . . . The Thirty Years' War proved beyond a shadow of a doubt that the last states to defend the ideal of a united Christian Europe were invoking that principle while in fact they aimed at maintaining or imposing their own supremacy. It was at Münster and Osnabrück that Christendom was buried. The tragedy was that nothing could replace it; and twentieth-century Europe is still bleeding in consequence (Daniel-Rops 1964, vol. 1, pp. 200–201).

In Christendom's stead, the expectation grew that, through pursuing a rationally grounded morality, finally and decisively one would step away from the religious disputes that not merely divided but also led to civil war, unrest, and carnage. Faith in faith was lost, but faith in reason remained and served as one of the major forces of secularization. The hope was that perpetual peace could be secured in secular terms within an international community of persons bound by a liberal rationality and a morality such as Kant's.

The crucial point is that the medieval faith in reason made plausible the Enlightenment's rationalist reaction to the Thirty Years' War and the British Civil War, so that it seemed that the appropriate response to the religious wars of the 17th century was to embrace reason alone and to abandon faith. The dominant culture of the Enlightenment as a consequence confidently rejected the Western medieval faith in faith and instead affirmed the modern Western faith in reason, including moral philosophy, presuming that morality would retain nearly the same canonical content when grounded in reason that it had possessed when grounded in faith. In particular, the hope, which was Kant's hope, was that one could substitute philosophical reason for God, so that one could appeal to one reason, one moral rationality, just as there had once been a recognition of and appeal to one God. The expectation was that general lineaments of

Christian morality would be preserved but grounded in reason and fully severed from Christianity. Moral philosophy could then reliably guide mankind to an enlightened age, while keeping the traditional morality of the West more or less intact, all of which would be supported through reason, not through faith. Modernity was Western Christianity secularized. As Vattimo put it:

> [T]he West is secularized Christianity and nothing else. In other words, if we want to talk about the West, Europe, modernity—which, in my argument, are held to be synonymous—as recognizable and clearly defined historical-cultural entities, the only notion we can use is precisely that of the secularization of the Judeo-Christian heritage (Vattimo 2002, p. 73).

Therefore, with Kant one finds the affirmation of traditional Christian morality articulated without Christ and purportedly grounded in reason. Kant continued the Scholastic project of the mid-13th century.

The universalist moral aspirations of ancient Greece, reborn in the Middle Ages, took on a fully secular character in late modernity, which through the Enlightenment's conceits led to the French Revolution with its claims regarding human equality, human dignity, and human rights. Had this project's intellectual goals been realized, all persons as free, equal, and interchangeable individuals would have implicitly been united in one moral community of rational moral agents, bound by a single moral rationality, collaborating through political structures guided and justified by that rationality, so that this canonical rationality would have been the ultimate source of the moral authority of the modern state. If the rationalist horn of Euthyphro's dilemma would have been fully vindicated, not just in the moral but in the political realm as well, a justification through sound rational argument would have been given for one particular, canonical, content-full understanding of the good, the right, and the virtuous, as well as for political authority. However, as already observed, this project fails in principle. In a life-world unable to find the foundations to secure a single canonical morality to guide life-style and death-style choices, there is not just demoralization and deflation of the secular ethos of sexuality, reproduction, and marriage, but the authority of the state is also brought into question. It is not just that canonical Western morality has been disestablished, but the moral legitimacy of the state as well. State power has come to substitute for failed expectations regarding the authority of reason to convey moral legitimacy. Morality, buttressed by moral philosophy, becomes a political agenda.

VIII. From Modernity to Post-Modernity: Setting the Stage for Contemporary Morality and Bioethics

Modernity looked to the future, confident in the bond between peace and a global secular universalist ethics that was expressed in the progressivist movements of the 19th century. Despite the bloodshed of the French Revolution, faith in moral rationality remained tied to a faith in rational progress towards a peaceful collaboration among all humans. There would be a liberation from the surd constraints of traditional Christianity. This secular faith in the emergence of an ever better world was broad in its compass:

> But the world is growing better. And in the Future—in the long, long ages to come—IT WILL BE REDEEMED! The same spirit of sympathy and fraternity that broke the black man's manacles and is today melting the white woman's chains will tomorrow emancipate the working man and the ox; and, as the ages bloom and the great wheels of the centuries grind on, the same spirit shall banish Selfishness from the earth, and convert the planet finally into one unbroken and unparalleled spectacle of PEACE, JUSTICE, and SOLIDARITY (Moore 1906, p. 328–9).

These progressive commitments and expectations were grounded in the secular morality of the Enlightenment and the French Revolution, which promised the triumph of the Enlightenment's ideals. There was the full expectation that one would secure the liberty and equality of all men and all women. As the 19th century drew to a close, there was also the sense that the whole fabric of Western European tradition was rotten, and that something quite new was coming.

Many had the sense of the end of the age. On the one hand, there had been dramatic developments in science, technology, and industry. On the other, the kingdoms, duchies, and principalities of Europe appeared secure. Yet, there was a sense that all was about to collapse.

> The term 'fin de siécle' originated in a play of 1888 by two obscure Parisian writers, but the name came to be applied to a cultural malaise in late nine-

teenth-century Europe. In its strictest sense, '*fin de siécle*' referred not just to the fact that the nineteenth century was drawing to a close, but it signified a belief on the part of the literate and voluble bourgeoisie that the end of the century would bring with it decay, decline and ultimate disaster (West 1994, p. 1).

This foreboding was particularly marked in Vienna, the capital of the last remnant of the fusion of disparate cultures and peoples in a Christian empire. There was a growing sense that the bond to the past was about to be broken.

Vienna in the *fin de siècle*, with its acutely felt tremors of social and political disintegration, proved one of the most fertile breeding grounds of our century's a-historical culture. Its great intellectual innovators—in music and philosophy, in economics and architecture, and, of course, in psychoanalysis—all broke, more or less deliberately, their ties to the historical outlook central to the nineteenth-century liberal culture in which they had been reared (Schorske 1980, p. xviii).

There was a premonition that a deep rupture was about to occur that would separate Europe from much of the past.

Even before the First World War there was a sense of foreboding, a feeling that Western culture, the bearer of the universalist dreams that had been fortified by the Enlightenment, was no longer secure. One finds, for example, Spengler's *The Decline of the West*, a work evidently engendered in part by Spengler's reaction to the Agadir Crisis (known to the Germans as the *Panthersprung* after the German gunboat Panther sent to the Moroccan port of Agadir), which involved a confrontation between Germany and Great Britain as France prepared to send troops to protect the Sultan of Morocco. This German international military confrontation, aimed at maintaining the balance of power, coincided with a 30% one-day drop in the German stock exchange. All of this brought Spengler in 1912 to undertake his *opus magnum*, the first volume of which was completed in 1914, although it only appeared in print four years later (Spengler 1918, 1922). Spengler among others contributed to the view that Western civilization was in its last stages.

In England, this sense of foreboding and coming change was reflected in
and abetted by the Bloomsbury Group, a coterie of intellectuals who met on
Thursday evenings at 46 Garden Square in London's Bloomsbury district (the
residence of Virginia Woolf). The Bloomsbury Group was a herald of the recognition that Western Christendom had become an empty shell and that a secular,
post-Christian age was taking shape with a new sense of morality.[40] It was tied
as well to the intellectual, saliently homoerotic, socialist as well as Marxist secret
club of the Cambridge Apostles, whose roots went into the early 19th century,
and which in the 20th century became a source of Communist spies and supported the virtues of "higher sodomy" (Deacon 1986; Sinclair 1986). As Sinclair observed, "The Apostles secretly and the Bloomsbury group openly were
cultural and sexual rebels. They were élitists whose views influenced an élite"
(Sinclair 1986, p. 23). Virginia Woolf (1882–1941), one of the central figures of
the Bloomsbury Group, recognized that this change in the dominant culture was
transforming how at least the leading intellectuals, along with the literary and
artistic communities, perceived the world (Holroyd 1967). There was a feeling
not simply that God was dead, but that human nature had changed.

> One evening in 1923, a strikingly elegant woman with a face of severe, almost
> classical beauty stood in front of a group of Cambridge students to deliver a
> lecture about modern literature, built around a sentence that was as arrest-
> ing as she was beautiful: "in or around December 1910, human character
> changed." The author of this grandiose claim was speaking about novels, but
> her statement applied to all the arts, and she was uniquely qualified to make
> such a statement, because already in 1910 she had been at the heart of one
> of Europe's most conspicuous artistic groups. She was, of course, Virginia
> Woolf (Blom 2008, p. 277).

Woolf pointed to what was a sea change in the character of literature and the
arts, as well as in the understanding of morality,[41] that occurred just prior to
the First World War. She had appreciated the secularization combined with the
demoralization and deflation of morality that would radically change the dominant culture and how we regarded ourselves.

As Tom Regan correctly observes, "Bloomsbury exercised a degree of power
in the artistic world that was disproportionate to the Group's size" (Regan 1986,

p. 8). It possessed remarkable influence, even at its periphery, extending for instance to T. S. Eliot,[42] who with his publication of *The Waste Land* in 1922 and with James Joyce's publication of *Ulysses* constituted the *annus mirabilis* of modernism. Leon Edel after the First World War makes a similar point about the importance of the Bloomsbury Group: "Bloomsbury individuals, publishing, writing, painting, active in economics and politics, exercise wide influence but are unaware of [their] collective power, which is considerable" (Edel 1979, p. 280). Woolf as a part of the Bloomsbury Group both reflected and enabled the public break of English intellectuals from Christianity. In part, the break was tied to an explicit setting aside of established sexual norms, anticipating the sexual cultural revolution of the 1960s. The Group flaunted its disregard for Christian sexual mores in a way that had just become possible. Only a decade after the conviction of Oscar Wilde (25 May 1895), Bloomsbury was at peace with provoking public outrage.

> For example, Vanessa Stephen was married to the wealthy coal heir Clive Bell, but had a child by the handsome Scottish-born painter artist Duncan Grant who was attracted to Vanessa's brother Adrian, but who also had a string of homosexual affairs with fellow Apostles Keynes and Strachey who had been engaged in a bitter tug-of-war over the Society's new acquisition Arthur Lee Hobhouse, who had fallen head over heels in love with Grant, who later formed a *ménage-a-trois* with Vanessa and Grant's new lover, David Garnett (Engel 2006, p. 309).

The world of Bloomsbury, which spanned the period from 1905 to 1920, left its imprint on the intellectual class of the time, so much so as to provoke the following lament: "The 'Cambridge-Bloomsbury milieu'—this 'ethos'—[as F. R.] Leavis [1895–1978] complained,[43] destroyed the best of Britain's intellectual empire decades before the death watch of its political counterpart" (Regan 1986, p. 8). English culture had become post-Christian. It was somewhere between 1908 and 1910 that Thomas Hardy wrote his poem, the "God's Funeral" (Wilson 1999, p. 3).

Bloomsbury marked a break from the past, so that one was no longer tied to an external reality as a criterion of truth, but to oneself alone, set within a framing narrative that was no longer Christian. It possessed as well a special focus on the sensual. As Charles Taylor observes regarding Bloomsbury,

> they radicalized the claims of ordinary human sensual desire against the supposedly "higher" demands of discipline or abstinence. For instance, Bloomsbury homosexuals threw off the restrictions of their society. They all "came out," not, indeed, before the general public—homosexual relations were still a criminal offence in those days—but in the society they frequented. They helped to set the climate of the latter half of the century, in England and elsewhere (Taylor 2007, p. 406).

Even more significant was their turn to immanence. "It was this immanentization which many people reacted to when they accused Bloomsbury of trivializing the human condition, of immuring themselves against deep and powerful forces, and reducing the issues of human life to what can be encompassed by individual feelings" (Taylor 2007, p. 406). This break in ethos was also associated with a profound change in the arts.

This break separated the early from the later work of Pablo Picasso (1881–1973),[44] the early from the later work of Wassily Kandinsky (1866–1944),[45] and the early from the later work of Paul Klee (1879–1940).[46] By 1910 there was the first exhibition of post-impressionist painting at Grofton Galleries in London with Desmond MacCarthy as the secretary. As Leon Edel reports, "Years later he would call the show 'the Art-quake of 1910'" (Edel 1979, p. 164). In 1911 *Der blaue Reiter* (The Blue Rider) group held its first exhibition, which was the same year as the first exhibition of cubist painting. In 1912 Kandinsky published *Über das Geistige in der Kunst* (Kandinsky 1912), defending an art that would no longer mirror reality or even record impressions of reality, but be purely constructive.

> . . . we are fast approaching a time of reasoned and conscious composition, in which the painter will be proud to declare his work constructional—this in contrast to the claim of the impressionists that they could explain nothing, that their art came by inspiration. We have before us an age of conscious creation, and this new spirit in painting is going hand in hand with thought towards an *epoch of great spirituality* (Kandinsky 1947, p. 77).

As the art movement of futurism appreciated, the transformation of contemporary Western culture was also due to technology, from telephones to fast cars, recasting not just the pace, but the very sense of ordinary life (Blom 2008). The changes have been all-encompassing. Ihab Hassan, in describing what is occurring, quotes the artist Jean Dubuffet (1901–1985): "I have the impression that a complete liquidation of all the ways of thinking, whose sum constituted what has been called humanism and has been fundamental for our culture since the Renaissance, is now taking place, or at least, going to take place very soon" (Hassan 1975, p. xiii). Modernity had collapsed into post-modernity.

One should also note that it was in May of 1910 that Igor Fyodorovich Stravinsky (1882–1971) met with Nicholas Roerich (1874–1947) to discuss initial plans for what became known as *Le Sacre du Printemps* or *The Rite of Spring*, with the subtitle "Pictures of Pagan Russia." In 1911, most of what remained was completed so that on March 8, 1913, Stravinsky signed and dated the finished orchestral score in Clarens, Switzerland. The premiere on May 29, 1913 (as an aside: the anniversary of the fall of New Rome, Constantinople), provoked a small riot, which forced the ballet dancer and choreographer Vaslav Nijinsky (1890–1950) to stand on a chair shouting numbers to the dancers. One must recall that Nijinsky a year earlier had danced his erotic interpretation of Claude Debussy's (1862–1918) *L'Après-midi d'un faune*.

> That boisterous evening rightly stands as a symbol of its era and as a landmark of this century. From the setting in the newly constructed, ultramodern Théâtre des Champs-Élysées, in Paris, through the ideas and intentions of the leading protagonists, to the tumultuous response of the audience, that opening night of *Le Sacre* represents a milestone in the development of "modernism," modernism as above all a culture of the sensational event, through which art and life both become a matter of energy and are fused as one. Given the crucial significance of the audience in this culture, we must look at the broader context of *Le Sacre* (Eksteins 1989, p. 16).

The cutting-edge artists of the time were often passionately committed to a pursuit of self-satisfaction that was set against the remaining fabric of traditional Christian morality. One might think of the ballet impresario and founder of the Ballets Russes, Sergei Pavlovitch Diaghilev (1782–1929).

Diaghilev's sexual proclivities were well known, and he made no attempt to mask them; quite the reverse. Stravinsky said later that Diaghilev's entourage was "a kind of homosexual Swiss Guard." Not surprisingly, a sexual tension pervaded the whole experience of the Ballets russes, among performers, managers, hangers-on, and audience. Some of the ballet themes were openly erotic, even sadomasochistic, as in *Cléopatre* and *Schéhérazade* (Eksteins 1989, p. 34).

All of this confirmed what Virginia Woolf metaphorically described as a change in "human character." Within intellectual circles, Christianity and traditional Christian culture had become publicly incredible. A post-Christian civilization was emerging.

Against the background of progressivist hopes, the carnage of the First World War was inconceivable. Yet it occurred. As Walker Percy recognized:

What theorists of the old modern age had to confront were the altogether unexpected disasters of the twentieth century: that after three hundred years of the scientific revolution and in the emergence of rational ethics in European Christendom, Western man in the twentieth century elected instead of an era of peace and freedom an orgy of wars, tortures, genocide, suicide, murder, and rapine unparalleled in history. The old modern age ended in 1914 (Percy 1987, p. 27).

What happened had not been inconceivable for Spengler. He recognized that all was about to change. Progressivist Enlightenment hopes would have to be reconsidered. The war's aftermath confirmed for many the cultural change Bloomsbury had both abetted and recognized. Yet, many attempted to redeem the slaughter by regarding the Great War as the war that would end all wars. This in the end only made things worse.

The 18th and 19th centuries' faith in reason, progress, and peace was seriously wounded on the battlefields of the First World War. "[T]he war was experienced by intellectuals as unrelieved horror, catastrophe, brutalization, subjection to matter, fear, loss of innocence and sensitivity, and a graveyard of dearly held prewar illusions" (Wohl 1979, p. 219). The faith in reason continued, but often in lame and distorted forms, such as the metaphysics that underlay the Soviet bloc.

After the First World War, everything in the dominant secular culture looked, and in a great measure was, profoundly altered. Empires had fallen, economies were in shambles, and revolutions were afoot. A robustly secular Germany had emerged. Civil war threatened and eventually became real in many European countries, including Spain. Some concluded that a post-Christian future would lie with either Hitler or Stalin. Berlin was threatened by a loss of a rule of law that endangered life and property. Core to this instability was the Spartacus League (*Spartakusbund*), which had been formed by Karl Liebknecht (1871–1919), Rosa Luxemburg (1871–1919), and others in the later part of 1914, and which became the German Communist Party (DKP). The Spartacus Uprising in Berlin (January 4–15, 1919) was a politically transforming event and included the killing of Karl Liebknecht, who had on November 9, 1918, proclaimed a Free Socialist Republic on the same day that the precursor to the Weimar Republic was announced, and Rosa Luxembourg by the Freikorps (a group of anti-Communist paramilitary units).

The result was that, given the dangers of Berlin, the German Republic became the Weimar Republic, the National Assembly meeting for the first time on 11 February 1919 in Weimar. There was also a Bavarian Soviet Republic proclaimed on April 6, 1919, which was ended on May 3, 1919, by the German army and the Freikorps. There was even a Bremen Soviet Republic proclaimed on January 10, 1919, which fell February 4, 1919, as well as a Ruhr Red Army, and short-lived revolutionary governments in Braunschweig, Kiel, and Wurzburg. A Soviet Republic was proclaimed in Hungary on March 21, 1919, and was ended by force on August 1, 1919. Belá Kun (1886–1938), who was influential in this short-lived republic, fled to Germany, where he became a leader in the German revolutionary March action (March 27, 1921). He then fled to the Soviet Union, where he was executed on August 29, 1938, during the purge. There was even an Irish Limerick Soviet (April 15–27, 1919).

In Germany and elsewhere, there was a lost generation marked by a deep cynicism. As Pierre Drieu la Rochelle (1893–1945) put it with regard to France, those who returned from the Great War

> embarked on a period of debauch. They spent their time in salons, restaurants, bars, and opium dens. They experimented with pederasty and slept

with one another's women out of boredom and in obedience to the law of novelty. They conceived no children, and in their sterility they bled France of the men needed to defend its frontiers and to restore its greatness. Their life was filled with frantic activity, but the reality behind their movement was "depressing immobility, idle contemplation, and sterile expectation" (Wohl 1979, p. 29).

The 1920s and 1930s in Europe were profoundly troubled times. The very fabric of society appeared unsure. Among the many consequences of these wide-ranging happenings was a disillusionment with reason, expressed in artistic movements such as Dada.[47] Even in America there was a lost generation (Nash 1970), to take the term coined by Edith Stein and then used by Ernest Hemingway. "'That's what you are. That's what you all are,' Miss Stein said. 'All of you young people who served in the war. You are a lost generation . . . exactly as the garage keeper said'" (Hemingway 1964, p. 29). The garage keeper had used the term *génération perdue*. It was a generation, many of whose members once again proclaimed the death of God. "We have grown used . . . to a Godless universe" (Krutch 1956, p. 78).

In the case of the Soviets, highly exaggerated claims were advanced regarding the capacities of reason, as for example were promised by dialectical materialism, and became integral to the dogma of the Soviet state. This led to the publication of the philosophical equivalent of theological manuals on dialectical materialism (Boguslavsky et al. 1978) and the supposed scientific prediction and description of a future utopia (Gilison 1975). A new rationalism was born. This faith in reason along with its commitment to the pursuit of secular justice and moral progress released powerful and destructive forces with the result that in the 20th century, secular states embraced a faith in philosophy and moral-philosophical rationality that justified the slaughter of millions in the pursuit of secular visions of justice and human flourishing. The hopes of the progressivists culminated in a bloody pursuit of justice, liberty, and equality. The promises of modernity were radically brought into question. As Michael Gillespie has put it,

The view of history as progress was severely shaken by the cataclysmic events of the first half of the twentieth century, the World Wars, the Great

Depression, the rise of totalitarianism, and the Holocaust. What had gone wrong? Modernity, which had seemed on the verge of providing universal security, liberating human beings from all forms of oppression, and producing an unprecedented human thriving, had in fact ended in a barbarism almost unknown in previous human experience. The tools that had been universally regarded as the source of human flourishing had been the source of unparalleled human destruction. And finally, the politics of human liberation had proved to be the means to human enslavement and degradation. The horror evoked by these cataclysmic events was so overwhelming that it called into question not merely the idea of progress and enlightenment but also the idea of modernity and the concept of Western civilization itself (Gillespie 2008, pp. 285–86).

Rather than bringing peace, secular moral rationality produced disagreement, conflict, and bloody war. Immanuel Kant's secularly pious axiom, "Seek ye first the kingdom of pure practical reason and its *justice*, and your end (the blessing of perpetual peace) will come to you of itself" (Kant 1996, p. 344, AK VIII.378), was shipwrecked on the bloody conflicts of the 20th century, which were driven by the pursuit of supposedly philosophically grounded visions of justice and human rights (e.g., the killings undertaken by Josef Stalin, Mao Zedong, and Pol Pot). The result was that it was becoming increasingly clear what should have been known in Greece in the 5th century before Christ, namely, that neither moral rationality nor the politically reasonable is one, but many, and that neither is the guarantor of peace and moral progress. At the high water of modernity, the West had "lost touch with the roots of [its] own modernity" (Berman 1982, p. 17).

The dominant secular contemporary culture with its new ethos, which is after God and after metaphysics, is also in an important sense after morality. It is not just that morality and bioethics cannot be what the Western moral-philosophical project had promised and failed to secure: a moral vision that would be established as canonical through intellectual reflection. In addition, given the failure of the moral-philosophical project, these developments invited a reconsideration of the authority of the secular state. What Athens had promised regarding a moral rationality independent of the Divine cannot be achieved.

What Jerusalem promised is against the secular ethos of our times and appears ever more scandalous and incredible. Indeed, the invocation of the Bible is seen to undermine the autonomy of citizens. "[T]he anchoring of thought in a divine text is intrinsically wrongheaded for a democratic polity of autonomous citizens, since it undermines the personal autonomy and competence needed for political decisions in any polity that is based on popular sovereignty" (Sajó 2009, p. 527). The West, by marrying Athens to Jerusalem, begat an intellectual framework that eventually led not just to the end of Christendom, but to the secularization of public discourse, and in turn to the loss of any foundational justification of the authority of the state, and along with it any justification of health care law and public policy. Against the background of Christendom, the authority of the secular state appears especially insipid. The Christian empire had ruled by the grace of God.

Through his victories at the battles at the Milvian Bridge on 28 October 312 and at Chrysopolis on 18 September 324, Constantine had established Christianity and created Christendom, the Christian empire. Although he sat as a catechumen at the First Ecumenical Council of Nicea in 325 and lived a far from saintly life, he was baptized on Ascension Thursday, 337, to die on that Pentecost and become St. Constantine the Great, Equal-to-the-Apostles. Christianity has its current compass because of him and his empire. Hundreds of millions turned from the errors of their way and became devout Christians. Because of him the subsequent history of Christianity and of Europe was placed within a Christendom that held for a millennium and a half with a Divine anointing of its authority (i.e., until the abdication of the last Tsar, St. Nicholas). Even Christendom's fundamental transformation in the West after the third Christmas Mass in 800, when Pope Leo III crowned Charles the Great emperor of the Western empire, left intact, indeed enhanced the view that the empire possessed a Divine sanction. By the crowning in 962 by Pope John XII of Otto the Great in Rome on the Feast of the Christchild's Presentation in the Temple (February 2), Western Christianity had clearly emerged as a distinct denomination, which Pope John XII blessed, while at the same time claiming authority over emperor and kings (Pope John XII was bludgeoned to death by an enraged cuckolded husband). The message was that the emperor ruled by the grace of God conferred by the papacy. The Western remnant of Christendom proved to be slow in dying, although Christendom is now securely dead, save for ambiguous remnants such as certain kingdoms with their empty established churches as in Denmark, England, and Norway. With the death of Christendom, there died as well in the West any hope of grounding state authority in God and, as modernity shattered into post-modernity, any hope of grounding the state's authority in reason. The now post-modern state is left with being anointed neither by God nor by reason, but only by and through force. This is the case, despite the fact that this force claims to be anointed by a supposed democratic consensus with which all in fact do not concur. The status of the state has become something like the status of a not-too-happy marriage within which one may find oneself: an arrangement that one accepts as a status quo because it is too costly at the moment to divorce. It is an acceptable *modus vivendi.*

We are returned to the reflections at the beginning of the first chapter. A culture after God is a novum so that the authority of its political structures and health care policy must be considered anew. Such a culture has never before existed. Even pagans recognized the presence of real spiritual powers and claimed divine authority for the state. What can one then say about the authority of the state after God, indeed after modernity's hope for a canonical secular rationality? Has the state—distantly analogous to sexual life-style choices—become a political life-style choice? The cultural characteristics that define post-modernity in great measure involve the recognition that all secular moralities, bioethics, and accounts of the politically reasonable are merely particular, merely socio-historically-conditioned moral and political narratives sustaining particular fabrics of moral and political intuitions floating as freestanding narratives within the horizon of the finite and the immanent. Unlike announcements of the moral and political requirements of God, which can be recognized even by an atheist as putatively grounded in a God's-eye perspective, although the claim will be considered by the atheist to be factually false,[48] secular moral and political accounts are in their content in principle thoroughly and necessarily contingent and plural, as well as historically conditioned.[49] Without a foundation, secular morality, bioethics, and accounts of political legitimacy are ultimately rootless. Post-modernity is the recognition of this state of affairs.

This state of affairs has wide-ranging implications regarding the content and the force of the claims advanced by the contemporary dominant secular culture on matters such as the legitimacy of social-democratic states, along with their claims regarding liberty, equality, fair equality of opportunity, and human rights, as well as tolerance, social justice, human dignity, and patient rights. There is still a hope on the part of many for a cosmopolitan culture of universal human rights and universal justice (Benhabib 2008). However, given the human condition, we are forced to rethink the possibility and meaning of morality. Unfortunately, we will find that the hoped-for moral authority of the state can at best be replaced by the authority of political power. Power is left to replace the force of reason as the authority of democracies. As Agnes Heller laments, "The condition of a common spirituality has already been named; it is called freedom. The political framework for its appearance had already been set: it is called democracy. Yet no spirit has yet filled this framework. As far as modernity is concerned, Moses is still wandering in the desert" (Heller 1990, p. 173). The aspirations of modernity, along with its morality, bioethics, and the authority of its states, are ill-founded.

IX. Living in the More-Than-Minimal State: The Political Authority of a Modus Vivendi

The secularization that transformed the dominant culture and its morality has recast how that culture can coherently regard the state and its authority. That is, what has happened with regard to secular morality and bioethics, indeed with regard to sexual life-style choices, has happened as well with respect to secular political authority. Neither can be shown by sound, secular, rational argument to be grounded in God's will[50] or in reason, or as in the case of the more-than-minimal state, in the will of the governed. Although a minimal state can in principle enjoy the consent of the governed, no one lives in a merely minimal state (Engelhardt 1986, 1996). No such polity exists anywhere on the face of the earth. Secular political authority in the states that do exist is thus without secular foundations beyond the force those states can impose. Again, if persons wish to collaborate peaceably and with common secular moral authority, they can in a minimal state secure a content-less secular ethics and bioethics grounded in the authority of those who agree through mutual consent to join in particular undertakings (Engelhardt 1986, 1996). However, this will only account for the minimal state, which only protects against unconsented-to touchings. The more-than-minimal state is without general secular moral authority.

Given the limits of secular moral rationality, those who do not share a common vision of the right, the good, and the virtuous (i.e., those who are moral strangers), if they wish to collaborate with common authority, can engage procedural means by which those willing persons can give moral authority to common undertakings and social structures such as contracts and markets (Engelhardt 1986, 1996). Such procedures cannot establish the moral rightness or moral worth of any of the particular procedures that might be embraced. Again, the meaning of any reference to the good, the right, and the virtuous is embedded in a particular framework so that crucial normative terms receive different intensions and extensions, as do space, time, mass, and energy in an Aristotelian versus an Einsteinian physics. There may be family resemblances, but there is no essence shared in common. As a consequence, the free market, which is only the outcome of arbitrary agreements, has more moral authority (i.e., the authority of permission) than democratic elections in which all do not concur, and IBM (for whom no one is compelled to work or to buy goods and/or services without their permission) more authority than Texas, the United States, or France, where all who participate do not in fact consent.[51] Nevertheless, one cannot in general secular terms establish the moral rightness or worth of such procedures just because they are grounded only in the will of those who consent. That is, the procedures by which one appeals to the permission of the participants cannot be shown in and of themselves to be canonically good or bad, right or wrong, virtuous or vicious.

In and of itself, the procedural morality and bioethics of relying on the permission of those who wish to collaborate in order to create a sphere of common moral authority cannot in general secular moral terms be shown to have a moral standing such that it would be wrong to refuse to enter into this practice, to embrace the appeal to individual permission as the source of authority. It is simply that, even if there is no sound, secular, rational argument for establishing as canonical any particular ranking of goods (i.e., for establishing any particular morality and bioethics), the practice of not using persons without their permission provides the only possibility of a secular web of common secular authority because it is grounded in the individual permission of those who wish for whatever reason to enter into this practice. Given moral diversity, consent to treatment as founded in the basic forbearance right not to be touched without one's permission becomes central to secular bioethics (in addition to being supported by the social-democratic affirmation of liberty). The practice of using persons only with their permission offers a general secular possibility for establishing a limited grounding for a content-less moral practice (i.e., content-less in not specifying as canonical a particular moral content, a particular thin theory of the good, a particular ranking or ordering of primary human goods, goals, and concerns). But one cannot establish the rightness or goodness of entering into this practice.

Again, individuals have priority in this sparse morality not because of an affirmation of, or any commitment to individuals or individualism. Instead, individuals are central because general secular moral authority, given its view of persons as individuals apart from history, social context, and sex, as well as given intractable moral pluralism, cannot be derived from a canonical, concrete, common, secular moral vision, but by default must be drawn from individual persons. When persons meet in a moral context in which they decide to collaborate, and do so without reference to God, as well as without a final canonical moral vision anchored in being or in reason as warranted by conclusive sound rational arguments, then they have only individual permission as a common source of authority. In such circumstances, when moral strangers collaborate they meet each other outside of, or considered apart from, any concrete moral communities, and apart from any canonical secular morality that could be established by reason, for such does not exist. They meet as naked moral strangers. In such circumstances, one is left in a secular context with drawing authority from individuals, because in a secular culture one cannot derive moral authority from God, and because moral rationality cannot provide through sound rational argument a grounding for guidance by reference to a canonical morality with its bioethics. By default, without God and without a conclusive, sound, secular, rational argument to establish a particular morality, a general secular moral authority can only be derived from the permission of individuals who agree to collaborate. Because the only social structures authorized by such a general secular moral authority in the absence of a sound rational argument to establish a canonical, content-full morality are those established through the permission of the individuals who freely join together, as in the market, through contracts, through corporations, and within minimal states, this default morality that binds moral strangers has an unavoidably libertarian and individualistic, not to mention generally vacuous character.

Again, the libertarian and content-less character of this default morality and the sparse bioethics it sustains (Engelhardt 1986, 1996) is not rooted in any value ingredient in, or attributed to, individual choice. This cardinal place of permission accounts in part for the salience of consent in secular morality. This general sparse secular morality involves, one should note, no commitment to living outside of a thick moral community. Further and quite crucially, these considerations highlight the limited scope of secular moral authority, including the plausibility of establishing the secular moral authority of the political structures of a more-than-minimal state. Authority is limited because of the plausible limits of the consent of persons to be governed by others. To appreciate the force of these limitations on the possibility of all citizens actually adequately giving consent to be governed by a more-than-minimal state, one need only apply to the state's acquisition of secular political authority through consent from those governed the same requirements now generally required for valid consent to participate in research involving human subjects. If such requirements for valid consent were applied to identify valid consent to be governed in a more-than-minimal state, then the consent to being or remaining a citizen would need to be informed and uncoerced, starkly underscoring the limits of secular political moral authority, including the deficient authority of democracies in which majorities repress minorities. In addition, if giving consent to be governed were like giving consent to be a subject of research, those asked to consent to a government should also be at liberty to withhold consent or withdraw consent (if one withdraws consent to be governed, may one retreat into one's own sovereign exclave?). Finally, and most importantly, not *all* citizens are likely to give consent, just as *all* possible participants in research do not actually consent.

We are therefore returned to where we began. Insofar as a secular polity would wish to enjoy the actual consent of the governed, it would need to be a minimal state, where a minimal state is a polity in which no one is used without his permission and where therefore the minimal state can presume universal consent to its authority in order to avoid persons acting as unreliable enforcers of justice and thus using others without their consent, namely, as means merely. Or to put the matter somewhat differently, the minimal state, the night-watch-man state can reasonably regard itself as enjoying the consent of the minimally governed, insofar as the persons involved agree to collaborate without the use of unconsented-to force, that is, with mutual permission. In this account of the minimal state, what is advanced is not a libertarian account that would set aside the thick, non-libertarian communities of moral friends. What is instead sought is a generally justifiable secular justification for the large-scale coopera-tion among moral strangers in the more-than-minimal state. The appeal to per-mission justifies only the market, contracts, and the minimal state, along with a bioethics, medical law, and health care policy that only affirms and protects forbearance rights. *The Foundations of Bioethics* (Engelhardt 1986, 1996) and *Viaggi in Italia* (Engelhardt 2011) confront the implausibility that any contem-porary governments, even democracies, as more-than-minimal states enjoy the uncoerced consent of all, or perhaps even the *uncoerced* consent of the majority of those governed.

To underscore this central point once again: the libertarian character of a defensible general secular morality and bioethics, as the morality and bioethics for moral strangers (Engelhardt 1986 and 1996), as a morality and bioethics for those meeting to collaborate in a context after God and after foundations, is fully compatible with the moralities and bioethics of concrete consensual moral communities whose commitments may be far from libertarian (e.g., the com-munism of monasteries). In voluntary, face-to-face communities (e.g., monas-teries or religions such as Orthodox Judaism and Orthodox Christianity), in which all participants actually consent to live within a particular moral vision, their lives are usually framed by a content-full morality and bioethics, where liberty is regarded as being far from the most important good, much less as the cardinal right-making condition. In addition, those within such a community meet as moral friends. The arguments in *The Foundations of Bioethics*, *Secular Humanism*, and *Viaggi in Italia* are not opposed to content-full moral and bio-ethical commitments that bind persons through their consent within particular, peaceable, consensual, moral communities, but concern instead the question of how moral strangers can enjoy common moral authority when they collaborate. The morality and bioethics available under these circumstances are woefully inadequate (Engelhardt 2000). Still, many have misconstrued *The Foundations, Secular Humanism*, and some of the essays in *Viaggi in Italia* as a libertarian manifesto that is hostile to robust, thick, inadequate moral communities. It would be wrong to regard the arguments in *The Foundations of Bioethics, Secular Humanism*, and/or *Viaggi in Italia* as attempts to secure a particular concrete libertarian morality, a particular community of libertarian moral friends.

As moral strangers, although we may meet in a circumstance deaf to God and after foundations, many still have numerous reasons to collaborate. In addition, as moral strangers, we have in permission a source by default for a sparse but nevertheless morally grounded ethics of collaboration. This political possibility allows for the justification of the minimal state, but not the more-than-minimal state. Again, no one lives in a minimal state where authority can actually be drawn from the consent of the governed. After God and after foundations, indeed after Christendom, the authority of the more-than-minimal state is therefore a great puzzle: its authority cannot in general secular terms be derived from God, reason, or common consent. How if at all can one understand the more-than-minimal state as possessing moral authority? And what kind of authority could it have? In our actual circumstances, we as moral strangers are left with fashioning a political structure for which we possess no common account of its authority, indeed without a common way in secular terms to regard the more-than-minimal state as having moral authority. If the more-than-minimal state has no commonly justifiable moral authority, but only political authority, what does this mean? How is the authority of the more-than-minimal state, which is tantamount to states as we know them, to be understood?

The multiplicity of incompatible accounts of the authority of the state and of the politically reasonable, each with its own basic premises and rules of evidence, is robust and intractable. This circumstance undermines the plausibility of any particular argument establishing a canonical moral authority for the more-than-minimal state or a canonical view of the politically reasonable. There cannot be a deliberative democracy, for a society is not a Socratic seminar bound by a common understanding of the morally rational or politically reasonable (Gutmann & Thompson 2004). Instead, the "authority" of the state develops like incomplete agreements in the market, which produce a *modus vivendi* when enough concur so as to maintain a particular political order. As Buchanan and

Tullock predict, "The relevant choice among alternative institutions reduces to that of selecting that set which effectively minimizes the costs (maximizes the benefits) of living in association" (Buchanan & Tullock 1965, p. 304). As a consequence,

> The origin of civil government and the major influences in its development may be almost wholly nonrational in the sense that explanation on a contractual basis is possible. Societies form governments and change governments for a variety of reasons, many of which remain mysterious and far below the level of objective, scientific analysis (Buchanan & Tullock 1965, p. 318).

What emerges is a de facto *modus vivendi*, which is not a contract. It is a temporary resting point accepted by enough persons so as to be stable. "We" agree as long as there are enough to impose an "agreement," a *modus vivendi*.

In the face of a plurality of diverse and incompatible accounts, Agrippa's *pente tropoi* apply not just to morality and bioethics, but also to attempts to justify the state's authority. One faces a crisis of authority for the state. The only state that can be grounded in the permission or consent of the governed is the minimal state. Yet, all states on the face of the earth are more-than-minimal states. One is brought to the unpleasant conclusion that, beyond appeals to rhetoric, indeed propaganda (e.g., early inculcation and indoctrination of the view that democratic states have a moral authority) as well as, and most importantly, institutionalized coercive force regarding which most may regard it to be prudent to submit as long as there is effective protection of life and property, the state has no established canonical secular moral authority for the force it wields. Against the background of Christendom, in which the king was anointed by the church and ruled by divine authority, claims of authority by secular democratic polities possess only the authority of force to which enough subjects are willing out of prudential concerns to acquiesce. As a result, the more-than-minimal state understood in general secular terms can at best be a political structure with which enough are willing for the time being to live peaceably so that life and property can remain secure. In this circumstance the state functions merely as a *modus vivendi*, because it lacks a grounding moral rationality or even the support of a canonical view of the politically reasonable. As George Tsai defines the state of affairs,

> A *modus vivendi* is a strategic compromise among contending groups in a society none of whom is in a position to impose its preferred way of life on the others without unacceptable costs and each of whom as a result adopts a policy of mutual accommodation as the best that it can hope to achieve under its circumstances (Tsai 2013, p. 794).

A particular state as a *modus vivendi* is at best a state that is for the time being practically tolerable.

The bad news is that the authority of the state cannot even be that of a *modus vivendi* in the strong sense in which *all* subjects have some interest in the state's continued functioning. Many may not have such an interest, but lack the power at this time to change things without harming their own interests. Consider instead Kozinski's *modus vivendi* as "a merely tolerable, self-interested, and non-principled concession of each citizen to the exigencies of contemporary historical reality 'providing the only workable alternative to endless and destructive civil strife'" (Kozinski 2010, p. 16, quoting Rawls 1993, p. 159). A *modus vivendi* as I use it recognizes that many who acquiesce in the government as it is are merely biding their time until an opportunity exists for a regime change, perhaps even if this requires civil war. That is, many may actually hold that strife would be worthwhile if the success of a revolution were only a bit more certain. The authority of the state consequently becomes the naked power of government and the benefits it imposes.

Once one recognizes that the state is only a *modus vivendi*, then it is also clear that there is no illegitimacy in principle involved in publicly advancing religious grounds for legislative acts, as long as this is compatible with the polity's stability (i.e., preserves the *modus vivendi*). Even constitutional decisions need not be based on secular public reason, as long as the decisions are compatible with the *modus vivendi*, thus preserving life and property (Perry 2001). This recognition is, to say the least, provocative.[52] After all, given the inability to establish a secular canonical account of either the morally rational or the politically reasonable, an appeal to the will of God has no less force than an appeal to moral or political intuitions.

When compelled by state force to live in a more-than-minimal state, many may still recognize the importance of limited constitutional frameworks that can as far as possible set boundaries to aspirations of both democracies and oligarchies. Because of a fear of arbitrary rule, including the tyranny of majorities, one can still envisage distinguishing among more or less onerous more-than-minimal states, even if they are all understood only to be *modi vivendi*. For example, one can prudently support constitutions that can constrain the tyranny of the majority, not merely the tyranny by the few. Given the threat of the despotism of the majority, constitutionally established limits on democratic rule will recommend themselves to many if not most in order to protect a secular polity from being used by the majority to impose in a totalizing fashion its own secular vision of the right, the good, and the virtuous. Limited constitutional structures erect constraints not just against religious fundamentalist aspirations, but against secular fundamentalist aspirations as well. In the face of intractable moral pluralism and in deafness to God, constitutionally limited governments can be a bulwark against a society that would otherwise leave little social space for substantive moral and religious diversity. However prudent this view will appear to many, there is no sound rational argument to give it canonical status. In general terms, it is at best a political life-style choice.

Because judgments regarding the proper character of the limits that should be placed on the government are dependent on granting particular basic premises and rules of evidence, substantive, indeed intractable disagreement on these matters will remain. Which is to say, even general secular moral considerations in favor of constitutionally limited governments float in the air without foundations. No matter how prudent and therefore attractive limited constitution structures may appear to many (including the author of this book), there is no conclusive secular moral rational argument to justify them. The authority of all more-than-minimal states is grounded neither in consent nor in conclusive sound rational argument. Therefore, states framed around constitutions that limit the political authority of majorities cannot morally vindicate the political authority they claim and exercise any more or less legitimately than the regime of Louis XVI of France. Again, this is the case because there is no one canonical moral view, but a plurality of incompatible views regarding what should count as a proper political constitution of government or what goods should be sought through government.

The failure of argument to establish as canonical any form of constitutionalism, including the liberal democratic state with its affirmation of equality and human rights, must once more be underscored. The reality of our intellectual situation goes so against the grain of the high-flown expectations born of the Enlightenment that many simply deny the limited character of philosophical reasoning and proceed as if its limitations did not exist. Against all evidence to the contrary, the proponents of liberal agendas of equality, human rights, and human dignity often resolutely hold "these truths" to be either self-evident or rationally established. They fail to recognize the socio-historically conditioned character of their claims. Bioethicists act as if they could establish moral and bioethical truth and as if they were experts regarding that truth. The view that bioethics is grounded in a common human morality is core to Beauchamp and Childress's highly influential textbook (Beauchamp & Childress 1979). This textbook, throughout its many editions, makes many such claims, which are examined in chapter six.

One is brought again to the conclusion, *pace* the contemporary secular religions or ideologies of democracy, limited democracy, and human rights, that the more-than-minimal state is at best a *modus vivendi*, a political structure with which enough of its citizens are willing to live so that for the time being the rule of law is possible in order to secure the protection of life and property. However, there is no canonical secular moral understanding that will allow one to know how to decide when a particular state will or will not be a more or less morally acceptable *modus vivendi*. Different persons and different moral communities at different times will have different and indeed incompatible understandings as to when a state is still an acceptable *modus vivendi*. Moreover, for persons living ever more resolutely within the horizon of the finite and the immanent, it will likely be immediate satisfaction that will be salient in such decisions, thus encouraging the seductive rhetoric of mass media democracies. At the most, there can be empirical judgments, educated guesses, regarding the likely political stability of some versus other forms of *modi vivendi*. The culture wars now also reflect disputes regarding the acceptability of a particular form of governance as a *modus vivendi*.

X. The Secular State after God

The loss of the hope that philosophy can supply governments, along with medical law and health care policy, with canonical direction and with a general secular moral authority confronts us with the different character of moral and political claims after God and without foundations. We are faced not just with the demoralization and deflation of morality and bioethics, but also with the frank moral delegitimization of the secular state. One has entered into a culture after God, after metaphysics, and after foundations, a normative territory structured by an atheistic methodological postulate, so that one has in principle lost a point of ultimate orientation or legitimization. Within this context, neither kings nor democratic majorities can claim a divine right, or a unique warrant grounded in reason, to rule. In the face of intractable moral and bioethical pluralism, there is no conclusive argument to establish as canonical any particular moral rationality or particular view of the politically reasonable. For its part, the state's secular claim to authority is reduced merely to the authority of possessing sufficient coercive force and rhetorical appeal to maintain rule of law, a *de facto* acceptable level of law and order.

The delegitimization of the state, the recognition that the state's authority is not justified by a canonical sense of the politically reasonable, much less of the morally rational, for such do not exist, strikes a deathblow not just to aspirations to a deliberative democracy, but as well to a rationalist vision of the legitimacy of democracy. In a culture after God, there is no divine right, or for that matter any canonical rational right, of majorities or of democratic constitutionalism. They boil down to the assertion that a majority may impose a democratic constitutionalism on its own terms, if this is integral to its particular vision of human flourishing. It is ironic that it is secular constitutionalists who, albeit guided by an atheist methodological postulate, nevertheless appeal to a God's-eye perspective to make such claims as: "The sovereignty of a people exercising its faculty of reasoning is the essence of the constitutionalism that necessitates secularism" (Sajó 2008, p. 629). There is an appeal to a particular God's-eye-like perspective, even though those appealing deny the claims of any actual ultimate perspective. They simply assert the priority of their particular political vision and account of human flourishing.

Not even the Roman empire under Diocletian (244–311, reign 286–305) presumed to act bereft of any ultimate approval by the transcendent. Quite to the contrary, the emperor was seen as, and regarded himself as, acting with the authority of Jupiter.[53] A secular culture can make no such claims. We are left with the secular state maintaining authority as long as its subjects are not willing through force to set that state aside. As a consequence, a state in general secular terms exists insofar as it is sufficiently accepted, at least *pro tempore*, as a *modus vivendi*. Secularization has disclosed not just a radically different and post-Christian morality and bioethics, but a quite post-Christian possibility for the state's authority, along with the authority of law and public policy. The appeal to force remains the only substitute for the failed appeal to reason. Indoctrination, propaganda, and coercion are the final cement of large-scale states.

Notes

[1]This chapter is in part drawn from the following lectures: "Religion, Politics, and the State: Rethinking Morality in Modern Secularized Societies," Politeia, University of Milan, January 30, 2012; "Bioethics after Foundations: Feeling the Full Force of Secularization," Secularization and Bioethics conference sponsored by Centro Evangelico di Cultura "Arturo Pascal" and Consulta di Bioetica Onlus in Turin, January 31, 2012; "The Deflation of Morality: Rethinking the Secularization of the West" at the University of Salento, Lecce, February 1, 2012, and "Religion, Politics, and the State in Modern Secularized Societies," presented to Comune di Napoli on February 6, 2012.

[2]This secular content is what James K. A. Smith characterizes as constituting Charles Taylor's secularism₁. "The priest, for instance, pursues a 'sacred' vocation, while the butcher, baker, and candlestick maker are engaged in 'secular' pursuits" (Smith 2014, pp. 20–21).

[3]Charles Taylor notes that one dimension of the secularization of the dominant culture of the West involves "a move from a society where belief in God is unchallenged and indeed, unproblematic, to one in which it is understood to be one option among others, and frequently not the easiest to embrace" (Taylor 2007, p. 3). To put the matter more strongly, in many circles belief in God has become a social embarrassment and its expression a faux pas.

[4]Taylor also observes a change in the character of public spaces, which is associated with secularization. "One understanding of secularity then is in terms of public spaces. These have been allegedly emptied of God, or of any reference to ultimate reality" (Taylor 2007, p. 2). They have at least been de-Christianized, whether or not one credits Thomas Luckmann's qualifications regarding a residual religion (Luckmann 1990).

[5]Max Weber affirms the *Entzauberung der Welt* by which the recognition of divine and angelic powers is exorcised. "That great historic process in the development of religions, the elimination of magic from the world which had begun with the old Hebrew prophets and, in conjunction with Hellenistic scientific thought, had repudiated all magical means to salvation as superstition and sin" (Weber 2001, p 61).

[6]Orthodox Christianity has maintained the ancient practice of persons taking blessed oil home to anoint themselves and their family members. Statkus reports that this custom was even recognized in the West in the first centuries.

In the early centuries Pope Innocent I (401–417) and other early writers seemed to give evidence in their writing to the ministry of sacred oil by lay people. According to these writings it seems to have been an accepted custom for lay people to anoint not only others but also themselves (Statkus 1951, pp. 25–26).

Kilker's criticism of this view is not convincing (Kilker 1926, p. 82).

[7]The move to a values discourse in Germany has been noted by Paul Edward Gottfried (1941–) (Gottfried 2007). It has been tied to a change in the character of political, indeed public discourse.

In "Der lange Marsch der CDU nach links," German political historian Karlheinz Weissmann presents an argument about "value conservatism" similar to mine in explaining the "leftward lurch" of the Christian Democrats on social and national questions under Helmut Kohl and even more under Merkel. According to Weissmann, in the 1970s the center-right CDU decided to exchange the defense of "structural conservatism," identified with the family, church, army, and nation, for a less confrontational "Wertekonservatismus," a position that signified a "dwindling of its conservative content" (Gottfried 2007, p. 163).

[9]Protagoras recognized that without a point of ultimate reference "Man is the measure of all things, of things that are that they are, and of things that are not that they are not" (Diogenes Laertius 2000, Protagoras IX.51, pp. 463, 465).

[9]For a critical assessment of the view that one should be intolerant of the "intolerant," see Carson 2013.

[10]Hegel appreciated that the intractable pluralism created by the Reformation helped secularize society through dividing the power of religion and thus enhancing the state. "Consequently, far from it being, or ever having been, a misfortune for the state if the Church is divided, it is *through this division alone* that the state has been able to fulfil its destiny as self-conscious rationality and ethical life" (Hegel 1991, §270, p. 302). See, also, Gregory 2012.

[11]The contemporary understanding of tolerance affirmed by the now-dominant secular culture is much more affirmatory of the object of tolerance than T. M. Scanlon appreciates (Scanlon 2003).

[12]One might consider the general account of the transformation of society given by John Milbank.

Both Durkheim and Weber categorize societies in terms of the relation of the individual to something social and universal, and this reflects the perspective of modern Western politics, whose prime concern is the 'bodily' mediation between the unlimited sovereignty of the State and the self-will of the individual. As a grid, or frame through which to view all societies, this perspective tends to occlude the fact that for many non-Western, or pre-modern societies, what matters is not the binary individual/society contrast, but the hierarchical ordering of different status group-ings, and the distribution of roles according to a complex sense of common value. Sociology, of course, registers this difference, but it does so *negatively*, in terms of the observation that organic and hierarchical societies exercise strong 'control' over the individual, as if the member of this traditional society were secretly shadowed by the presence of the modern, self-determining subject. In consequence, the relation of the individual to the whole—which defines only *modern* politics—is seen as the universal site of the social, and it follows that all the complex rituals, hierarchies, and religious views which go to make up the stratified, organic society can be 'explained' in terms of the functional maintaining of strong control of the whole over the indi-vidual parts. Such 'explanation' is only regarded as more than tautology because the normative perspective of modernity allows one to think that there is always a dimen-sion of pure 'social action,' pure 'social power,' occurring between the individual and the social, and separable from its ritual, symbolic or linguistic embodiment. But 'a social whole' apart from the interactions of the various norms and strata is a reifying abstraction, and there is no 'social action' definable or comprehensible apart from its peculiar linguistic manifestation, the inexplicability of the particular symbolic system (Milbank 2006, 103–104).

[13]Moses Maimonides in commenting on the prerogative of kings to have concubines remarks: "The Oral Tradition states that he may take no more than eighteen wives. The figure eighteen includes both wives and concubines" (Maimonides 2001, p. 518).

[14]For a statement of the Orthodox Christian condemnation of fornication, see Jubilee Bishops' Council 2000, X.6, pp. 43–44.

[15]Orthodox Christianity embraced the theological rather than the philosophical horn of the dilemma Plato poses in the *Euthyphro*. If one understands the choice, *grosso modo*, as between holding that the holy can be understood in terms of the right, the good, and the virtuous, or that the right, the good, and the virtuous can only be understood in terms of the holy, Orthodox Christianity affirms the latter. See Engelhardt 2000, §4.

[16]For Kant, Christianity is to be evacuated of transcendent force and be left only with moral meaning. "The Christian principle of morality is not theological and thus heterono-mous, being rather the autonomy of pure practical reason itself" (Kant 1956, p. 133). How-ever, as Hegel shows, the content of the moral reason does not follow from reason, but is constituted within a particular socio-historically conditioned context. See G. W. F. Hegel, *Grundlinien der Philosophie des Rechts*, §150.

[17]The ancient Church maintained the practice of celebrating Liturgy over the relics of martyrs. See, for example, Canon XX of Gangra (A.D. 340) and Canon VII of Nicea II (A.D. 787) (Doig 2008, p. 89; Freeman 2011, p. 13).

[18]For a defense of the radical recasting of the roles of the sexes and the understanding of the family, see the feminist arguments of Susan Okin (1989).

[19]The 1960s and 1970s were awash with a literature that celebrated sexual lust in its own right. Consider, for example, Shiraishi 1975. In addition, one might think of Patti Smith's *Witt*, especially her poem "Rape" (Smith 1973, p. 24). Here belongs also some of the poetry of Leonard Cohen. Consider, for example, the poem "the 15-year-old girls" (Cohen 1972, p. 97).

[20]For an account of "hooking-up" as a successful strategy for ambitious secularized women, see, for example, "Hearts of Steel: Single Girls Master the Hook-up" in Rosin 2012, pp. 17–46. See also Bogle 2008.

[21]Although 67.4% of women who did not complete high school had a child outside of marriage, only 8.3% of mothers who completed at least college had an illegitimate child (Rector 2010, p. 4). There is a strong positive connection between poverty and having a child outside of wedlock, so that only 26% of non-poor families have children that are not from a marital union, 71% of poor families have children that are not from a marital union (Rector 2010, p. 5). Another way to present the association between poverty and illegitimacy is to note that in 2008 single parents had a poverty rate of 36.5%, while married couples with children had a poverty rate of 6.5% (Rector 2010, p. 1).

[22]For a picture at the beginning of the 1960s of the generation that was seeking to lose itself and rebel against established norms of traditional Western Christian culture, see *Beatitude Anthology* 1960.

[23]Woodstock involved a rejection of traditional mores and an invitation to a new post-moral order. It took place as a music festival held publicly on acreage belonging to Max Yasgur's dairy farm near Bethel, New York. See also Heelas 1996.

[24]The number of children born outside of a traditional marriage has increased from slightly over one out of twenty to slightly over four out of ten. This demographic development has recast the very life-world of marriage and reproduction (Hamilton, Martin, & Ventura 2012).

[25]Birth rate in 1960: http://www.nationmaster.com/graph/hea_bir_rat_cru_per_1000_peo-crude-per-1-000-people&date=1960; birth rate in 2012: http://www.indexmundi.com/g/g.aspx?c=it&v=25; out-of-wedlock births in 1960: http://demoblography.blogspot.com/2007/06/percentage-of-out-of-wedlock-births-in.html; out-of-wedlock births in 2012: http://www.catholicculture.org/news/headlines/index.cfm?storyid=16264 [accessed November 5, 2015]

[26]Birth rate in 1960: http://www.nationmaster.com/graph/hea_bir_rat_cru_per_1000_peo-crude-per-1-000-people&date=1960; birth rate in 2013: http://www.indexmundi.com/united_states/birth_rate.html; out-of-wedlock births in 1960: http://www.cdc.gov/nchs/data/databriefs/db18.htm; out-of-wedlock births in 2011: http://www.cdc.gov/nchs/fastats/unmarry.htm [accessed November 2, 2015]

[27]Concerns about the supposedly drastic and imminent threats from overpopulation became a focus of intellectual discussions during the mid-1960s. Prominent was Paul Ehrlich's (1932–) book, *The Population Bomb*, which painted the picture of an imminent threat of starvation and unraveling of some of the structures of civilization (Ehrlich 1968). In this, he was criticized by Julian Simon (1932–1998) (Simon 1981; Myers & Simon 1994). Sentiments such as those affirmed by Paul Ehrlich led to further apocalyptic predictions of the environmental

consequences of an uncontrolled population increase, as in the report prepared for the Club of Rome. See Meadows et al. 1974. For a similar example, see Council 1980–1981. For a recent review of some of these matters, in particular the debate between Paul Ehrlich and Julian Simon, see Sabin 2013.

[28]The involvement of Christian clergy in the deconstruction of traditional Christian mores has been significant. One might think of recent examples of the contribution to this chaos made by Rt. Rev. John Shelby Spong, the Episcopal bishop of Newark, NJ (Spong 1988). In this genre, one would need also to place the work of the Episcopal minister and clinical pastoral care educator at New York Presbyterian Hospital, Columbia University, Raymond J. Lawrence, Jr. (Lawrence 1989, 2007).

[29]For a recent study of the financial consequences of marrying early or late, see Hymowitz et al. 2013.

[30]Regarding the inequality of men and women, Kay Hymowitz remarks: "As women move into their thirties and forties, they remain less enticing to younger men than men of that age are to younger women. Men who at 23 may have felt like the class dork find their stride by 30. Women are on the opposite trajectory. Sexism? Evolution? It doesn't really matter; it's not going away" (Hymowitz 2011, p. 19).

[31]Kay Hymowitz, for example, remarks concerning contemporary men: "Between his lack of familial responsibilities, his relative affluence, and an entertainment media devoted to his every pleasure, the single young man can live in pig's heaven" (Hymowitz 2011, p. 19).

[32]Regarding children living in non-traditional families, the data indicate significant risks.

> Neglect and abuse is [sic] particularly associated with the presence of new 'partners' of the mother. Step-fathers, or 'live-in' and visiting boyfriends, constitute the most powerful risk factor for child maltreatment, being hugely over represented as perpetrators of severe physical abuse, sexual abuse and child killing. The behaviour of the mother is also affected by the presence of new 'partners': those mothers living with a 'partner' after divorce were reported as more aggressive than those living with the father in a study of adolescents from comprehensive schools in South Wales. If the most safe family environment is one where both biological parents are married to each other, then the most unsafe of all family environments is where the mother is living with someone who has neither a biological or [sic] tie to her child (Morgan 2000, p. 42).

[33]One might think of the case of Hasidic women who consciously set about raising the next generation of committed religious Jews (Fader 2009).

[34]Women who describe themselves as "not at all religious" were much more likely to have an illegitimate birth than those who described themselves as "very religious." Among whites, the difference was one-third the rate of illegitimacy among Hispanics and one-half the rate among blacks (Abrahamse 1988).

[35]Here I draw on the contrast between the two senses of will employed by Kant: *Wilkür*, free choice as choice prescinded from reference to the norms that should guide and direct

rightly-ordered choice, and *Wille* as choice in accord with norms in conformity to the will of God, granting that for Kant the will of God is a discursively rational will (Silber 1960).

[36]Laocoön warns the Trojans regarding the Greek gift of the Trojan horse: "I fear the Greeks, even when bearing gifts." Virgil's *Aeneid* II.49.

[37]Against the background of the universalist aspirations of the liberal-democratic commitments of the Enlightenment, the selection of the Jews as the Chosen People (Deuteronomy 7:6–8) is at best scandalous.

[38]The general positive impression of Socrates is due to the high esteem in which he was held by Plato and which may not be fully justified. Diogenes Laertius gives a somewhat different picture in *Lives of Eminent Philosophers*, Book II, §5.

[39]St. Paul's remark in Galatians that "there is neither Jew nor Greek, slave nor free, male nor female, for you are all one in Christ Jesus" [3:28] is often interpreted as affirming equality in the sense of the interchangeability of men and women. This of course is a wrong reading, for traditional Christianity, along with St. Paul, is gender-essentialist. The point made by St. Paul is that men and women, Jews and Greeks, slaves and free are all equally called to salvation.

[40]Bloomsbury was in many ways the equivalent of the Paris salon of the 18th century.

> That world [of Bloomsbury] began in 1905, when, after the death of their father Leslie, the Stephen children—Virginia, Vanessa, Thoby, and Adrian—moved from Kensington to 46 Gordon Square in the London area known as Bloomsbury, where Thoby introduced his Cambridge friends to his sisters. . . . Uncommon in their collective power, the Bloomsberries were unusual also for the intensity and depth of their shared passions, for their loves and loyalties, the latter often challenged by the former. Strachey loses Grant to Keynes. Clive Bell loses Vanessa to Fry. Fry loses Vanessa to Grant. Vanessa shares Grant with David Garnett. As an anonymous wit has said, in Bloomsbury "all the couples were triangles" (Regan 1986, pp. 7–8).

For brief sketches of the members of the Bloomsbury Group, as well as of some of its close associates, see Spalding 1997.

[41]Richard Rorty describes these momentous changes prior to the Great War.

> The big change in the outlook of the intellectuals—as opposed to a change in human nature—that happened around 1910 was that they began to be confident that human beings had only bodies, and no souls. The resulting this-worldliness made them receptive to the idea that one's sexual behaviour did not have much to do with one's moral worth. . . . For these reasons, the biggest gap between the typical intellectual and the typical nonintellectual is that the former does not use "impurity" as a moral term (Rorty 1999, pp. 168–169).

[42]As an indication of the broad connections of the Bloomsbury Group, consider Virginia Woolf's diary entry for Monday, October 28, 1918: "as I write this, the post brings a letter from Eliot asking to come & see us" (Woolf 1977, vol. 1, p. 210).

[43]Frank Raymond Leavis was an influential British literary critic who taught for many years at Cambridge.

[44]Consider the difference between Picasso's self-portrait of 1906 and *Les Demoiselles d'Avignon* from the end of 1906 or early 1907.

[45]One might contrast Kandinsky's *Arab Cemetery* of 1909 with his *Black Lines* of 1913.

[46]Compare Klee's *Baumgruppe* of 1899 and his *Sonne im Hof* of 1913.

[47]The Erste Internationalle Dadamesse was held on Lützowufer in Berlin on 30 June 1920. As with much that followed the Great War, Dada had roots before and during the war.

The most radical artistic response to the war came from a group of people who made a complete break with traditional loyalties and gathered in neutral Zürich in 1915 to found there the Dada idea—if one can speak of this nihilistic manifestation as an idea. The cohort had an international flavor but its core was German. Among the protagonists were Hugo Ball, Richard Huelsenbeck, Hans Richter, Hans Arp, and the Rumanian Tristan Tzara. In histrionic and epigrammatic barbs against the orgy of self-destruction Europe was involved in, they denied all meaning, even their own. The only sense was nonsense, the only art anti-art. *Bevor Dada da war, war Dada da*—before Dada was there was Dada there. Richard Huelsenbeck encouraged the "aimless of the world" to unite (Eksteins 1989, p. 210).

[48]Immanuel Kant as an atheist recognized the cardinal importance of a God's-eye perspective. A Divine command account of morality can at least in principle be appreciated even by atheists as involving an unconditioned perspective, even if there be no agreement about the existence or content of that perspective.

[49]Again, since there is no sound rational argument that can establish a particular, content-full, secular morality as canonical, all secular morality has a socio-historically contingent, that is, a socio-historically constituted and constructed character. This is the case in that secular morality has no foundations beyond a cluster of mutually supporting intuitions sustained by a particular narrative, all suspended within the horizon of the finite and the immanent. In contrast, the commands of God at least make reference to a God Who breaks into history. Because these commands, these norms, are contingent on His will, they are grounded not in sound rational argument, but in the will of the transcendent Creator Who is the final reference point for all that is.

[50]In a culture after God, its members will not credit St. Paul's declaration that even secular governments have authority from God in the maintenance of the rule of law (Romans 13:1–4).

[51]For more on the comparative authority of governments versus corporations, see Engelhardt 1996, esp. pp. 174, 176, 178.

[52]The literature bearing on the appropriateness of religious discourse in the public space and public forum is extensive. See, for example, Audi 1998; Audi & Wolterstorff 1997; Ungureanu 2008; and Weithman 2002.

[53]It should be noted that Emperor Constantine's arch in Rome shows him with his back towards Jupiter. See, for example, Van Dam 2008, p. 67.

References

Abrahamse, Allan. 1988. *Beyond Stereotypes: Who Becomes a Single Teenage Mother?* Santa Monica, CA: Rand Corporation.

Akerlof, George A., Janet Yellen, & Michael L. Katz. 1996. An analysis of out-of-wedlock childbearing in the United States, *Quarterly Journal of Economics* 61.2: 277–317.

Allen, Elizabeth S. & David C. Atkins. 2012. The association of divorce and extramarital sex in a representative U.S. sample, *Journal of Family Issues* 33.11(November): 1477–1493.

Alvaré, Helen. 2013. Constitutional abortion and culture, *Christian Bioethics* 19.2 (August): 133–149.

Anonymous. 2013. *Wall Street Journal* 261, #21 (January 26/27): D1.

Audi, Robert & Nicholas Wolterstorff. 1997. *Religion in the Public Sphere*. Lanham, MD: Rowman & Littlefield.

Bartholomew, Patriarch. 1997. Joyful light, address at Georgetown University, Washington, DC, October 21. Available at: evlogeite.com/?page_id=16

Beatitude Anthology. 1960. San Francisco: City Light Books.

Beauchamp, Tom L. & James F. Childress. 1979. *The Principles of Biomedical Ethics*. New York: Oxford.

Benhabib, Seyla. 2008. *Another Cosmopolitanism*, ed. Robert Post. New York: Oxford University Press.

Berger, Peter L. 1969. *The Social Reality of Religion*. London: Penguin.

Berman, Marshall. 1982. *All That Is Solid Melts Into Air*. New York: Simon and Schuster.

Bishop, Bill. 2009. *The Big Sort: Why the Clustering of Like-minded America is Tearing us Apart*. Boston: Mariner Books.

Blom, Philipp. 2010. *A Wicked Company*. New York: Basic Books.

Blom, Philipp. 2008. *The Vertigo Years: Change and Culture in the West, 1900–1914*. New York: Basic Books.

Bloom, Harold. 1992. *The American Religion: The Emergence of the Post-Christian Nation*. New York: Simon & Schuster.

Bogle, Kathleen A. 2008. *Hooking Up*. New York: New York University Press.

Boguslavsky, B. M., V. A. Karpushin, A. I. Rakitov, V. Y. Chertikhin, & G. I. Ezrin. 1975. *ABC of Dialectical and Historical Materialism*, trans. Lenina Ilitskaya. Moscow: Progress Publishers.

Brooks, David. 2000. *Bobos in Paradise: The New Upper Class and How They Got There*. New York: Simon & Schuster.

Brown, Helen Gurley. 1965. *Sex and the Office*. New York: Pocket Books.

Brown, Helen Gurley. 1962. *Sex and the Single Girl*. New York: Bernard Geis Associates.

Buchanan, James M. & Gordon Tullock. 1965. *The Calculus of Consent*. Ann Arbor, MI: University of Michigan Press.

Carson, D. A. 2013. *The Intolerance of Tolerance*. Grand Rapids: Wm. B. Eerdmans.

Cherlin, Andrew. 2010. *The Marriage-Go-Round: The State of Marriage and the Family in America Today*. New York: Vintage Books.

Cohen, Leonard. 1972. *The Energy of Slaves*. New York: Viking Press.

Connolly, William. 1999. *Why I Am Not a Secularist*. Minneapolis: University of Minnesota Press.

Council on Environmental Quality and the Department of State. 1980–1981. *The Global 2000 Report to the President*, 3 vols. Washington, DC: U.S. Government Printing Office.

Cox, Harvey. 1966. *The Secular City*. New York: Macmillan.

Daniel-Rops, Henri. 1963. *The Church in the Seventeenth Century*, trans. J. J. Buckingham. Garden City, NY: Doubleday.

Dawkins, Richard. 2006. *The God Delusion*. New York: Houghton Mifflin.

Delkeskamp-Hayes, Corinna. 2013. Introduction, *Christian Bioethics* 19.2 (August): 115–129.

Delkeskamp-Hayes, Corinna & Tibor Imrényi. 2013. Claims, priorities, and moral excuses: A culture's dependence on abortion and its cure, *Christian Bioethics* 19.2 (August): 198–241.

Diogenes Laertius. 2000. Protagoras, in *Lives of Ancient Philosophers*, vol. 2 (pp. 321–367), trans. R. D. Hicks. Cambridge, MA: Harvard University Press.

Dreyfus, Hubert & Sean Dorrance Kelly. 2011. *All Things Shining: Reading the Western Classics to Find Meaning in a Secular Age*. New York: Free Press.

Duffy, Eamon. 1992. *The Stripping of the Altars*. New Haven, NJ: Yale University Press.

Edel, Leon. 1979. *Bloomsbury: A House of Lions*. London: Penguin Books.

Edin, Kathryn & Timothy J. Nelson. 2013. *Doing the Best I Can*. Berkeley, CA: University of California Press.

Ehrenhalt, Alan. 1995. *The Lost City: The Forgotten Virtues of Community in America*. New York: Basic Books.

Ehrlich, Paul. 1968. *The Population Bomb*. New York: Ballantine Books.

Eliot, T. S. 1982. *The Idea of a Christian Society*. London: Faber & Faber.

Eksteins, Modris. 1989. *Rites of Spring*. Boston: Houghton Mifflin.

Engel, Randy. 2006. *The Rite of Sodomy: Homosexuality and the Roman Catholic Church*. Export, PA: New Engel Publishing.

Engelhardt, H. T., Jr. 2011. *Viaggi in Italia: Saggi di bioetica*, eds. & trans. Rodolfo Rini & Maurizio Mori. Florence: Le Lettere.

Engelhardt, H. T., Jr. 2010a. Moral obligation after the death of God: Critical reflections on concerns from Immanuel Kant, G.W.F. Hegel, and Elizabeth Anscombe, *Social Philosophy & Policy* 27.2: 317–340.

Engelhardt, H. T., Jr. 2010b. Kant, Hegel, and Habermas: Reflections on 'Glauben und Wissen', *The Review of Metaphysics* 63.4: 871–903.

Engelhardt, H. T., Jr. 2000. *The Foundations of Christian Bioethics*. Salem, MA: Scrivener Publishing.

Engelhardt, H. T., Jr. 1996. *The Foundations of Bioethics*, 2nd ed. New York: Oxford University Press.

Engelhardt, H. T., Jr. 1991. *Bioethics and Secular Humanism*. Philadelphia: Trinity International Press.

Engelhardt, H. T., Jr. 1986. *The Foundations of Bioethics*. New York: Oxford University Press.

Eppler, Erhard. 1975. *Ende ohne Wende*. Stuttgart. Kohlhammer.

Fader, Ayala. 2009. *Mitzvah Girls*. Princeton, NJ: Princeton University Press.

Fan, Ruiping (ed.). 2011. *The Renaissance of Confucianism in Contemporary China*. Dordrecht: Springer.

Fan, Ruiping. 2010. *Reconstructionist Confucianism: Rethinking Morality after the West*. Dordrecht: Springer.

Fan, Ruiping. 1997. Self-determination vs. family determination. Two incommensurable principles of autonomy, *Bioethics* 11: 309–322.

Fernandez-Villaverde, Jesus, Jeremy Greenwood, & Nezih Guner. 2012. From shame to game in one hundred years, pp. 1–61. economics.sas.upenn.edu/~jesusfv/fgg.pdf

Finer, Lawrence B. 2007. Trends in premarital sex in the United States, 1954–2003, *Public Health Reports* 122 (January-February): 73–78.

Florida, Richard. 2011. *The Rise of the Creative Class Revisited*. New York: Basic Books.

Freeman, Charles. 2011. *Holy Bones Holy Dust*. New Haven, CN: Yale University Press.

Fukuyama, Francis. 1999. *The Great Disruption*. New York: Free Press.

Gaylor, Anne Nicol. 1975. *Abortion is a Blessing*. Psychological Dimensions.

Gilison, Jerome M. 1975. *The Soviet Image of Utopia*. Baltimore: Johns Hopkins University Press.

Gillespie, Michael A. 2008. *The Theological Origins of Modernity*. Chicago: University of Chicago Press.

Goldin, Claudia & Lawrence F. Katz. 2000. The power of the pill: Oral contraceptives and women's career and marriage decisions, *Journal of Political Economy* 110.4: 730–770.

Gorovitz, Samuel & Alasdair MacIntyre. 1976. Toward a theory of medical fallibility, *Journal of Medicine and Philosophy* 1.1: 51–71.

Goss, Charles W. 1908. *A Descriptive Bibliography of the Writings of George Jacob Holyoake*. London: Crowther & Goodman.

Gottfried, Paul Edward. 2007. *Conservatism in America*. New York: Palgrave.

Greenwood, Jeremy & Nezih Guner. 2010. Social change: The sexual revolution, *International Economic Review* 51.4 (November): 893–923.

Gregory, Brad S. 2012. *The Unintended Reformation: How a Religious Revolution Secularized Society*. Cambridge, MA: Belknap Press.

Grogan, Pat. 1985. *Abortion is a Woman's Right*. New York: Pathfinder Press.

Gutmann, Amy & Dennis Thompson. 2004. *Why Deliberative Democracy?* Princeton, NJ: Princeton University Press.

Hamilton, Brady, Joyce Martin, & Stephanie Ventura. 2012. Births: Preliminary data for 2011, *National Vital Statistics Report* 61.5 (October 3): 1–18.

Harris, Sam. 2005. *The End of Faith*. New York: W. W. Norton.

Hassan, Ihab. 1975. *Paracriticism*. Urbana, IL: University of Illinois Press.

Haworth, Abigail. 2013. Why have young people in Japan stopped having sex? *The Guardian* (October 19). Available: www.theguardian.com/world/2013/oct/20/young-people-japan-stopped-having-sex

Heelas, Paul. 1996. *The New Age Movement*. Oxford: Blackwell.

Hegel, G.W.F. 1991. *Elements of the Philosophy of Right*, ed. Allen W. Wood, trans. H. B. Nisbet. Cambridge: Cambridge University Press.

Hegel, G.W.F. 1977. *Faith & Knowledge,* trans. Walter Cerf and H.S. Harris. Albany: State University of New York Press.

Hegel, G.W.F. 1968. *Jenaer kritische Schriften*, in *Gesammelte Werke*, vol. 4. Hamburg: Meiner.

Heller, Agnes. 1990. *Can Modernity Survive?* Berkeley: University of California Press.

Hemingway, Ernest. 1964. *A Moveable Feast: Sketches of the Author's Life in Paris in the Twenties.* New York: Charles Scribner's Sons.

Himmelfarb, Gertrude. 1999. *One Nation, Two Cultures.* New York: Vintage Books.

Himmelfarb, Gertrude. 1995. *The De-moralization of Society: From Victorian Virtues to Modern Values.* New York: Alfred A. Knopf.

Hite, Shere. 1977. *The Hite Report.* New York: Dell.

Hollinger, David A. 1996. *Science, Jews, and Secular Culture.* Princeton, NJ: Princeton University Press.

Holyoake, George. 1896. *The Origin and Nature of Secularism.* London: Watts & Co.

Holyoake, George. 1871. *The Principles of Secularism*, 3rd ed. London: Austin & Co.

Hutchison, William R. 1989. *Between the Times: The Travail of the Protestant Establishment in America, 1900–1960.* New York: Cambridge University Press.

Hymowitz, Kay S. 2011. *Manning Up: How the Rise of Women Has Turned Men into Boys.* New York: Basic Books.

Hymowitz, Kay, Jason Carroll, W. Bradford Wilcox, & Kelleen Kaye. 2013. *Knot Yet: The Benefits and Costs of Delayed Marriage in America.* http://nationalmarriageproject.org/wp-content/uploads/2013/04/KnotYet-FinalForWeb-041413.pdf

James, E. L. 2012. *Fifty Shades of Gray.* New York: Vintage.

James, E. L. 2012. *Fifty Shades Darker.* New York: Vintage.

James, E. L. 2012. *Fifty Shades Freed.* New York: Vintage.

John Paul II. 1998. *Fides et ratio.* Vatican City: Libreria editrice vaticana.

Jubilee Bishops' Council of the Russian Orthodox Church. 2000. The Orthodox Church and society: The basis of the social concept of the Russian Orthodox Church. Belleville, MI: Firebird.

Kandinsky, Wassily. 1947. *Concerning the Spiritual in Art*, trans. Michael Sadleir. New York: George Wittenborn.

Kandinsky, Wassily. 1912. *Über das Geistige in der Kunst.* Munich: Piper-Verlag.

Kant, Immanuel. 1996. Toward perpetual peace, in *Practical Philosophy*, ed. and trans. Mary J. Gregor (pp. 315–351). Cambridge: Cambridge University Press.

Kant, Immanuel. 1956. *Critique of Practical Reason,* trans. Lewis White Beck. Indianapolis: Bobbs-Merrill.

Kilker, Adrian. 1926. *Extreme Unction.* Washington, DC: Catholic University of America Press.

Kinsey, Alfred C., Wardell B. Pomeroy, Clyde E. Martin. 1948. *Sexual Behavior in the Human Male.* New York: Saunders.

Kinsey, Alfred C., Wardell B. Pomeroy, Clyde E. Martin, & Paul H. Gebhard. 1953. *Sexual Behavior in the Human Female.* New York: Saunders.

Kirchenamt der EKD. 2013. *Zwischen Autonomie und Angewiesenheit: Familie als verlässliche Gemeinschaft stärken.* Munich: Gütersloher Verlagshaus.

Klinenberg, Eric. 2013. *Going Solo: The Extraordinary Rise and Surprising Appeal of Living Alone.* New York: Penguin Books.

Kozinski, Thaddeus J. 2010. *The Political Problem of Religious Pluralism.* Lanham, MD: Rowman & Littlefield.

Krutch, Joseph W. 1956 [1929]. *The Modern Temper.* New York: Harcourt, Brace & World.

Laborde, Cécile. 2008. *Critical Republicanism: The Hijab Controversy and Political Philosophy.* New York: Oxford University Press.

Lake, Kirsopp (trans.). 1965. The martyrdom of Polycarp, in *The Apostolic Fathers,* vol. 2 (pp. 307–345). Cambridge, MA: Harvard University Press.

Lawrence, Raymond J., Jr. 2007. *Sexual Liberation: The Scandal of Christendom.* Westport, CT: Praeger.

Lawrence, Raymond J., Jr. 1989. *The Poisoning of Eros.* New York: Augustine Moore Press.

Lewis & Short. 1879. *A Latin Dictionary.* Oxford: Clarendon Press.

Liturgikon, The. 1994, 2nd ed. Englewood, NJ: Antakya Press.

Locke, John. 1983 [1689]. *A Letter Concerning Toleration,* ed. James H. Tully. Indianapolis: Hackett.

Longman, Phillip. 2004. *The Empty Cradle.* New York: Basic Books.

Luckmann, Thomas. 1990. Shrinking transcendence, expanding religion? *Sociological Analysis* 30: 127–136.

MacMullen, Ian. 2007. *Faith in Schools? Autonomy, Citizenship, and Religious Education in the Liberal State.* Princeton, NJ: Princeton University Press.

Maguire, Daniel C. 2001. *Sacred Choices.* Minneapolis: Fortress Press.

Maimonides, Moses. 2001. *Mishneh Torah,* trans. Eliyahu Touger. New York: Moznaim Publishing.

Marcuse, Herbert. 1955. *Eros and Civilization*. Boston: Beacon Press.

Martin, Bernice. 1981. *A Sociology of Contemporary Cultural Change*. Oxford: Basil Blackwell.

Martin, Joyce, Brady Hamilton, Stephanie Ventura, Michelle Osterman, Elizabeth Wilson, & T. J. Mathews. 2012. Births: Final data for 2010, *National Vital Statistics Reports* 61.1 (August 28): 1–72.

Masters, William H. and Virginia E. Johnson. 1994. *Heterosexuality*. New York: HarperCollins.

Masters, William H. and Virginia E. Johnson. 1979. *Homosexuality in Perspective*. New York: Bantam Books.

Masters, William H. and Virginia E. Johnson. 1974. *The Pleasure Bond*. New York: Bantam Books.

Masters, William H. and Virginia E. Johnson. 1970. *Human Sexual Inadequacy*. New York: Little, Brown.

Masters, William H. and Virginia E. Johnson. 1966. *Human Sexual Response*. New York: Little, Brown.

Mayer, Susan. 1998. *What Money Can't Buy: Family Income and Children's Life Changes*. Cambridge, MA: Harvard University Press.

McConnell, Michael W. 1993. God is dead and we have killed Him?: Freedom of religion in the post-modern age, *Brigham Young University Law Review* 1993.1: 163–188.

Meadows, Donella H. et al. 1974. *The Limits to Growth: A Report for the Club of Rome's Project on the Predicament of Mankind*, 2nd ed. Englewood, NJ: Universe.

Milbank, John. 2006. *Theology and Social Theory: Beyond Secular Reason*, 2nd edition. Oxford: Blackwell Publishing.

Mommsen, Theodor. 1858. *Die römische Chronologie*. Berlin: Weidmannsche.

Moore, J. Howard. 1906. *The Universal Kinship*. London: George Bell.

Morgan, Patricia. 2000. *Marriage-Lite: The Rise of Cohabitation and its Consequences*. London: Institute for the Study of Civil Society.

Moynihan, Daniel Patrick. 1965. *The Negro Family: A Case for National Action*. Washington, DC: U.S. Department of Labor.

Murray, Charles. 2012. *Coming Apart*. New York: Crown Forum.

Myers, Norman & Julian L. Simon. 1995. *Scarcity or Abundance? A Debate on the Environment*. New York: W.W. Norton.

Nash, Roderick. 1990 [1970]. *The Nervous Generation: American Thought, 1917–1930*. Chicago: Ivan R. Dee.

Nozick, Robert. 1974. *Anarchy, State, and Utopia.* New York: Basic Books.

OECD. 2011. *Education at a Glance 2011: OECD Indicators.* Paris: OECD Publishing.

Okin, Susan. 1989. *Justice, Gender, and the Family.* New York: Basic Books.

Owen, J. Judd. 2001. *Religion and the Demise of Liberal Rationalism.* Chicago: University of Chicago Press.

Paris, Ginette. 1992. *The Sacrament of Abortion*, trans. Joanna Mott. New York: Spring Publications.

Pearlstein, Mitch. 2011. *From Family Collapse to America's Decline: The Educational, Economic and Social Costs of Family Fragmentation.* Lanham, MD: R&L Education.

Percy, Walker. 1987. *The Message in the Bottle.* New York: Farrar, Straus and Giroux.

Perry, Michael J. 2001. Why political reliance on religiously grounded morality does not violate the establishment clause, *William and Mary Law Review* 42: 663–683.

Rawls, John. 1999. *The Law of Peoples: The Idea of Public Reason Revisited.* Cambridge, MA: Harvard University Press.

Rawls, John. 1993. *Political Liberalism.* New York: Columbia University Press.

Rawls, John. 1985. Justice as fairness: Political not metaphysical, *Philosophy and Public Affairs* 14.5 (Summer): 223–251.

Rector, Robert. 2010. Marriage: America's greatest weapon against child poverty, *Backgrounder* 2465 (September 16): 1–16.

Regan, Tom. 1986. *Bloomsbury's Prophet.* Philadelphia: Temple University Press.

Reich, Wilhelm. 1963. *The Sexual Revolution*, trans. Theodore Wolfie. New York: Farrar, Straus and Giroux.

Roberts, Alexander & James Donaldson (eds.). 1994. *Ante-Nicene Fathers.* Peabody, MA: Hendrickson Publishers.

Root, Michael. 2013. Reforming the German family, *First Things* 237 (November): 19–21.

Rorty, Richard. 2011. *An Ethics for Today.* New York: Columbia University Press.

Rorty, Richard. 1999. *Philosophy and Social Hope.* New York: Penguin.

Rorty, Richard. 1991. *Objectivity, Relativism, and Truth.* New York: Cambridge University Press.

Rosin, Hanna. 2012. *The End of Men: And the Rise of Women.* New York: Riverhead.

Sabin, Paul. 2013. *The Bet.* New Haven, CN: Yale University Press.

Sajó, András. 2008. Preliminaries to a concept of constitutional secularism, *International Journal of Constitutional Law* 6.3-4: 605–629.

Sajó, András. 2009. The crisis that was not there: Notes on A reply. I•CON 7.3: 515–528.

Scanlon, T. M. 2003. *The Difficulty of Tolerance*. New York: Cambridge University Press.

Schillebeeckx, Edward. 1969. Silence and speaking about God in a secularized world, in *Christian Secularity*, ed. Albert Schlitzer (pp. 156–180). Notre Dame, IN: University of Notre Dame Press.

Schneewind, J. B. 1998. *The Invention of Autonomy: A History of Modern Moral Philosophy*. New York: Cambridge University Press.

Schorski, Carl. 1980. *Fin-de-siècle Vienna*. New York: Vintage.

Shiraishi, Kazuko. 1975. *Seasons of Sacred Lust*, ed. Kenneth Rexroth. New York: New Directions.

Silber, John R. 1960. The ethical significance of Kant's Religion, in *Immanuel Kant, Religion Within the Limits of Reason Alone*, trans. T. M. Greene and H. H. Hudson (lxxix–cxxxiv). New York: Harper & Row.

Simon, Julian. 1981. *Ultimate Resource*. Princeton, NJ: Princeton University Press.

Smith, James K. A. 2014. *How (not) to be Secular: Reading Charles Taylor*. Grand Rapids, MI: Wm. B. Eerdmans Publishing.

Smith, Patti. 1973. *Wĩtt*. New York: Gotham Book Mart.

Sowerby, Scott. 2013. *Making Toleration*. Cambridge, MA: Harvard University Press.

Spalding, Frances. 1997. *The Bloomsbury Group*. London: National Portrait Gallery.

Spengler, Oswald. 1922. *The Decline of the West*. vol. 2: *Perspectives of World-History*, trans. Charles Atkinson. London: George Allen & Unwin.

Spengler, Oswald. 1918. *The Decline of the West*. vol. 1: *Form and Actuality*, trans. Charles Atkinson. London: George Allen & Unwin.

Spong, John Shelby. 1988. *Living in Sin?* San Francisco: Harper & Row.

Statkus, Francis J. 1951. *The Minister of the Last Sacraments*. Washington, DC: Catholic University of America Press.

Taylor, Charles. 2007. *A Secular Age*. Cambridge, MA: Belknap Press.

Tsai, George. 2013. Lamentable necessities, *The Review of Metaphysics* 66.4 (June): 775–808.

Ungureanu, Camil. 2008. The contested relation between democracy and religion: Towards a dialogical perspective? *European Journal of Political Theory* 7: 405–429.

Van Dam, Raymond. 2008. *The Roman Revolution of Constantine*. Cambridge: Cambridge University Press.

Vattimo, Gianni. 2011. *A Farewell to Truth*, trans. William McCuaig. New York: Columbia University Press.

Vattimo, Gianni. 2004. *Nihilism and Emancipation*, ed. Santiago Zabala, trans. William McCuaig. New York: Columbia University Press.

Vattimo, Gianni. 2002. *After Christianity*, trans. Luca D'Isanto. New York: Columbia University Press.

Warner, Michael, Jonathan VanAntwerpen, & Craig Calhoun (eds.). 2010. *Varieties of Secularism in a Secular Age*. Cambridge, MA: Harvard University Press.

Weber, Max. 2001. *The Protestant Ethic and the Spirit of Capitalism*, trans. Talcott Parsons. New York: Routledge.

Weithman, P. J. 2002. *Religion and Obligations of Citizenship*. Oxford: Oxford University Press.

West, Shearer. 1994. *Fin de Siècle*. Woodstock, NY: Overlook Press.

Wheeler, Leigh Ann. 2012. *How Sex Became a Civil Liberty*. New York: Oxford University Press.

Wilson, A. N. 1999. *God's Funeral*. New York: W. W. Norton.

Wohl, Robert. 1979. *The Generation of 1914*. Cambridge, MA: Harvard University Press.

Wolff, Robert Paul, Barrington Moore, Jr., & Herbert Marcuse. 1965. *A Critique of Pure Tolerance*. Boston: Beacon Press.

Woolf, Virginia. 1977. *The Diary of Virginia Woolf*, 3 vols., ed. Anne Olivier Bell. New York: Harcourt Brace Jovanovich.

Zabala, Santiago. 2005. A religion without theists or atheists, in Richard Rorty and Gianni Vattimo, *The Future of Religion* (pp. 1–27), ed. Santiago Zabala. New York: Columbia University Press.

Zucca, Lorenzo. 2009. The crisis of the secular state—A reply to Professor Sajó, *International Journal of Constitutional Law* 7.3: 494–514.

CHAPTER FOUR

Fides et ratio, the Western Medieval Synthesis, and the Collapse of Secular Morality and Bioethics[1]

I. Western Christianity: A Faith in Reason

There is a crisis at the roots and in the substance of secular morality and bioethics. This crisis is a function of excessive, indeed false expectations regarding metaphysics and moral philosophy, as well as a loss of a God's-eye perspective. Unwarranted philosophical expectations grounded in the philosophical synthesis that shaped the emergence of Western Christianity at the beginning of the second millennium produced a metaphysics that promised philosophically to prove the existence of God and to justify a canonical moral philosophy. The contemporary West inherited an unfounded faith that reason could supply what faith had previously warranted. Among other things, this peculiarly Western European project of moral philosophy promised a rationally warranted account of morality that would provide a canonical moral *lingua franca*, a moral discourse accessible to all. This has failed. As a consequence, state power, albeit only the power of a *modus vivendi*, has been invoked to substitute for the power of reason and/or a canonical morality.

Among post-Christian Western Europeans, the expectation persisted that there is one content-full canonical morality, and that it can be warranted through sound rational argument. Such expectations regarding the possibility of a rationally justifiable secular canonical morality, which were defended by philosophers such as Immanuel Kant (1724–1804), Jeremy Bentham (1748–1832), and John

Stuart Mill (1806–1873), are expressions of this faith. As we have seen, this ethnically particular faith began to collapse in the 19th century as the inadequacies of its grounding assumptions became clear, so that by the end of the 20th century many appreciated that this faith lacked an adequate basis. The difficulty for a purported canonical secular morality, or for that matter for a purported canonical bioethics, is that it has now become clear that there is an intractable plurality of moral rationalities. The presence of intractable moral pluralism is a challenge to both secular morality and the Western Christian morality that grew out of Roman Catholicism. In order to put this state of affairs into context, one must appreciate that the original Christianity did not have such a faith in moral philosophy. It was not committed to the view that sound rational argument can establish a canonical morality. Nor did it seek to substitute state power for the power of reason, although it did anoint the Christian state.

II. Knowing God versus Knowing about God: The Encounter with Transcendence

Christianity did not begin in the arms of philosophy. Christ did not walk through Palestine preaching natural law. The early Church was not a philosophical seminar. The Apostles did not embrace the bond of *fides et ratio*, faith and reason. The Christianity of the first half-millennium marginalized pagan Greek philosophical faith in reason. This Christianity turned to Jerusalem, not to Athens. Although this Church took terms and distinctions from pagan Greek philosophers, it did not ground its theology in their philosophy. Quite to the contrary, as Tertullian records, this Church maintained a critical distance from and suspicion of philosophy.

> Writing to the Colossians, he [St. Paul] says, "See that no one beguile you through philosophy and vain deceit, after the tradition of men, and contrary to the wisdom of the Holy Ghost" [Col 2:8]. He had been at Athens, and had in his interviews (with its philosophers) become acquainted with that human wisdom which pretends to know the truth, whilst it only corrupts it, and is itself divided into its own manifold heresies, by the variety of its mutually repugnant sects. What indeed has Athens to do with Jerusalem? What concord is there between the Academy and the Church? what between heretics

and Christians? Our instruction comes from "the porch of Solomon" [Acts 3:5] who had himself taught that "the Lord should be sought in simplicity of heart" [Wis 1:1]. Away with all attempts to produce a mottled Christianity of Stoic, Platonic, and dialectic composition! We want no curious disputation after enjoying the gospel! With our faith, we desire no further belief. For this is our palmary faith, that there is nothing which we ought to believe besides (Tertullian 1994, "On Prescription Against Heretics" VII, p. 246).

In the same spirit, St. John Chrysostom (*c.* 347–407) made his famous remark regarding the Greek pagan philosophers.

[Christians are n]ot like Plato, who composed that ridiculous *Republic*, or Zeno, or if there be any one else that hath written a polity, or hath framed laws. For indeed, touching all these, it hath been made manifest by themselves, that an evil spirit, and some cruel demon at war with our race, a foe to modesty, and an enemy to good order, oversetting all things, hath made his voice be heard in their soul (Chrysostom 1994c, Homily I on the Gospel of St. Matthew, vol. 10, p. 5).

The Christians of the first centuries lived in a canonical morality grounded not in philosophy but in an experience of the living God Who commands.

This moral epistemology of Christianity is reflected in the way in which the Church of the first centuries understood the first and second chapters of St. Paul's Letter to the Romans. St. John Chrysostom recognized that St. Paul in the second chapter of Romans was not embracing the moral epistemology that lies at the roots of much Greek moral philosophy and that as a consequence lies at the basis of much of secular bioethics, as well as of Roman Catholic natural-law theory. Western Christian moral epistemology, which developed in the second millennium, among other things held that, even apart from an at least minimally religiously rightly-ordered life, one could by natural reason reliably discern between right and wrong actions. The Christians of the West by the early second millennium no longer engaged in serious ascetical discipline, including strenuous fasting and all-night vigils, as a necessary condition for moral theology or theology in general, so that moral theology became primarily an intellectual and academic, rather than a liturgical and ascetic undertaking. An epiphany of this change is the morbidly obese Thomas Aquinas. Given the Fall, natural reason, as the early Church appreciated, is a fallen reason. It is not philosophical rationality, but a noetic knowing, a knowing that can only be engaged when one is free from the domination of the passions so that it becomes possible, through an ascetical-liturgical life, for one to do theology, to know God.[2]

St. John Chrysostom saw that in the first chapter of St. Paul's letter to the Romans St. Paul was underscoring that, if one's life is distorted by false worship, if one worships the creature rather than the Creator, one will perceive wrongly the norms that should guide conduct.[3] In addition, one will be beset by misguiding passions, further distorting one's life.[4] There will be a cascade of perversions. The works of the law (*ta erga tou nomou*) in one's heart will not be distorted only if one lives a morally and liturgically rightly-ordered life. Only then will one's knowing not be misguided. Given one's nature as a being called to be a god by grace (St. Athanasius, *De incarnatione verbi dei* 54.3), one can by this nature begin to know what one ought to do, but only through right worship and right action, which maintains the rightly-ordered character of that nature, for we are beings that by nature are called to worship God and be united with Him. Again, this knowledge is achieved only insofar as one turns rightly to God. In commentary on chapter 2 of Romans[5] St. John Chrysostom underscored:

> But by Greeks he [St. Paul] here [Rom 2:12–16] means not them that worshipped idols, but them that adored God, that obeyed the law of nature, that strictly kept all things, save the Jewish observances, which contribute to piety, such as were Melchizedek and his, such as was Job, such as were the Ninevites, such as was Cornelius (Chrysostom 1994b, Homily V on Romans, vol. 11, p. 363).

The Church of the first centuries did not expect that pagans could reliably embrace the equivalent of a Christian morality and bioethics. In particular, there was no view that secular moral philosophy could of itself bring one to the norms for right action, for "God made foolish the wisdom of this world" (I Cor 1:20).[6] Among the many consequences of this state of affairs is that the early Church knew that there is no neutral moral-philosophical standpoint that can blunt the collision of traditional Christianity with non-Christian morality and the non-Christian bioethics of the contemporary post-Christian, indeed secular culture.

There is an important similarity between the position of the Christianity of the first millennium and the position embraced by Orthodox Jews. In particular, traditional Christians, along with Orthodox Jews, recognize a fully transcendent God Who commands, Who has been experienced, and Who gives precedence to the holy over the good, to the personal over the universal. The God's-eye perspective of the early Church of Orthodox Christians is not a perspective that discloses general moral principles, universal ideas, or abstract norms, but one that reveals the perspective of the Persons of the Trinity. The God's-eye perspective of Orthodox Christians and Orthodox Jews is not that of an anonymous judge, but that of a personal Father Who turns to persons as persons. Unlike with Plato's universalist vision of justice, everything is personal. For example, God declares in Exodus, "I will be gracious to whom I will be gracious. I will have compassion on whomever I will have compassion" (Ex 33:19). It is this perspective that allows King David, a murderer and adulterer but also the ancestor of Christ, to state: "Against Thee alone have I sinned and done evil in Thy sight" (Ps 50). This paradigm places centrally an acknowledgement of the personal God Who commands, Who has mercy, and Who forgives, not an independent morality and the values that such a morality might affirm.

Because the root of Christian and Jewish moral norms is in God's commandments and not in independent values and/or views of the virtuous life, strictly speaking, for Orthodox Jews and traditional Christians, there are no Judeo-Christian values. That is, life is not to be oriented by reference to things or by states of affairs that have intrinsic value apart from reference to God, in terms of Whom desires and values must be oriented. Otherwise, one comes to love the creature (e.g., the values) independently of a proper orientation to the Creator, with the result that one has a distorted view of what one should value and desire. Unlike the discursive secular values that aspire to be a moral *lingua franca*, there are instead the laws given to the sons of Noah, which are different from the laws given to the Jews. God's commandments, unlike values, create a personal relationship between the One Who commands, and the one who is commanded. By a command, God establishes a personal injunction as to how one should approach Him. Values in contrast can be dispassionately and impersonally contemplated. A command from God enters personally into one's life.

In this important sense, Orthodox Christians and Jews do not have a morality. That is, morality is not an independent normative framework between God and man, which philosophers can define, shape, contemplate, and expound. Nor is morality a fabric of moral norms that would benefit from a critical philosophical re-assessment. There is instead a recognition of the God Who gave 7 laws to the sons of Noah and 613 laws to the Jews. Of course, these different laws have implications for what values one might appropriately affirm or reject, as well as what goods one should pursue. But as already argued, the norms for behavior embraced by Orthodox Jews and Orthodox Christians are not grounded in a moral-philosophical foundation, vision, or account of values, but rather in an encounter with a fully transcendent, incomprehensible, personal God. A very distant and imperfect way of thinking about this relationship with God is that of the black hole at the heart of our galaxy, around which all the galaxy's stars revolve, but of which nothing is empirically known within its Schwarzschild horizon. The West entered the second millennium just as the original Christian moral paradigm in the West was being transformed by a synthesis of Aristotelian, Platonic, Stoic, and Christian understandings of reality and morality. It was this shift in the meaning of behavioral norms and in the character of theology, not just the generation of new dogmas, that created Western Christianity. The second millennium in the West produced a radically new life-world.

III. The Creation of Western Christianity

Already with Blessed Augustine of Hippo (A.D. 354–430), Western Christianity had begun to take on an identity of its own and to erect a new vision of Christianity. Augustine was widely influential in the West because he was the only one of the four Latin Fathers (with St. Jerome, St. Ambrose, and St. Gregory the Dialogist) who wrote extensive philosophical-theological works. Most importantly, he had a discursive philosophical sensibility, thus often writing as a philosopher. Last but not least, the church of North Africa and Augustine spoke to a wide range of theological issues that shaped Western Christian views regarding (1) priestly celibacy, (2) the moral status of early abortion, (3) the nature of the

Trinity, (4) the morality of lying, and (5) the meaning of free choice. As a result, under Augustine's influence a new Christianity began to take shape.

A very particular feature of Western Christianity was priestly celibacy. Already at the First Council of Nicaea in 325 there was a proposal that celibacy be imposed on all priests. Socrates Scholasticus gives the following record of the discussions at Nicea:

> It seemed fit to the bishops to introduce a new law into the Church, that those who were in holy orders, I speak of bishops, presbyters, and deacons, should have no conjugal intercourse with the wives whom they had married while still laymen. Now when discussion on this matter was impending, Paphnutius having arisen in the midst of the assembly of bishops, earnestly entreated them not to impose so heavy a yoke on the ministers of religion: asserting that "marriage itself is honorable, and the bed undefiled"; urging before God that they ought not to injure the Church by too stringent restrictions. "For all men," said he, "cannot bear the practice of rigid continence; neither perhaps would the chastity of the wife of each be preserved": and he termed the intercourse of a man with his lawful wife chastity (Scholasticus 1994, p. 18).

Socrates Scholasticus' report is confirmed by Sozomen.[7] Although the proposal of celibacy was rejected by Nicea I, the church of Carthage at a council in 418 or 419 in Canon IV forbade bishops, priests, and deacons from having sexual intercourse with their wives. "It is decided that Bishops, Presbyters, and Deacons, and all men who handle sacred articles, being guardians of sobriety, must abstain from women" (Nicodemus & Agapius 1983, p. 607). The priesthood was considered incompatible with marital sexuality, even though Canon LI of the 85 Apostolic Canons deposes any priest who does not marry, save for reasons of asceticism or health. In the West, however, the view was developing that the priesthood was incompatible with the marriage bed, even though Christianity teaches that the marriage bed is undefiled (Heb 13:4).

The requirement of celibacy for priests by Christians in the West eventually prompted a condemnation from Constantinople. In particular, Canon XIII of the Quinisext Council (the Council in Trullo, 692) states:

Since we have learned that in the church of the Romans it is regarded as tantamount to a canon that ordinands to the deaconry or presbytery must solemnly promise to have no further intercourse with their wives. Continuing, however, in conformity with the ancient canon of apostolic rigorism and orderliness, we desire that henceforward the lawful marriage ties of sacred men become stronger, and we are nowise dissolving their intercourse with their wives, nor depriving them of their mutual relationship and companionship when properly maintained in due season, so that if anyone is found to be worthy to be ordained a Subdeacon, or a Deacon, or a Presbyter, let him nowise be prevented from being elevated to such a rank while cohabiting with a lawful wife. Nor must he be required at the time of ordination to refrain from lawful intercourse with his own wife, lest we be forced to be downright scornful of marriage, which was instituted by God and blessed by His presence, as attested by the unequivocal declaration of the Gospel utterance: "What therefore God hath joined together, let no man put asunder" (Mt 19:6); and the Apostle's teaching: "Marriage is honorable, and the bed is undefiled" (Heb 13:4), and: "Art thou bound unto a wife? Seek not to be free" (I Cor 7:27). . . . If, therefore, anyone acting contrary to the Apostolic Canons require any person who is in sacred orders—any Presbyter, we mean, or Deacon, or Subdeacon—to abstain from intercourse and association with his lawful wife, let him be deposed from office. Likewise, if any Presbyter or Deacon expel his own wife on the pretext of reverence, let him be excommunicated; and if he persist, let him be deposed from office (Nicodemus & Agapius 1983, pp. 305–6).

The Church of the Councils affirmed that marital sexuality is blessed by God, and that this blessing did not depart from the marriage bed of a priest and his wife. The imposition of priestly celibacy was recognized as against the Tradition and the canons.

The West, however, persisted in its condemnation of a married priesthood, a condemnation renewed by Popes Gregory VII (1073–1085), Urban III (1085–1087), and Pascal II (1099–1118), although until at least the 12th century and somewhat beyond priests continued to marry and live openly with their wives in the West, especially in outlying lands such as England. The result was a very unstable state of affairs for priests and their wives, marked by considerable persecution. For example,

> The London council of 1102 had forbidden under heavy penalties the marriage of the clergy. . . . But the king continued to make a financial matter of it and 'received large sums from the priests for license to live as before.' . . . It seems certain that a large number of the parish clergy and even the higher clergy openly continued their intercourse with women. [Given the opposition of Rome,] [t]he legislation [often] merely substituted an illicit for a legal relationship (Poole 1955, p. 183).

> The parish priest . . . was usually married, or at least 'kept a hearth-girl (focaria) in his house who kindled his fire but extinguished his virtue' and kept 'his miserable house cluttered up with small infants, cradles, midwives, and nurses' (Poole 1955, pp. 224–225).

It was not until the First Lateran Council (A.D. 1123), considered by Roman Catholics to be their Ninth Ecumenical Council, that the marriage of clergy was apparently forbidden by Canon 21, although the canon is missing from some texts of the council.

Finally, in what Roman Catholics considered their Tenth Ecumenical Council, Lateran II (A.D. 1139), they proclaimed in its seventh canon:

> Adhering to the path trod by our predecessors, the Roman pontiffs Gregory VII, Urban and Paschal, we prescribe that nobody is to hear the masses of those whom he knows to have wives or concubines. Indeed, that the law of continence and the purity pleasing to God might be propagated among ecclesiastical persons and those in holy orders, we decree that where bishops, priests, deacons, subdeacons, canons regular, monks and professed lay brothers have presumed to take wives and so transgress this holy precept, they are to be separated from their partners. For we do not deem there to be a marriage which, it is agreed, has been contracted against ecclesiastical law. Furthermore, when they have separated from each other, let them do a penance commensurate with such outrageous behaviour (Tanner 1990, vol. 1, p. 198).

It is worth noting that the canon treats wives and concubines on a par. The requirements of celibacy have over the centuries caused mischief and, among other things, helped occasion the Reformation.

There were other moral points of conflict. The Church originally recognized, as Orthodoxy today still appreciates, abortion's categorical prohibition. Augustine accepted the prohibition but revised what should count as an abortion. Given Augustine's commitments to discursive reflection, he came to regard the Christian prohibition of abortion in terms of its involving the killing of a person. This led Augustine to hold that an early abortion was not the equivalent of murder, because the early embryo was not ensouled and therefore not a person ("Quaestionum in Heptateuchum," ii, 80, Patrologia Latina, XXXIV, 626). Augustine thus contributed directly to the philosophical character of the Western Christian struggle with its appreciation of the Christian prohibition of abortion.

The prohibition of abortion exists from the very beginning of the Church. For example, the *Didache*, a work probably from the latter part of the first century, lists the following prohibitions:

Thou shalt do no murder; thou shalt not commit adultery; thou shalt not commit sodomy; thou shalt not commit fornication; thou shalt not steal; thou shalt not use magic; thou shalt not use philtres; thou shalt not procure abortion, nor commit infanticide; thou shalt not covet thy neighbour's goods; thou shalt not commit perjury, thou shalt not bear false witness; thou shalt not speak evil; thou shalt not bear malice. Thou shalt not be double-minded nor double-tongued, for to be double-tongued is the snare of death. Thy speech shall not be false nor vain, but completed in action. Thou shalt not be covetous nor extortionate, nor a hypocrite, nor malignant, nor proud, thou shalt make no evil plan against thy neighbour. Thou shalt hate no man; but some thou shalt reprove, and for some shalt thou pray, and some thou shalt love more than thine own life (The Didache 1965, pp. 311, 313, II.2–7).[8]

The original prohibition was independent of any view of when ensoulment occurs. St. Basil the Great reaffirmed the Orthodox position regarding abortion as a *sui generis* prohibition when he stated: "She who has deliberately destroyed a fetus has to pay the penalty of murder. And there is no exact inquiry among us as to whether the fetus was formed or unformed" (St. Basil 1955, vol. 2, p. 12).[9] This categorical prohibition of abortion accords with one of the laws given to the sons of Noah.[10] However, the Western church recapitulated the distorting effect of philosophical reflections, as had occurred previously with the Alexandrian school of theology, which had also been dominated by philosophical concerns that nested Origen's teaching within speculations, leading to their condemnation. Roman Catholic moral-philosophical reflections regarding abortion focused Roman Catholic thought on the question of when the soul enters the embryo.

Given the influence of Aristotelian philosophy on Roman Catholicism, especially given Aristotle's argument that the rational soul enters the body only after conception (40 days for males and 80–90 days for females [*De Generatione Animalium* 2.3.736a–b and *Historia Animalium* 7.3.583b]), beginning in the 13th century Western theologians such as Thomas Aquinas held that early abortion was not the equivalent of the taking of a human life.[11] The consequence was that in Western canon law early abortion was not treated as murder[12] from 1234[13] to the revision of canon law in 1917 that went into effect on 19 May 1918 (Denzinger 1965, p. 704), save for the period between 1588–1591 (Sixtus 1588). The underlying dogma supporting the recognition that early abortion is murder was once more firmly in place for Roman Catholics as of at least 1854.[14] The point is that Augustine took one of the major steps to conforming Western Christianity's morality to the requirements of moral philosophy, which meant that dogma was changed as philosophical fashions changed. The transformation of Western Christian moral theology into a form of moral philosophy, or at least into a moral theology bound by constraints and moved by goals set by moral philosophy, had been accomplished by the late 13th century.

Other defining dogmas of Western Christianity can also be connected with Augustine. Contrary to the Nicene-Constantinopolitan Creed (the Latin text of which regarding the Holy Spirit reads, "ex Patre procedentem"; *Conciliorum* 1962, p. 20) and to John 15:26 ("When the Advocate comes, whom I will send to you from the Father, the Spirit of truth who proceeds from the Father, he will testify on my behalf"), Augustine argued for the novel position that the Holy Spirit proceeds not just from the Father but also from the Son, because of which the term *filioque* (and from the Son) was inserted into the Creed (Augustine, *de*

Trinitatem Book XV, §27.48). The result was that the West lost the appreciation of the truth that all comes from one Person, the fully transcendent Father. A quite different way of turning to and experiencing God emerged that had its origin in philosophical-theological reflection, rather than in theological experience. The West no longer experienced all coming from the Father Who begets the Son and gives procession to the Holy Spirit.

Also unlike the Church of the Apostles and the early Fathers,[15] Augustine held that telling a falsehood with the intention to deceive was always forbidden. "Mendacium est locutio contra mentem ad fallendum prolata (S. Aug. contra Mendacium c.4)" (Génicot 1902, vol. 1, §413, p. 390). In this he framed a novel moral understanding of how, among other things, one ought to act in defending the innocent (Ramsey 1985). When the Nazis come to the door looking for Jews, the Orthodox tell the most effective lie possible in order to defend them, rather than to craft some statement of the truth that one hopes will deceive. In contrast with Augustine, St. John Cassian the Just Roman (360–432) states:

> Holy men and those most approved by God employed lying, so as not only to incur no guilt of sin from it, but even to attain the greatest goodness; and if deceit could confer glory on them, what on the other hand would the truth have brought them but condemnation? Just as Rahab, of whom Scripture gives a record not only of no good deed but actually of unchastity, yet simply for the lie, by means of which she preferred to hide the spies instead of betraying them, had it vouchsafed to her to be joined with the people of God in everlasting blessing. But if she had preferred to speak the truth and to regard the safety of the citizens, there is no doubt that she and all her house would not have escaped the coming destruction, nor would it have been vouchsafed to her to be inserted in the progenitors of our Lord's nativity, and reckoned in the list of the patriarchs, and through her descendants that followed, to become the mother of the Saviour of all (Cassian 1994, vol. 11, p. 465).

Contrary to Augustine, Christianity had recognized that one ought to tell a falsehood with the intention to deceive in order to protect life, preserve chastity, and avoid idolatry and blasphemy.

Last but not least, Augustine also laid the basis for the Western doctrine of original sin, which eventually led to the Calvinist dogma of predestination.[16] Were human nature fully corrupt, could one ever freely turn to God's redemptive grace, or must one receive special grace in order to ask for grace and thus be predestined?

All of these developments contributed to Christianity in the West taking on a novel character that set it apart and eventually separated it and the bioethics it would produce from the Christianity of the first centuries. The character of the Christianity of the West already had a distinctly different texture, beginning at least with the creation of a rival Western Christian empire as a consequence of Pope Leo III crowning Charles the Great as emperor after the third Mass on Christmas, 800. As James Bryce aptly puts it, "The coronation of Charles is not only the central event of the Middle Ages, it is also one of those very few events of which, taking them singly, it may be said that if they had not happened, the history of the world would have been different" (Bryce 1959, p. 41). This act of coronation effectively divided what had been one Christian empire, one Christendom. Of course, Fyodor Dostoevsky places the defining change earlier with the Donations of Pepin (A.D. 745, 756), by which the pope was established not only as priest, but also king, as the ruler of a secular state.[17] In any event, the crowning did create an effective, though not complete, separation of the West from the original vision of a united Christendom.

The West by the mid-9th century in its views regarding priestly celibacy, the status of the early embryo, the nature of God (i.e., the Trinity), the morality of lying, the meaning of free choices, and the authority of the pope of Rome was becoming manifestly different from the original Christianity of the first seven councils. Western Christianity had changed the traditional Wednesday fast to Saturday, and employed unleavened bread for the Eucharist, even though the Gospels and St. Paul's Letter to the Romans say that Christ took *artos*, a loaf of bread, not unleavened bread.[18] Areas of the West had begun no longer to abstain from fish, eggs, and dairy on days of fasting. Also, men were at least nominally required to be celibate if they became priests. These theological differences, combined with the *filioque* and the growing papal claims to universal jurisdiction, led to the excommunication in A.D. 867 of Pope Nicholas I (*c.* 800–867, elected

858) by St. Photios the Great (*c.* 810–*c.* 893, patriarch 858–867 and 877–886), and finally to Rome being removed from the diptychs in 1009.

A new understanding of church had arisen. It continued to grow through the dialectic of the roles of king and priest. On this point, Pope Gregory VII, Hildebrand (*c.* 1015–1083, elected 1073), transformed Western Christianity further. Western Christianity became an ecclesial community with an imperial papacy that claimed the authority to depose kings and emperors, which claims brought Heinrich IV to submission at Canossa in 1077. Struggles between pope and emperor continued, through which the temporal power of the pope came to eclipse that of the emperor. Finally, out of the dialectic of the struggle with King Philip IV of France (1268–1314, crowned 1285), papal claims of robust spiritual and temporal authority were articulated by Pope Boniface VIII in 1302 in his bull *Unam sanctam* including authority over all sovereigns of the world. Ironically, this occurred just before the papacy moved to France in 1305 with Pope Clement V. By the Fourth Lateran Council (A.D. 1215) and the Second Council of Lyons (A.D. 1274), the Roman Catholic dogma of the pope's universal original jurisdiction had created an ecclesial structure that was non-conciliar and in which the pope was in an important sense the one and only bishop with full episcopal authority. (This assertion of consummate episcopal authority was expressed, for example, when Pope Paul VI signed Vatican II's "Declaration on the Relationship of the Church to Non-Christian Religions" [*Nostra aetate*], as well as other declarations, as "I, Paul, Bishop of the Catholic Church" [Abbott 1966, p. 668].) But by the end of the 13th century, papal authority had reached a zenith.

The papacy maintained the upper hand in Western Europe, although this became difficult when, after 1378, there was both a pope of Rome and one of Avignon, and even more complicated with three popes after a pope was installed in Pisa as of 1409. As a consequence, the papacy spent much of its social and spiritual capital on the Avignon papacy (1309–1376) and then on the feuding of two and subsequently three separate, sparring popes of Rome (Urban VI, 1378–1389; Boniface IX, 1389–1404; Innocent VII, 1404–1406; Gregory XII, 1406–1415), of Avignon (Clement VIII, 1378–1394; Benedict XIII, 1394–1415), and of Pisa (Alexander V, 1409–1410; and John XXIII, 1410–1415).[19] The monarchical papacy was not set aside by the Conciliar movement, which temporarily asserted the authority of ecumenical councils at the Council of Constance (1414–1418), and which reduced the number of concurrent popes from three down to Martin V of Rome, who was elected in 1417. In important ways, the West remained crippled after the Council of Ferrara-Florence (Ferrara 1438–1439, Florence 1439, Rome 1439–1445, which continued the Council of Basil of 1431). Less than eighty years after the Council of Ferrara-Florence, the West shattered irrevocably as the Reformation began. The result was the emergence of a distinctively new ecclesial structure.

The most significant change defining the character of the new Western Christianity with major implications for the emergence of a morality and bioethics anchored in moral-philosophical hopes was a change in the character and understanding of theology. The early Renaissance of pagan Greek learning effected by Charles the Great had achieved a subtle but eventually monumental change in how the West regarded theology. Charles's interest in encouraging learning in the West led to the establishment of his Palatine School in Aachen, as well as cathedral schools throughout the Western empire. By the 12th century, there were strong anticipations of the Scholastic philosophical synthesis that would finally be forged in Paris in the 13th century. One might in particular think of the intellectual community that developed in Chartres. But it was in Paris where already in the 12th century anticipations of this synthesis of faith and reason were manifest. By the 12th century, Paris possessed a *de facto* university that had emerged from the cathedral school of Notre Dame and could boast such members as Peter Lombard (*c.* 1096–1164), the author of *Libri Quattuor Sententiarum*. In 1208, the University of Paris existed formally. It was in this environment that a full-fledged synthesis of faith and reason, of *fides et ratio*, was articulated, engendering a theology guided by philosophical rationality. Philosophy, which had been introduced as the handmaid of theology, became a ruling mistress.[20] Combined with a new ecclesiology and new doctrines (e.g., purgatory and indulgences), along with the changes in the character of day-to-day life (e.g., the presence of an officially celibate priesthood and changes in the fasts), this new theological perspective constituted a paradigm change in what it is to be the Church.

Western Christianity and its history are complex. Not all Western Christianity has labored in the shadow of Aristotle. For example, the Franciscan William of Ockham (*c.* 1288–*c.* 1348), who both studied and taught at Oxford, along with the *via moderna* he embraced and transformed, understood that the God Who lives is the God Who commands, and that He is not constrained by limits that philosophers might seek to establish. When William of Ockham fled Avignon and Pope John XXII in 1328 for the protection of Emperor Ludwig (reigned 1328–1347), who promised to protect William with his sword if William would protect him with his pen, Ockham had rejected a critical element of the 13th-century philosophical synthesis. The *via moderna* movement as Ockham affirmed it recognized the radical transcendence of God. The movement appreciated that the Lawgiver is eternal, although not His law.[21] Moreover, it understood that His law does not flow from, nor is it justified through, secular moral rationality. Therefore, God's law cannot be constrained by the moral requirements of a philosophically grounded natural law.

Supporters of this *via moderna*, and those who in general embrace the theocentric horn of Euthyphro's dilemma, can appropriately be characterized as authentic fundamentalists, given their recognition of the radically transcendent character of God and the grounds for His moral requirements, which sets them beyond the demands of Rawls's notion of the politically reasonable. They reject the secular culture's claims regarding the priority of its secular moral vision, along with its view of the morally rational and/or of the politically reasonable. They constituted a full reaction against the Thomistic Aristotelianism of the mid-13th century. This *via moderna* was ironically closer to the theological position of the ancient Church than the so-called *via antiqua* that emerged in the 12th and 13th centuries in the West.

Because of Western Christian medieval theology's defining engagement with moral philosophy, and despite the *via moderna* and its consequences, including its influence on Martin Luther (1483–1546), morality and eventually even bioethics for Roman Catholicism emerged in the West as a third thing between God and man. Morality, at least for modernity and the Enlightenment, became what it had been for most Greek philosophers, namely, a fabric of norms that were supposedly derivable from and justified by philosophy apart from a recognition of God. The Western Middle Ages (apart from the *via moderna*, especially with William of Ockham) in general embraced the rationalistic horn of Euthyphro's dilemma, holding that God affirmed the good, the right, and the virtuous because they are so and are independent of Him, rather than holding that the good, the right, and the virtuous can only be such insofar as they are directed to the Holy. The embrace of the rationalist horn lies at the roots of modernity and contemporary secularity. It made it seem plausible that one can know the nature of the moral life apart from God, leading to the view that moral philosophy can be approached as a fully secular undertaking. This in turn led to the view that a secular culture could be a rightly directed moral culture. Indeed, it is not hyperbole to say that contemporary secularity, along with contemporary bioethics, was made possible by Western Christianity's faith in moral philosophy, which served as a necessary bridge from the world of the Middle Ages to modernity, and from the Enlightenment—through the failure of the Western moral-philosophical project—to contemporary post-modern secularity. This faith in discursive reason promised to make moral philosophy the master of morality.

The contemporary character of the secularization of the West, including its secular bioethics, thus has important, albeit complex, roots in the Western Christian High Middle Ages. Against the background of the history of ideas so far laid out, the question is how closely these developments are tied to Western culture and Western Christianity. Could things have been different? Is the contemporary world necessarily secular? Is it the necessary outcome of history? How closely is the contemporary secularity of the West tied to Western Christianity's dialectic of faith and reason? Because of the dominance of Western culture and power, how closely is the secularity of the dominant global culture tied to the rationalism and subsequent secularization of the West? Could the history of the West have been different?

IV. Could Things Have Been Otherwise?
A Brief Exploration of Islam's Rejection of an
Aristotelian Transformation of Traditional Belief

Contemporary Muslim culture, along with its dominant view of morality and bioethics, stands in stark contrast with the dominant secular culture of the West. While there has been an increasing secularization of Western Christian culture, and though the history of Islamic thought is complex (Fakhry 2004; Hourani 1985), there has if anything been a desecularization of the Muslim cultural sphere. Islam has remained relatively immune to secularization, and, save for Turkey with Mustafa Kemal Atatürk (1881–1938), immune to aggressive, state-supported secularization. The kemalist ideology, which Atatürk engendered, surely did reach beyond the boundaries of Turkey and even influenced Iran until Ayatollah Khomeini (1902–1989) and the traditionalist revolution of 1979. Among other things, kemalism shaped nasserism, the secularist movement founded by Gamal Abdel Nasser (1918–1970), which led to the execution of Sayyid Qutb (1906–1966) of the Egyptian Muslim Brotherhood. However, despite these significant secularist movements, Muslim countries have not been secularized in the ways that have transformed Western Europe and the Americas. In short, while there has been secularization, it has been trivial in comparison with what has occurred in the West. Over the last half-century, there has even been a desecularization of the dominant culture within the Muslim cultural sphere. This Muslim counter-example to the seemingly inexorable march of secularization is rooted in a number of factors. Only one will be explored in any detail here, namely, the crucial role played by Abu Hamid Muhammad ibn Muhammad al-Ghazali (1058–1111) in bringing into focus forces that established a powerful hermeneutic of suspicion regarding the role of philosophy in theology. Al-Ghazali recognized in Greek philosophy, which had been tied to the secularization of 5th century Athens, a threat to the integrity of the Muslim faith. Through al-Ghazali, philosophy, but especially moral philosophy, in particular the moral theology shaped by Greek philosophy, was brought into question as a threat to appreciating the importance, character, and content of revelation.[22]

By the early 9th century, a vibrant interest in Aristotle had developed as a part of a Renaissance of Greco-Roman learning in the Levant, in particular in Baghdad. The philosopher Abu Ya'qub al-Kindi (c. 801–873) followed by Abu Nasr al-Farabi (c. 870–950) produced extensive commentaries on Aristotle that were influencing Muslim religious thought with views derived from pagan Greece. These cultural developments by the late 10th century had already begun significantly to transform Muslim theology and religious understanding, as would happen later in 13th-century Western Christianity. The impact was significant. By the dawn of the 11th century, the philosopher and physician Avicenna (Ibn Sina, A.D. 980–1037) was applying Aristotelian views to a range of matters, including theology. Avicenna did not directly deny the claims of the

Koran, even though he held that philosophy could through reason establish its own truths (Avicenna, n.d.). Muslim culture influenced by Aristotle was pressed to accept a new set of philosophical truths, which were held to be independent of, and often in tension if not in contradiction with, the dogmas of the Muslim faith.

The crucial turn away from what would have been a Muslim Scholasticism was set in motion in the mid-9th century when a reaction began to develop against the Mu'tazilites, whose view was that the Koran was created at the time of its revelation, embedded in its particular socio-historical context, and subject to philosophical critical analysis. The Mu'tazilites supported a rational theology (*kalam*), philosophical disputations (*gadal*), and more generally philosophy (*falsafa*). Among other things, the Mu'tazilites held that sacred precedent was not sufficient to establish Muslim law. This all began to change in Baghdad with the caliphate of Ja'far Mutawakkil (822–861, reigned beginning in 847), after which the legal tradition of the Hanbalites with their rejection of the philosophical analysis of the Koran gained ascendancy. The law was to be followed, not critically reassessed by scholars (i.e., there was a rejection of *ijihad*, interpretation). Ahmad ibn Hanbal (780–855) opposed the view of the Mu'tazilites, and the Hanbalites succeeded in largely transforming Islamic culture into one grounded on a strict interpretation of its jurisprudence. The Mu'tazilites were also opposed by the Ash'arite school founded by Abu Hasan al-Ash'ari (873–935). At the age of forty, al-Ash'ari broke from the Mu'tazilite school and its rationalist theology, rejecting philosophical reflections on the demands of the Muslim religion. The Ash'arite school affirmed a thoroughgoing voluntarism with regard to God and a determinacy with regard to human will and all reality. Indeed, reality was regarded as created every moment anew by the will of God. For the Ash'arites, reality had no rational structure.

Al-Ghazali took a step beyond that of the Ash'arites, who, though they rejected a philosophical critique of Muslim belief, still used philosophy to defend Muslim views. In the summer of 1095, al-Ghazali rejected the philosophy of Aristotle and philosophy in general, turning to embrace what he took to be the authentic core of Muslim faith. Admittedly, Islam has many faces, some of which are still shaped by philosophy.[23] Nevertheless, al-Ghazali achieved a watershed appreciation of the threat to traditional religious belief from Greek pagan philosophy. Al-Ghazali's rupture from the secular thought of his day was driven by his concern to free the Muslim faith from the threat of being recast in terms not dictated by God, but by Greek pagan philosophy. Al-Ghazali realized that if philosophy became integral to theology and culture (as it would in Western Christianity), then the faith could be, indeed would be, recast in philosophy's terms. Al-Ghazali recognized that a philosophical shift in cultural paradigm threatened to marginalize traditional Muslim religious commitments.

This realization led al-Ghazali to erect a set of commitments that have served to protect the Muslim faith and culture against secularization through philosophy's reshaping the character of faith. In particular, due to al-Ghazali, important elements of Muslim culture have internalized a hermeneutic of suspicion against the pagan Greek philosophers, who had begun to influence major segments of society in late-11th-century Baghdad. The influences of Greek pagan philosophical thought had been so substantial and broadly in place that they had already established a dialectic of faith and reason, of *fides et ratio*, through which discursive rationality was transforming and secularizing the Muslim faith, as had also already begun with Christianity in the West. But given the response of al-Ghazali, this process was reversed and this transformation did not occur. Put more generally, al-Ghazali returned Islam to the theocentric pole of Euthyphro's dilemma.

The criticism mounted against Greek philosophy by al-Ghazali was multifaceted. In his monumental *The Incoherence of the Philosophers*, al-Ghazali penned a response to the transformation of faith and practice threatened by the influence of pagan views of God and reality. In particular, he faulted philosophers because of their rejection of revealed religious truth and of an experience of or encounter with God. As he argued, those in the Levant influenced by Greek philosophy no longer recognized what it was to acknowledge the transcendent God, Who is not the god of philosophers.

(2) I have seen a group who, believing themselves in possession of a distinctiveness from companion and peer by virtue of a superior quick wit and intelligence, have rejected the Islamic duties regarding acts of worship, disdained religious rites pertaining to the offices of prayer and the avoidance of prohibited things, belittled the devotions and ordinances prescribed by

the divine law, not halting in the face of its prohibitions and restrictions. On the contrary, they have entirely cast off the reins of religion through multifarious beliefs, following therein a troop "who rebel away from God's way, intending to make it crooked, who are indeed disbelievers in the hereafter" [Quran 11:19] (Al-Ghazali 2000, pp. 1–2).

Al-Ghazali was committed to preventing Islam from being recast in terms external to its faith. He acted to focus Muslims anew on what it is to accept a God Who reveals Himself.

One of his major points of response was in harmony with a critique made by St. John Chrysostom and others, namely, that the pagan philosophers had not established a canonical morality or metaphysics that could trump the demands of faith, but had instead produced a cacophony of diverse accounts.

(7) ... I took it upon myself to write this book in refutation of the ancient philosophers, to show the incoherence of their belief and the contradiction of their word in matters relating to metaphysics; to uncover the dangers of their doctrine and its shortcomings, which in truth ascertainable are objects of laughter for the rational and a lesson for the intelligent—I mean the kinds of diverse beliefs and opinions they particularly hold that set them aside from the populace and the common run of men (Al-Ghazali 2000, p. 3).

Greek philosophy had promised a unified moral and metaphysical vision. This promise, al-Ghazali recognized, had not been kept, nor could it be kept. Rather than Greek philosophy establishing a unified moral and metaphysical vision, philosophy disclosed an intractable plurality of moral and metaphysical positions. Against this scandal of the failure of Greek philosophy to secure a canonical moral and metaphysical vision, al-Ghazali turned to what he took to be a God Who discloses Himself in a written text.

Al-Ghazali set in motion a critical rejection of the role of Greek philosophy in Muslim religious thought that continued long after his death. This critical rejection of pagan philosophical influences reversed the career of one of the most important intellectuals and scholars of the 12th century in the Muslim cultural domain, a man who had been influenced by Greek thought and who attempted to reshape the Muslim faith: the polymathic philosopher, physician, judge, and astronomer Averroes (Ibn Rushd, 1126–1198). Averroes had gone further than Avicenna in holding that philosophy provided the clearer and more cultivated presentation of matters in areas of theological truth. Indeed, following Averroes, it was held that the truths of philosophy were independent of, and not necessarily identical with, the truths of the faith grounded in the Koran. In response to al-Ghazali's *The Incoherence of the Philosophers*, Averroes published *The Incoherence of the Incoherence* (Averroes 2008). Al-Ghazali's rejection of this doctrine of "double truth," that there were truths of philosophy that existed independent of and apart from the truths of faith, strengthened the reaction against the project of accommodating Muslim belief to the demands of philosophy. Among other things, this reaction forced Averroes to leave Cordoba and die in exile in Morocco. The Jewish thinker Moses Maimonides (A.D. 1135–1204), who also was heavily influenced by Greek thought, abandoned Cordoba under similar pressure. He died in Cairo.

Al-Ghazali recognized that Greek philosophy could not authoritatively disclose the nature of God or His requirements, from which insight he developed a complex appreciation of the danger to faith from embedding faith and theology within a philosophical framework. As a consequence, a Muslim scholasticism did not develop as it did in the Christian West, where Scholasticism transformed Christianity. The position of al-Ghazali regarding the dangers of pagan philosophy has strong family resemblances with the *via moderna*, William of Ockham, and Orthodox Christianity, which in its Ninth Ecumenical Council (1341, 1347, 1351) condemned philosophy. Metropolitan Hierotheos summarizes the Council:

> In the whole text of the "Synodikon of Orthodoxy" it is seen clearly that philosophy is condemned. Both the way in which philosophy refers to and presents God and the conclusions to which it comes are condemned. And of course, in speaking of philosophy, we mean metaphysics as it was developed by Plato, Aristotle and other, later philosophers. . . . Yet it is not these works of the philosophers that are anathematised, but the fact that the teachings of the philosophers are preferred to the Faith, and that philosophy is used to distort the truth of the Church. It is not forbidden to study the works of the ancient Greeks, that is, of the pagans, but those Christians are reproached

who follow and accept their futile theories. Anathema is pronounced "on those who accept the Greek teachings, not on those who only cultivate them for culture, but on those who also follow these futile doctrines of theirs." And as we said before, those are censured who prefer "the foolish so-called wisdom of the profane philosophers" to the orthodox teaching (Hierotheos 1998, pp. 226–227).

The West in contrast came ever more to embrace the Scholasticism that Aristotle had helped engender. Unlike Islam and Orthodox Christianity, beginning in the 12th but especially in the 13th century, Western Christianity framed an intellectual edifice of thought that placed Christian faith and theology within a philosophical framework. Secular bioethics would later emerge within this rationalist framework. The Scholasticism that developed eventually produced a culture that supported a turn to secular modernity and to the Enlightenment, so that a secular culture came to be dominant in the West. Orthodox Christians escaped this Scholastic transformation. Al-Ghazali rescued Islam from this fate and contributed a critical basis on which later traditionalist Muslim movements could build.

Others like al-Ghazali recognized that, were philosophy to be core to theology, belief in God would be rendered into a theological philosophy cast in secular terms. Muhammad ibn 'Abd al-Wahhab (1703–1792), for example, in the spirit of al-Ghazali also argued for a return to the original principles of the Muslim faith. The Wahhabists, to which al-Wahhab gave issue, have supported the Hanbalists, totally rejecting any philosophical exegesis or re-interpretation of the Koran. They have become a major element of contemporary Muslim fundamentalism and desecularization (al-Uthaymin 2009). In particular, Wahhabism has gained wide influence and this movement has become an important religious force because of the commitment and support of the kingdom of Saudi Arabia. Wahhabism along with other currents of traditionalism has succeeded, for better and often for worse, in generally protecting the Muslim cultural domain from the secularization that has transformed, indeed radically changed the West. Among other things, al-Ghazali and his followers immunized their faith against the dialectic of *fides et ratio* that in the end reshaped, secularized, and disestablished Western Christianity by recasting belief and morality in terms of the requirements of a secular, indeed pagan philosophy. The Muslim cultural domain thus was able to avoid the secularization that defines the once Christian West.

It was the Christian West in transition to being post-Christian that produced the secular morality and bioethics that emerged in America in the 1970s. This development of bioethics was preceded by secular reflections on the contributions of medicine to the health of the state (Castro 1614; Rau 1764; Frank 1779) and on professional medical ethics (Gregory 1770; Percival 1803). In the shadow of the Enlightenment, a space opened for secular medical-ethical discourse and reflection. It was the beginning of a medical ethics for a culture after God. In contrast, the dominant life-world of the Muslim cultural sphere has resisted the Western European demoralization and deflation of morality and bioethics. Its bioethics remains embedded within a religious framework.

V. From a Faith in Reason to a Commitment to a Political Agenda

We are brought back to the themes addressed at the end of chapter three: the Hegelian relocation of morality (and eventually bioethics) within the perspective of the state that exists because of the West's secularization. While Islam located the state within the demands of obligations to God through the re-establishment, to various degrees, of sharia in many contemporary Muslim countries, the West has been confronted with the ungrounded character of the liberal morality and bioethics that took shape from the Enlightenment and the French Revolution. Confronted with the collapse of the Western moral project, the West is now marked by the force of the turn recognized by Hegel and through which the liberal moral commitments of the Enlightenment and the French Revolution have become the substance of a social-democratic account of the politically reasonable. The power of the state has been invoked to substitute for the failed power of reason so as to secure a quasi-morality and the remaining hopes of bioethics. A political agenda has come to substitute for a moral agenda.

This state of affairs has produced a secular jihad against traditional religious belief and practices in general, and against Christian and Muslim traditional belief and practice in particular. The neo-conservative American adventures into the Levant are an expression of this policy agenda. If the Soviet commitment to an atheistic society and public policy is regarded as the second wave of aggressive secularization following the French Revolution, the European Union has epitomized the third wave. The result has been the emergence of truly secular fundamentalist states, states in which a secular ideology is established with the same totalizing force as a religion is established within a religious fundamentalist state (Engelhardt 2010a, 2010b). The next chapter addresses the secular fundamentalist state, a phenomenon born of the West's attempt to define society in secular terms. The focus in chapter five is on how this is expressed in an attempted secular transformation of bioethics and the health care professions in the West. For this now-dominant secular culture, the pursuit of its moral agenda has been recast into a political agenda. The secularization of bioethics and of the professions is integral to the redefinition of the life-world of social-democratic polities. The disestablishment of Western Christendom and the collapse of the moral-philosophical project have led in turn to the establishment of the secular fundamentalist state with its commitment to purge the public forum, and indeed the public space, of any mention of, much less orientation to, God. This political agenda involves cleansing the public culture from all reference to the transcendent, to ultimate meaning. This religious cleansing requires the secularization of morality, bioethics, health care, and the health care professions. The West had no al-Ghazali to protect it from radical secularization.

Notes

[1]This chapter has been developed from a lecture, "The Deflation of Morality: Rethinking the Secularization of the West," given originally at the University of Salento, Lecce, Italy, on 1 February 2012. Distantly ancestral versions of some of the material in this chapter were also given as lectures: "Religion, Politics, and the State: Rethinking Morality in Modern Secularized Societies," Politeia, University of Milan, January 30, 2012, and "Religion, Politics, and the State in Modern Secularized Societies," Comune di Napoli, February 6, 2012.

[2]In Orthodox Christianity, the ascetic life is recognized as a necessary condition for doing theology in the strict sense. In describing the journey towards union with God, the journey of theology, Metropolitan Hierotheos states: "The stage of illumination constitutes the first dispassion. A characteristic trait of this level is the knowledge of beings; the 'theoria' of the causes of beings and the participation in the Holy Spirit. The benefits of illumination are the purification of nous by the divine grace, which consumes the heart like fire; the noetic

revelation of the 'eye of the heart' and the birth of the Word within the nous, expressed in noble sense. In other words, in this state man acquires knowledge of God and unceasing noetic prayer. Moreover, man comes to know things human and divine and experiences the revelation of the mysteries of the kingdom of Heaven" (Hierotheos 1994, p. 50).

³ As St. Paul emphasizes, if one worships the creature rather than the Creator, one's life will be distorted. "For this reason [worshipping the creature rather than the Creator] God gave them up to degrading passions. Their women exchanged natural intercourse for unnatural, and in the same way also the men, giving up natural intercourse with women, were consumed with passion for one another. Men committed shameless acts with men and received in their own persons the due penalty for their error. And since they did not see fit to acknowledge God, God gave them up to a debased mind and to things that should not be done" (Romans 1:26–28).

⁴ As St. Paul argues regarding those who did not worship the Creator: "for though they knew God, they did not honor Him as God or give thanks to Him, but they became futile in their thinking, and their senseless minds were darkened" (Romans 1:21).

⁵ The passage in Romans 2 about the law written in our hearts reads: "When gentiles, who do not possess the law, do instinctively what the law requires, these, though not having the law, are a law to themselves. They show that what the law requires is written on their hearts, to which their own conscience also bears witness; and their conflicting thoughts will accuse or perhaps excuse them" (Romans 2:14–15).

⁶ St. John Chrysostom, for example, underscores the noetic knowledge of a true theologian such as St. John the Evangelist. Regarding him, Chrysostom says: "For when a barbarian and untaught person utters things which no man on earth ever knew," this "affords another and a stronger proof that what he says is divinely inspired, namely, convincing all his hearers through all time; who will not wonder at the power that dwells in him?" (Chrysostom 1994a, Homily II.4 on the Gospel according to St. John, vol. 14, p. 5). Chrysostom combines this account of St. John the Evangelist's noetic knowledge with a criticism of philosophy.

> The human soul is simply unable thus to philosophize on that pure and blessed nature; on the powers that come next to it; on immortality and endless life; on the nature of mortal bodies which shall hereafter be immortal; on punishment and the judgment to come; on the enquiries that shall be as to deeds and words, as to thoughts and imaginations. It cannot tell what is man, what the world; what is man indeed, and what he who seems to be man, but is not; what is the nature of virtue, what of vice (Chrysostom 1994a, Homily II.3, vol. 14, p. 5).

⁷ At the Council of Nicea (A.D. 325),

> . . . Paphnutius, the confessor, stood up and testified against this proposition; he said that marriage was honorable and chaste, and that cohabitation with their own wives was chastity, and advised the Synod not to frame such a law, for it would be difficult to bear, and might serve as an occasion of incontinence to them and their wives; and he reminded them, that according to the ancient tradition of the church, those who were unmarried when they took part in the communion of sacred orders, were

required to remain so, but that those who were married, were not to put away their wives. Such was the advice of Paphnutius, although he was himself unmarried, and in accordance with it, the Synod concurred in his counsel, enacted no law about it, but left the matter to the decision of individual judgment, and not to compulsion (Sozomen 1994, "The Ecclesiastical History" §XXIII, vol. 2, p. 256).

[8]Prohibitions against abortion and infanticide are recorded as well in "The Epistle of Barnabas," a 2nd-century work. "Thou shalt not procure abortion, thou shalt not commit infanticide" (Barnabas 1965, p. 403, XIX.5).

[9]The editor of the translation of St. Basil's remarks notes: "By a 'formed' fetus is meant one in which the rational soul has already been infused; by an 'unformed' fetus is understood one in which the rational soul has not yet been infused. The distinction between the formed and the unformed fetus is recognized in Exodus 21:22–23 (LXX)" (St. Basil 1955, vol. 2, p. 12).

[10]Orthodox Jews recognize a prohibition of abortion that applies to the Gentiles. The Jews knew that seven laws had been given to Noah and his sons. "Seven precedents were the sons of Noah commanded: social laws; to refrain from blasphemy; idolatry; adultery; bloodshed; robbery; and eating flesh cut from a living animal." R. Hanania b. Gamaliel said: Also not to partake of the blood drawn from a living animal (Sanhedrin 56a). A Jewish court, giving a gloss on the prohibition against bloodshed, at the time of Christ held "[A son of Noah is executed] even for the murder of an embryo. What is R. Ishmael's reason?—Because it is written, Whose sheddeth the blood of man within [another] man, shall his blood be shed. What is a man within another man?—An embryo in his mother's womb" (Sanhedrin 57b).

[11]Thomas Aquinas's arguments regarding the rational soul entering only some time after conception involve restatements of Aristotle's position. See *Summa Theologica* I, 118, art. 2, as well as II, II, 64, art. 8. See also Aquinas commenting on Aristotle's *Politics* and Aristotle's proposed use of abortion: Aquinas 1875a, vol. 26, p. 484, Book VII, Lectio XII. Aquinas also addressed this issue in his Commentary on the Sentences of Peter Lombard: Aquinas 1875b, vol. 11, p. 127.

[12]For the history of the development in canon law of a distinction between the metaphysical and moral significance of early versus late abortion, see Corpus Juris Canonici Emendatum et Notis Illustratum cum Glossae: decretalium d. Gregorii Papae Noni Compilatio (Rome, 1585), *Glossa ordinaria* at book 5, title 12, §20, p. 1713.

[13]On the 5th of September, 1234, Pope Gregory IX declared in his bull, *Rex pacificus*, that his *Corpus Iuris Canonici* was the official code of canon law for Roman Catholics. Gregory IX's decretals incorporated material from Gratian's collection of canon law, the *Decretum Gratiania* or *Concordia discordantium canonum*. This code distinguished between early abortion, which does not involve an ensouled fetus, and later abortion when the fetus is ensouled.

[14]The Roman Catholic debate as to when the rational soul enters the body after conception both influenced and was influenced by Roman Catholic reflections on the date to be set for the conception of Mary, the mother of God. This was tied as well to the novel Roman Catholic doctrine of the immaculate conception. The view at first was that "Before the creation of Mary's soul, that which was to become her body shared the common lot; but before the creation of her soul *Mary* did not yet exist" (Nicolas 1958, p. 333). In the early 18th century,

the feast for the conception of Mary the mother of God was in Roman Catholicism set nine months before her birthday (December 8). On September 8, 1854, Pope Pius IX declared "infallibly" that Mary the mother of God was conceived immaculately, that is, without the consequences of the sin of Adam, *in primo instanti suae conceptionis* (Denzinger 1965, *Bulla Ineffabilis Deus*, p. 562), indicating that ensoulment took place at the time of conception. The distinction between early and late abortion had been effectively undermined.

[15]For a discussion of Augustine's crucial role in developing the Western Christian view that lying is always forbidden, see Ramsey 1985.

[16]Because Augustine of Hippo misread the Greek in Romans 5:12 ("Therefore, even as through one man sin entered into the world, and death through sin, thus death passed to all men, on account of which all have sinned" [*Orthodox New Testament* 1999, vol. 2, p. 98]), Augustine held that all men had inherited from Adam not just corruption, death, and through death an estrangement from God, but the guilt of Adam's sin as well. Augustine therefore contends:

> I see the apostle has most plainly taught us: That owing to one man all pass into condemnation who are born of Adam unless they are born again in Christ, even as He has appointed them to be regenerated, before they die in the body, whom He predestinated to everlasting life, as the most merciful bestower of grace; whilst to those whom He has predestinated to eternal death, He is also the most righteous awarder of punishment, not only on account of the sins which they add in the indulgence of their own will, but also because of their original sin, even if, as in the case of infants, they add nothing thereto (Augustine 1994, vol. 5, p. 361).

For a further account of the ancient Church's (as well as Orthodox Christianity's) account of original sin, see Romanides 2002.

[17]Dostoevsky criticized and condemned the radical transformation of Christianity in the West, which he saw as connected to the pope's becoming a civil ruler, thus assimilating kingship to priesthood. He appreciated the moral and theological consequences of Western Christendom's attempt directly to wield political power. "[T]he State is eliminated and the Church is raised to the position of the State. It's not simply Ultramontanism, it's arch-Ultramontanism! It's beyond the dreams of Pope Gregory the Seventh!" (Dostoevsky 1949, p. 57).

[18]With regard to the use of leavened bread in the Eucharist, see Matthew 25:26, Mark 14:22, Luke 22:19, and I Corinthians 11:23. The Greek word *artos* at the time of Christ identified a loaf of wheat bread.

[19]There are good reasons to hold that Pope John XXIII of the 15th century, who was supported by Emperor Sigismund (1368–1437) and who convoked the Council of Constance, should be considered the rightful pope of the Latins. This would mean that Pope John XXIII of the 20th century should be referred to as the so-called Pope John XXIII.

[20]Peter Damian (1007–1072) and Gerard of Czanad (†1046) engaged the phrase "handmaid of theology" (*ancilla dominae*) so as to put philosophy in a subordinate place. Their goal was not to expand the role of philosophy, but the very opposite, namely, to contain philosophy's aspirations to guide theology. Peter Damian, after all, understood that the dogmas

of Christianity are the revelation of a fully transcendent God, Who, Damian held, could undo or annihilate the past, should He wish (Copleston 1962, vol. 2.1, p. 167). The metaphor "handmaid of theology" was introduced into Christian reflection by Clement of Alexandria (ca. 150–215) in *The Stromata*, Book I, §5. For Clement, philosophy in its strict sense meant love of the wisdom of God. Clement had borrowed the metaphor "handmaid of theology" from an earlier usage by Philo the Jew (20 B.C.–A.D. 50).

[21] Again, the early Church and Orthodox Jews recognized that God at different times gave different laws to different persons, as for example in the case already noted of 7 laws being given to Noah and his sons, and 613 laws being given through Moses to the Jews. Indeed, Christ himself uses the language of divine command when He states, "a new commandment I give to you: that you love one another. Just as I have loved you, you also should love one another" (John 13:34).

[22] For overviews of Islam's response to philosophy, see Reilly 2010.

[23] For a brief introduction to the complex history of the interaction of Greek philosophy with the Muslim faith, see al-Ghazali 1999, Fakhry 2001, Griffel 2009, Nasr & Leaman 1996.

References

Abbott, Walter M. (ed.). 1966. *The Documents of Vatican II*. New York: Herder and Herder.

al-Ghazali. 2000. *The Incoherence of the Philosophers*, trans. Michael E. Marmura. Provo, Utah: Brigham Young University Press.

al-Ghazali. 1999. *Al-Ghazali's Path to Sufism*, trans. R. J. McCarthy. Louisville, KY: Fons Vitae.

al-Uthaymin, Abd Allah Salih. 2009. *Muhammad ibn 'Abd al-Wahhab: The Man and his Works*. New York: L. B. Tauris.

Aquinas, Thomas. 1875a. *Aristoteles Stagiritae: Politicorum seu de Rebus Civilibus*, in *Opera Omnia*. Paris: Vives.

Aquinas, Thomas. 1875b. *Commentum in Quartum Librum Sententiarium Magistri Petri Lombardi*, in *Opera Omnia*. Paris: Vives.

Augustine. 1994. *St. Augustine's Anti-Pelagian Writings*, trans. Peter Holmes & Robert E. Wallis, in *Nicene and Post-Nicene Fathers*, First Series, vol. 5, ed. Philip Schaff. Peabody, MA: Hendrickson.

Averroes. 2008. *The Incoherence of the Incoherence*, trans. Simon Van Den Bergh. London: E.J.W. Gibb Memorial Series.

Avicenna. n.d. *Avicenna on Theology*, trans. A. J. Arberry. Dubai: Kitab al-Islamiyyah.

Barnabas. 1965. The Epistle of Barnabas, in *Apostolic Fathers*, vol. 1 (pp. 305–333), trans. Kirsopp Lake. Cambridge, MA: Harvard University Press.

Basil, St. 1955. *Letters*, trans. Sister Agnes Clare Way, 2 vols. Washington, DC: Catholic University of America Press.

Bryce, James. 1959. The coronation as a revival of the Roman empire in the West, in *The Coronation of Charlemagne*, ed. Richard E. Sullivan (pp. 41–49). Boston: D. C. Heath.

Cassian, John. 1994. Second conference of Abbot Joseph, trans. Edgar Gibson, in *Nicene and Post-Nicene Fathers*, Second Series, vol. 11 (pp. 460–474), eds. Philip Schaff & Henry Wace. Peabody, MA: Hendrickson.

Castro, Rodericus. 1614. *Medicus-Politicus: sive de officiis medicopoliticis tractatus*. Hamburg: Frobeniano.

Chrysostom, St. John. 1994a. *Nicene and Post-Nicene Fathers*, vol. 14: *Homilies on the Gospel of Saint John*. Peabody, MA: Hendrickson Publishers.

Chrysostom, St. John. 1994b. *Nicene and Post-Nicene Fathers*, vol. 11: *Homilies on the Acts of the Apostles and the Epistle to the Romans*. Peabody, MA: Hendrickson Publishers.

Chrysostom, St. John. 1994.c *Nicene and Post-Nicene Fathers*, vol. 10: *Homilies on the Gospel of Saint Matthew*. Peabody, MA: Hendrickson Publishers.

Conciliorum Oecumenicorum Decreta. 1962. Freiburg im Breisgau: Herder.

Copleston, Frederick. 1962. *The History of Philosophy*. Garden City, NY: Image Books.

Denzinger, Henricus (ed.). 1965. *Enchiridion Symbolorum*. Freiburg in Breisgau: Herder.

Didache, The. 1965. In *Apostolic Fathers*, vol. 1 (pp. 337–409), trans. Kirsopp Lake. Cambridge, MA: Harvard University Press.

Dostoevsky, Fyodor. 1949. *The Brothers Karamazov*, trans. Constance Garnett. Garden City, NY: International Collectors Library.

Eliot, T. S. 1982. *The Idea of a Christian Society*. London: Faber and Faber.

Engelhardt, H. T., Jr. 2010a. Religion, bioethics, and the secular state: Beyond religious and secular fundamentalism, *Notizie di Politeia* 26.97: 59–79.

Engelhardt, H. T., Jr. 2010b. Political authority in the face of moral pluralism: Further reflections on the non-fundamentalist state, *Notizie di Politeia* 26.97: 91–99.

Fakhry, Majid. 2001. *Averroes*. Oxford: Oneworld.

Fakhry, Majid. 2004. *A History of Islamic Philosophy*, 3rd ed. New York: Columbia University Press.

Frank, Johann Peter. 1779. *System einer vollständigen medicinischen Polizey.* Mannheim: C.F. Schwan.

Génicot, Eduardus. 1902. *Theologiae Moralis.* Lovanii: Polleunis et Ceuterick.

Gregory, John. 1770. *Observations on the Duties and Offices of a Physician.* London: Strahan.

Griffel, Frank. 2009. *Al-Ghazali's Philosophical Theology.* New York: Oxford.

Hierotheos, Metropolitan of Nafpaktos. 1998. *The Mind of the Orthodox Church,* trans. Esther Williams. Levadia, Greece: Birth of the Theotokos Monastery.

Hierotheos, Bishop of Nafpaktos. 1994. *Orthodox Spirituality,* trans. Effie Mavromichali. Levadia, Greece: Birth of the Theotokos Monastery.

Hourani, George. 1985. *Reason and Tradition in Islamic Ethics.* Cambridge: Cambridge University Press.

Nasr, Seyyed Hossein & Oliver Leaman (eds.). 1996. *History of Islamic Philosophy.* New York: Routledge.

Nicodemus & Agapius, Sts. (eds.). 1983. *The Rudder,* trans. D. Cummings. New York: Luna Printing.

Nicolas, Marie-Joseph. 1958. The meaning of the immaculate conception in the perspectives of St. Thomas, in *The Dogma of the Immaculate Conception* (pp. 327–345), ed. E. D. O'Connor. Notre Dame, IN: University of Notre Dame Press.

Orthodox New Testament. 2000. Buena Vista, CO: Holy Apostles Convent.

Percival, Thomas. 1803. *Medical Ethics.* Manchester: Russell.

Poole, Austin Lane. 1955. *From Domesday Book to Magna Carta,* 2nd ed. Oxford: Clarendon Press.

Ramsey, Boniface. 1985. Two traditions on lying and deception in the ancient church, *Thomist* 49: 504–533.

Rau, Thomas. 1764. *Gedanken von dem Nutzen und der Nothwendigkeit einer medizinischen Policeyordnung in einem Staat.* Ulm: Stettin.

Reilly, Robert R. 2010. *The Closing of the Muslim Mind.* Wilmington, DE: ISI Books.

Romanides, John S. 2002. *The Ancestral Sin,* trans. George S. Gabriel. Ridgewood, NJ: Zephyr Publishing.

Scholasticus, Socrates. 1994. The ecclesiastical history of Socrates Scholasticus, trans. A. C. Zenos, in *Nicene and Post-Nicene Fathers,* Second Series, vol. 2 (pp. 1–178), ed. Philip Schaff. Peabody, MA: Hendrickson.

Sixtus V, Pope. 1588. *Contra procurates, Consulentes, et Consentientes, quorunque modo Abortum Constitutio.* Florence: Georgius Marescottus.

Sozomen. 1994. The ecclesiastical history of Sozomen, trans. Chester Hartranft, in *Nicene and Post-Nicene Fathers*, Second Series, vol. 2 (pp. 179–427), eds. Philip Schaff & Henry Wace. Peabody, MA: Hendrickson.

Tanner, Norman P. (ed.). 1990. *Decrees of the Ecumenical Councils*, vol. 1. Washington, DC: Georgetown University Press.

Tertullian. 1994. *Latin Christianity: Its Founder, Tertullian*, in *Ante-Nicene Fathers*, vol. 3, eds. Alexander Roberts & James Donaldson. Peabody, MA: Hendrickson Publishers.

CHAPTER FIVE

Bioethical Conflicts: Obligations to God versus Obligations to the Secular State[1]

I. Moral Conflict in a Post-Christian Culture: The Case of Conscientious Objection

Morality and bioethics are battlefields of disagreement. This chapter explores these disputes by attending to one of the cardinal battles in the culture wars: the refusal of traditional Christian physicians and health care professionals to provide forms of treatment that they recognize as forbidden by God. Such refusals, often characterized in milder terms as matters of conscientious objection, undermine the authority of the dominant secular culture and its view of the public professions. In a secular society, such refusals are thus provocative because they (1) underscore as moral choices what the dominant secular culture demands be regarded as life-style and/or death-style choices, (2) impede the provision of legally established health care services, and (3) violate what are increasingly considered to be human claim rights to those services, such as the right to receive an abortion.

As chapter two shows, the conflicts of the contemporary culture wars are not just disputes about particular normative issues. They are more importantly conflicts regarding the character and force of morality itself. In particular, the cardinal conflicts turn on the dominant secular culture's demoralization and deflation of traditional morality and bioethics, where demoralization has now become integral to a secular social-democratic political agenda. Against this background, refusals to provide medical services that support life-styles that the secular culture has accepted underscore not just an alternative moral or bioethical vision, or simply a rejection of the demoralization of traditional morality demanded by the dominant secular culture. They are in addition reactionary political acts that threaten to remoralize the public space. They refuse to accept the definitive judgment of the state regarding health care policy.

II. Medical Professionalism and the Secular Fundamentalist State

This conflict of cultures, along with moralities and bioethics, is in part a function of the dominant secular culture's affirming autonomy not just as a source of authority, but in addition as a cardinal directing value or goal. This involves not only endorsing respect for forbearance rights, but treating as canonical a particular content-full vision of proper free choice. One is held to be obliged freely to choose in conformity with very particular understandings of freedom. The result is that morally condemning autonomously chosen, peaceable, secularly accepted life-styles and death-styles is considered to be immoral because it involves a failure to accept others as free and equal sources of moral authority and personal moral truth. In addition, the condemnation of such secularly accepted life- and death-style choices in the dominant secular culture is regarded as a failure properly to appreciate the dignity and value of autonomous choices. One is not just to tolerate but to accept and affirm a bioethics of peaceable, autonomous, secular, life- and death-style choices of others. Finally, a failure to accept what traditional Christians hold to be wrong choices involves in part an affirmation of a supposed special priority of personal liberty.

Public professions as a consequence have come to be vested with the secular moral obligation both to respect the forbearance rights of others and to accord others not just a right to respect, but also to recognize their claim rights to autonomy and to offer social support for the dignity of their life-styles and death-styles, as well as the place of personal liberty. Traditional Christian health care professionals, along with their bioethics, are therefore condemned for their failure to support secularly accepted life-style choices, including homosexual life-styles. As a provocative example, one might imagine a physician's comparing for an adolescent patient the health risks of a male homosexual life-style with those of heavy smoking. Such an adverse judgment of a politically, that is, legally, accepted life-style (i.e., a homosexual life-style) will be construed as a form of morally prohibited intolerance and professional malfeasance. Indeed, traditional Christianity's "intolerance" of such life-styles, if voiced publicly, is judged to be an instance of hate speech, because such statements bring into question the moral rectitude of those exercising politically legitimate rights of self-determination in the choice of peaceable, personal life-styles and death-styles.

As we have already seen in chapter two, the dominant secular culture's commitment to a content-full view of autonomous choice requires that one acknowledge rights to mutual, positive, moral recognition not only of one's person, but of one's personal choices. This mutual, positive, moral recognition not only prohibits adversely characterizing as immoral permitted sexual life-style and death-style choices, but also requires basic professional support of secularly permitted life-styles and death-styles. That is, the dominant secular culture demands that medical professionalism and its bioethics be built around basic secular moral commitments to the advancement of very particular views of liberty, equality, human dignity, and social justice, which leads to a demand not just for moral affirmation of such life-styles, but their support through publicly recognized professions. A secular understanding of medical professionalism is then also used to advance a prohibition against Christian physicians refusing to provide medical services they know to be forbidden by God.

Medical professionalism is not univocal in meaning. The dominant secular culture seeks to establish in law and public policy its own vision of proper medical professionalism. Consider, for example, four different ways in which one can understand medical professionalism.

1. Medical professionalism as the ethos established by a free association of physicians pursuing goals to which the members, and by participation their patients, commonly agree—In this libertarian account of professionalism, the authority and rectitude of the physicians' collaborative practice of medicine is derived from the concurrence of the physicians involved and the patients who choose them as their physicians. No particular understanding of the good, the right, or the virtuous is presupposed. Instead, an understanding of medical professionalism is created through the free interaction of physicians and their patients.

2. Medical professionalism as constituted through a particular history and tradition—Although one might attempt to derive what is right in medicine, what the goods of medicine are, and what constitute the virtues of a good physician from medicine as a practice (Pellegrino & Thomasma 1988, 1981), this is not possible. This is the case in part because physicians at different times and in different places have placed different moral concerns in different rankings, thus giving different moral content to medicine as a practice. Medical professionalism in every place and epoch always has a particular socio-historically conditioned character, because medical professionalism is, at least in part, the product of a particular history set within a particular culture. One might think, for example, of the various Hippocratic traditions of medical professionalism.

3. Medical professionalism as religiously defined—Most religions possess norms limiting and directing how physicians should practice medicine. One might think of the different obligations, for example, of Orthodox Christian in contrast to Orthodox Jewish physicians.[2] In the case of both Orthodox Christian and Orthodox Jewish physicians, they will understand themselves as bound by obligations to God, which may go against societal norms and the wishes of others, as well as against particular secular socio-historically constructed understandings of medical professionalism. Health care professionals who are committed to traditional religious belief (here in particular one will find Orthodox Christians) will find themselves obliged to follow a professionalism at odds with the dominant secular understandings.

4. Medical professionalism as defined by the contemporary dominant secular culture—The culture wars of the late 20th and early 21st centuries have in part been shaped by a conflict as to what norms should be established at law and public policy to guide the practice of medicine, thus defining the character of proper medical professionalism.

These conflicts, involving incompatible views of medical professionalism, are shaped by substantively disparate views of reality, morality, and bioethics. Over against a medical professionalism that develops through the association of physicians, one that is grounded in a particular tradition, or one that derives its moral commitments from the health care professional's obligations to God, the contemporary secular vision of professionalism and its proper bioethics is rooted in the robust laicism that lies at the basis of the public policy of contemporary secular fundamentalist states.[3] This secular understanding of medical professionalism is not grounded in autonomy as permission, but in a very particular political-moral vision of the proper content and value of autonomy that requires particular choices to be made, directed by very particular understandings of liberty, equality, and human dignity. Within a society shaped by the contemporary dominant secular culture, the most strident conflicts will be between medical professionalism as secularly versus religiously defined. In this conflict, there will often be no place for compromise.

The now-dominant secular culture after God with its morality and bioethics is crucially tied to the emergence of secular fundamentalist states. Such states are committed to establishing polities that are after Christ and after God (Engelhardt 2010a, 2010b). The term secular fundamentalist state is used to identify a polity that imposes on its society a particular secular moral vision with the same zeal as a religious fundamentalist state imposes a particular religion (Engelhardt 2010c, 2010d). It frames its laws, institutions, public fora, professions, and discourse in conformity with a particular secular understanding of appropriate conduct, including a particular secular understanding of morality and of the politically reasonable. Such a state supports through state funds only its own particular secular understanding of morality and health care professionalism, so that the professions and the institutions under its control conform to the secular moral and political understanding it endorses. The secular fundamentalist state also refuses to support competing secular and religious understandings and institutions, while requiring that the discourse of the public forum and of the public space be secular in terms that it defines. As a consequence, the secular fundamentalist state requires professions, professionals, and institutions in the public space (e.g., physicians and nurses in hospitals, if not all licensed physicians and nurses) to conform in their professional functions to the dictates of the established secular-philosophical orthodoxy. In a secular fundamentalist state, civil society is shaped, directed, and constrained by the requirements of the secular fundamentalist state's established secular ideology, so that intermediate institutions insofar as possible are also recast in terms of the established secular orthodoxy (e.g., churches if they act politically will lose tax-exempt status).

The result has been a marginalization of Christian discourse and Christian moral claims regarding obligations to God. Given the laicist character of the secular state, Christian discourse and Christian moral claims have been placed within a very limited private sphere outside the public gaze, just as garbage dumps are hidden discretely outside the city limits. In particular, the dominant secular ideology has displaced, if not transformed, the role of religious discourse, religious institutions (e.g., churches), and religiously affiliated institutions (e.g., religiously affiliated hospitals), while advancing and giving salience to its own particular secular cultural commitments and institutions. Through the force of the secular fundamentalist state, the established laicist ideology has relegated the religious concerns of believers within the secular fundamentalist state to a circumscribed and shrinking sphere of privacy (Engelhardt 2010a, p. 72).

The emergence of secular-fundamentalist states has created a social context that is assertively hostile to traditional Christians appearing in the public space *as* Christians. The discourse and commitments of Christianity have been excluded from the public forum altogether, as well as, as far as possible, from the public space. For example, "Merry Christmas" is to be replaced as far as possible with "Happy Holidays." However, post-traditional Christians may not fully recognize how different the moral discourse of secular-fundamentalist states is from the moral discourse and moral claims of traditional Christianity. This is the case because, among other things, post-traditional Christians have themselves embraced the secular discourse of human rights, human equality, human dignity, and social justice, which discourse is not originally Christian but is grounded in the secular morality that became salient after the French Revolution. Such post-traditional Christians have recast their own moral discourse in terms of a secular idiom.

III. A Profound Gulf: Why There Is No Common Ground

Traditional Christian physicians and health care professionals, including pharmacists (e.g., who will be obliged not to fill a prescription for an abortifacient), are culturally disruptive because traditional Christian physicians publicly affirm obligations to God. These obligations include not merely refusing to provide medical interventions they recognize to be forbidden by God, but also recognizing that they are in addition obliged to refuse even to refer patients to those who would provide such services. The prohibition against referral is grounded in the circumstance that, if one recognizes that an action is categorically prohibited, one may not even refer persons to those who will provide that forbidden service. Thus, if one recognizes that killing the innocent is wrong (e.g., abortion and physician-assisted suicide), one must not only refuse to kill the innocent, but one must also refuse to refer to expert murderers and assassins for those seeking to have the innocent be killed. In this regard, traditional Christian health care professionals will be socially disruptive because such professionals will define themselves openly and publicly over against important moral requirements of the dominant secular culture. Last but not least, if the refusal on the part of health care professionals to provide particular health care interventions, or even to refer for them, is phrased in terms of an obligation to God, such refusals will violate the claimed secular normativity of public discourse. Such refusals introduce religious claims into the public space and undermine the priority of the established secular moral order, along with its view of medical professionalism.

Refusing to provide and, even worse, refusing to refer for services traditional Christians know to be forbidden, but which the secular state has rendered legal and has transformed into morally legitimate life-style and death-style choices, are thus significant offenses against the norms of an officially secular culture and its polity. They constitute salient acts of non-cooperation with the secular state. In such an officially secular culture established by a secular state, there is in addition a special animus against Christian norms, images, and discourse, in that these secular states have self-consciously affirmed a laicist separation between state and Christianity. By erasing the separation of state and secular ideology, these states endorse a union of state and ideology. Such states seek to define themselves through norms that are self-consciously after Christianity by defining public life, public professions, and public institutions in a totalizing, secular fashion that sets aside what had been a Christian public culture. This transformation of public life, public professions, and public institutions is often carried out in the name of defending purported secular obligations to honor human rights, secularly defined. The force of these developments is expressed in pressure brought to bear on Christian physicians either to violate their obligations to God or to leave their profession.

This secularization of the professions is pursued through giving priority to professional norms as public standards, while reducing moral claims to mere personal or private preferences. The secular culture attempts to establish a higher-order moral account that endorses the priority of secular professional ethics over "private" moral concerns. The goal is to have secular professional ethics trump other moral obligations, including one's obligations to God. "Selfless" secular professionalism and secular social justice are thus invoked as objective moral norms that require health professionals to violate their "private" obligations to God (i.e., not to be involved in the insemination of unmarried women, the use of donor gametes even within a marriage, abortion, including the filling of prescriptions for abortifacients, physician-assisted suicide, and euthanasia), which are redescribed as merely "personal" concerns. Thus, the commitment to honor one's obligations to God is characterized as a self-centered, selfish focus on private matters or private religious "feelings" that are inferior in their force and that conflict with, and are overridden by, public secular social obligations that one possesses as a health care professional (Cantor 2009). A separation of the private from the public is invoked so as to quarantine religious obligations within a sphere of merely private moral feelings and concerns. In this way, obligations to God not to perform certain acts are reduced to mere matters of personal taste. They are regarded as life-style choices involving private values and private moral feelings that should be courageously overridden on behalf of society. Of course, from the perspective of the traditional Christian medical professional, neither God nor obligations to God are a private matter or a matter of "feelings," but reflect the deep character of reality. Nothing could be more public than religious moral norms. Traditional Christians and the defenders of the secular fundamentalist state will in short not even agree on a common description of what is at stake.

Christian professionals, by announcing that the provision of particular services is profoundly wrong, implicitly accuse others of acting wrongly. That is, when Christian health care professionals refuse to honor requests for legally recognized health care services such as the insemination of unmarried women, the use of donor gametes for third-party-assisted reproduction within marriage, treatment for sexual dysfunction in homosexual couples, *in vitro* fertilization and embryo transfer for lesbian couples, abortion, physician-assisted suicide, and euthanasia, such refusals are considered not just to offend against the proper claim rights of others, indeed against social justice, but also implicitly and improperly to accuse others of immoral behavior when making peaceable life- and death-style choices that are held in the secular culture to be licit choices. As a consequence, those who refuse to provide or refer for forbidden services are judged to be acting immorally in imposing their own "personal morality" and bioethics on non-consenting others within a normatively secular public space, as well as acting in an improperly judgmental fashion. They are regarded as acting to impose their views on others, in that it is assumed that medical professionals in a secular society have a duty to provide those services. Such refusals are also seen as dangerous to the secular public order in impeding the exercise of the legally established entitlements of others to established medical service that should be readily provided by publicly licensed health care professionals.

The result is a conflict of moralities, bioethics, and visions of proper health care professionalism. This conflict is driven by the secular fundamentalist state's requiring that, save in very limited circumstances, Christian physicians, nurses, pharmacists, and other health care professionals, hospitals, and health care institutions practice and provide health care in conformity with the secular fundamentalist state's established secular bioethics and its vision of medical professionalism (Meyers & Woods 1996). The secular ethos also attempts to acquire additional moral weight for its intrusions by invoking support from the emerging web of secular human rights claims. For example, the refusal of traditional Christian physicians to be involved in abortion, including pharmacists refusing to fill prescriptions for abortifacients, is as a result regarded as a violation of the human rights of women to control reproduction (Bunch 1990; Margolin 2008; Zampas & Gher 2008). They are seen as part of a religious war against women.

Against this background, one can better appreciate Julian Savulescu's claim that Christian health care professionals should either provide medical interventions that they know to be forbidden by God or cease being health care providers: "If people are not prepared to offer legally permitted, efficient, and beneficial care to a patient because it conflicts with their values, they should not be doctors" (Savulescu 2006, p. 295). Gianni Vattimo for similar reasons takes a stance like Savulescu's: "[G]ynecologists with a conscientious objection to performing abortions seem to me . . . like a policeman with an aversion to carrying firearms, they should find another job" (Vattimo 2004, p. 106). Savulescu and Vattimo give voice to the view that Christian health care professionals are first and foremost practicing within a secular profession. They are to be professionals who in their moral lives are fully absorbed into a secular professional role. The commitment of health care professionals to their secularly defined professionalism is to be exhaustive of their public persona.

The secular transformation of the professions is meant to locate professional roles fully within the commitments and expectations of a secular culture and its understanding of public social roles. At the minimum, this requires medical professionals in their professional practice never to allow duties to God to trump secular professional obligations. Most particularly, Christian physicians are not to conduct themselves like the unmercenary physicians of antiquity, who as saints remain models for contemporary Christian health care professionals. The Holy Unmercenaries were martyred for locating their professional role as physicians fully within their commitments as Christians. As Christian physicians, they asked their patients to repent, to convert, to be baptized, and to be saved as a part of becoming their patients.[4] These exemplars of proper Christian medical professionalism realized that as a part of their role as physicians they should pray with and help dying patients to prepare for going before Christ's dread judgment seat.[5] With the Holy Unmercenaries one can recognize the profound and intractable conflict between these two radically different views of reality, morality, and medical professionalism presented in the collision of traditional Christianity with the secular culture.

In summary, the dominant secular culture through its realization in the secular fundamentalist state is committed to establishing in public policy a set of secular professional norms and a secular ideal of medical professionalism that prohibits Christian physicians, health care professionals, and health care institutions from refusing to provide and/or from refusing to refer for legally established health care services. The secular political agenda is as far as possible to totalize the character of the secular culture in establishing the secular culture in all publicly visible conduct. Refusals to provide services thus go against the commitments of the dominant secular culture and of the secular fundamentalist state.

1. First, refusals to provide and to refer for customary and secularly morally accepted medical services constitute a refusal to accept the secular culture's demanded demoralization of the moral significance of legally permitted life-style and death-style choices. Because the secular culture seeks thoroughgoingly to accomplish this demoralization through treating as matters of private choice secularly accepted peaceable decisions involving sexual preferences, reproductive preferences, and preferences regarding how one wishes to die, including whether to use physician-assisted suicide or euthanasia, the refusal of Christian health care professionals to provide health care services supportive of such secularly accepted peaceable life-style and death-style choices is held to involve an improper moralizing and intolerance, as well as a failure to maintain required secular medical professionalism.[6]

2. Second, for the dominant secular culture, refusals to provide legally established medical services due to an overriding obligation to God violate the secular character of the public space. Openly announcing that as a physician or health care professional one has an obligation to God that requires the non-provision of legally established health care services constitutes a failure from the standpoint of the secular state to recognize the asserted required secular character of public professions, institutions, and public discourse. The intrusion of Christian moral and bioethical commitments into the secular public space is a matter of particular concern for the secular state, because the now-dominant secular culture sees itself not just historically, but also normatively as after Christendom. It is after Christianity in the sense of being focused on the removal of Christian norms from public visibility: from the perspective of the now-dominant secular culture, Christianity and its norms are to be rendered normatively past.

3. Last and quite importantly, claims of rights of conscientious objection, not to mention claims of obligations to God, are considered unjustified by the secular fundamentalist state in being constraints on the secular liberty

and secular human rights of others. Refusals to provide legally established services are judged from the standpoint of the secular-fundamentalist state and its mores to constitute unjustified limitations on the established civil liberties of others, who are held within the secular culture to have a warranted expectation that they will have unimpeded access to legally approved services from state-licensed professionals.

After Christendom, in the ruins of Christendom, commitments to traditional Christian morality and bioethics are monumentally politically incorrect. Within the now-dominant secular culture, Christian physicians and nurses are not to be free to define themselves as *Christian* physicians and nurses. Instead, in a secular society they are publicly to have only a professional role congruent with secular social norms.

IV. Some Further Reflections on Kant: Rights of Conscience as Non-negotiable

The controversies and conflicts engendered by Christian physicians who refuse to provide particular health care services because they recognize those services to be forbidden by God show the foundational incompatibility between the normative understandings of traditional Christianity and those of the dominant secular morality. They underscore the basis for an ongoing conflict with the secular state and its establishment of an ethos of the secularly politically reasonable. On the one hand, the dominant secular morality, sustained by a secular vision of the secularly politically reasonable, cut off from any foundations, seeks a thoroughgoing demoralization of traditional Christian moral commitments, so that, regarding a wide range of issues, strong moral obligations, including strong bioethical obligations, are held not to exist. On the other hand, traditional Christians recognize themselves as having obligations to the transcendent God, which cannot be overridden, and which obligations make impossible the acceptance of this demoralization of traditional Christian morality upon which the dominant secular culture insists. For those who affirm the secular ethos, substantive moral concerns have disappeared regarding a range of issues. For the traditional Christian, the obligations are as strong as ever. The two moral, metaphysical, and political visions are incompatible and in profound conflict.

Those in controversy share insufficient common grounds in terms of which a compromise could be effected.

This gulf is not unique. Or rather, this gulf can even in part be recognized by Kantians. There is at least a somewhat similar foundational disagreement separating Kantian moralists and bioethicists from the morality and bioethics of the dominant secular culture. Kant clearly wished to resist not only the demoralization of traditional morality into life-style and death-style choices, but also the deflation of morality. One should recall that Kant would not accept as a morality the mere pursuit of the good considered apart from right-making conditions in terms of which one could judge moral agents to be blameworthy or praiseworthy. Although Kant was by no means a traditional Christian and probably was actually an atheist, he defended the full force of traditional Christian morality. In this, he was a thoroughly non-post-modern man who held at all odds a view supporting the full claims of morality. The difference between deontological and teleological moral visions is profound, though not as profound as the chasm separating traditional Christians from the secular culture. This latter gulf has the added dimension of being anchored in the will of the living and fully transcendent God. Nevertheless, the secular contrast can aid in appreciating the depth of the disagreements separating traditional Christianity from the now-dominant secular culture.

John Rawls captures well the distinction between deontological and teleological moral claims, which distinction undergirds a cardinal dimension of moral pluralism.

[In] teleological theories: the good is defined independently from the right, and then the right is defined as that which maximizes the good. More precisely, those institutions and acts are right which of the available alternatives produce the most good, or at least as much good as any of the other institutions and acts open as real possibilities (a rider needed when the maximal class is not a singleton). . . . It is essential to keep in mind that in a teleological theory the good is defined independently from the right. This means two things. First, the theory accounts for our considered judgments as to which things are good (our judgments of value) as a separate class of judgments intuitively distinguishable by common sense, and then proposes the hypothesis that the right is maximizing the good as already specified. Second, the theory enables one to judge the goodness of things without referring to what is right. . . . [In contrast,] a deontological theory [is] one that either does not specify the good independently from the right, or does not interpret the right as maximizing the good (Rawls 1971, pp. 24, 25, 30).

The result is that a deontologist ought not to violate core right-making conditions, no matter what the consequences: *fiat justitia, pereat mundus*. Although Kant lacks a consistent terminology, he can reasonably be interpreted as a deontologist committed to a right-making condition that is prior to the good, and not reducible to the good, thus constituting a stark contrast between the Kantian account of morality and the morality of teleologists such as Jeremy Bentham (1748–1832) and John Stuart Mill (1806–1873), but most significantly the now-dominant secular morality. Deontological duties are to bind regardless of their consequences.

This interpretation of Kant, which displays the deep differences separating deontological and teleological understandings of morality, is nested in Kant's solution to the third antinomy (whether humans should be regarded as free or as determined), which solution requires embedding morality in rationality. As a consequence, right-making conditions and wrong-making conditions define what is right, and alternatively, what is wrong, by reference to Kant's account of what constitutes a rational choice. For this reason, moral choices and therefore bioethical choices are to be made apart from any consideration of their consequences. That is, the rightness of moral and bioethical choices for Kant exists independently of consequences and is instead a function of the rationality of moral choice itself. Moreover, rightly constituted choices are not determined by the causal nexus within which they are made. This allows Kant to say that "Reason, irrespective of all empirical conditions of [an] act, is completely free" (Kant 1964, p. 477, A555=B583). Kant sees this focus on the character of rational choice to be a condition that all self-conscious agents should recognize as inescapably binding. According to Kant, we must acknowledge that "every being which cannot act otherwise than under the idea of freedom is thereby really free in a practical respect" [Kant 1959, p. 66, AK IV.448]. In this context, Kant affirms that morality is concerned with categorical, not with hypothetical imperatives.

"The categorical imperative would be one which presented an action as of itself objectively [i.e., rationally] necessary, without regard to any other end" (Kant 1959, p. 31, AK IV.415). Kant's position can thus be interpreted as embracing a right-making condition that is deontological and that therefore contrasts profoundly with teleological accounts, thereby underscoring an unbridgable gulf within secular moral thought. The conflict is beyond compromise.

There are grounds, however, to interpret Kant's account of morality in non-deontological terms. For example, Kant claims that persons are "that which constitutes the condition under which alone something can be an end in itself ... [such that persons have] not merely a relative worth, i.e., a price, but an intrinsic worth, i.e., *dignity*" (Kant, AK IV.435). Kant also holds, "Nothing in the world—indeed nothing even beyond the world—can possibly be conceived which could be called good without qualification except a *good will*" (Kant 1959, p. 9, AK IV.393). In such passages, Kant appears to ground his account of morality in the over-riding intrinsic good of persons and/or of the good will, not in a right-making condition, *sensu stricto*.

Despite the unclarities, Kant's final grounding of morality is as a fact of reason: "So act that the maxim of your will could always hold at the same time as a principle establishing universal law. . . . The consciousness of this fundamental law may be called a fact of reason, since one cannot ferret it out from antecedent data of reason, such as the consciousness of freedom . . . " (Kant 1956, pp. 30, 31, AK V.30, 31). It is therefore not inconsistent with Kant's arguments to interpret his moral account as grounded in a rightly-ordered reason that constitutes a right-making condition independent of consequences, so that the goodness of the good will and the intrinsic worth of persons lies in their being able to act rightly. Kant can thus be interpreted as affirming a deontological condition, a right-making condition, rather than a cardinal or intrinsic good, so that the rightness of moral acts lies not simply in their goodness. The goodness of persons as moral agents is thus grounded in the right-making character of reason, so that the right is prior to the good, and the right is independent of the good. In any event, this moral vision contrasts profoundly with that of teleological accounts in general and utilitarian accounts in particular, in which the righteousness of an action depends on its consequences. Kant's right-making conditions are framed from his God's-eye perspective, so that Kant holds these conditions not to be socio-historically-conditioned, but to bind persons independently of history, race, gender, and species. These sparse right-making conditions are to obligate persons as such.

The gulf separating the morality and bioethics of the dominant secular culture from that of traditional Christianity thus has an analogue in Kant's account of morality, which would also require physicians not to provide or refer for physician-assisted suicide, euthanasia, or the treatment of the sexual dysfunction of homosexuals. This is what one would expect, in that Kant wished to provide a rational foundation for the substance of Christian morality. In contrast, the morality of the dominant secular culture is constituted out of a set of norms nested in a freestanding fabric of moral intuitions supported by a narrative located and articulated fully within the horizon of the finite and the immanent, and which is therefore both demoralized and deflated in its moral significance. It has no strong right- or wrong-making conditions, and its goods are always context-conditioned. The ultimate standing of the morality and bioethics of the dominant culture is that which is conveyed by the secular fundamentalist state. In contrast, Kantian morality like traditional Christianity has a set of norms taken to be nested in an objective canonical perspective. Kant's arguments seek to support moral claims that he held were neither demoralized nor deflated, constituting what the dominant secular culture would characterize as an uncompromising and morally judgmental, indeed fundamentalist position. Kant is the last great moral-philosophical fundamentalist. The very meaning of Christian and of Kantian morality is other than that of the dominant secular culture. A Kantian bioethics is incompatible with the now-dominant secular bioethics. The Kantian relic of Christianity gives grounds for a substantive battle in the culture wars.

V. The Strangeness of Moral Strangers

Moral strangers are persons with whom one has no common way to resolve moral and bioethical disputes either through sound rational argument and/or by an appeal to a commonly recognized authority. Such a gulf separates traditional Christians (and for that matter Kantians) from the secularists of the now-dominant secular culture. Each experiences and understands reality in a fundamentally different fashion. Because all is seen with different frameworks of meaning, there will inevitably be conflicts between traditional Christianity's and the dominant secular culture's understanding of proper conduct and bioethics, even more so than with a Kantian morality and bioethics. The dominant secular culture insists on containing and re-interpreting the meaning of all action within the horizon of the finite and the immanent. Only if this immanent containment is enforced is one free to engage in peaceable life-style and death-style choices as one wishes. Otherwise, one will sense the claims of the transcendent God Who is beyond the horizon of the finite and the immanent. The disagreements due to the presence of persons who are moral strangers to the now-dominant secular culture threaten the peace of the established culture. Traditional Christian health care professionals, along with other traditional religious believers, will find themselves obliged to go against the constraints set by the now-dominant secular culture. Traditional Christians are troublemakers.

Notes

[1]This chapter grew out of a lecture, "Religion, Politics, and the State: Rethinking Morality in Modern, Secularized Societies," given at Politeia, University of Milan, Milan, Italy, January 30, 2012, and at Instituto Banco di Napoli, Naples, Italy, February 3, 2012.

[2]In contrast with Orthodox Christianity, which forbids all abortion, Orthodox Judaism holds that there is an obligation on the part of Jews to perform a direct abortion in order to save the life of the mother. "If a woman is in hard travail, one cuts up the child in her womb and brings it forth member by member, because her life comes before that of [the child]. But if the greater part has proceeded forth, one may not touch it, for one may not set aside one person's life for that of another" (*Oholoth* 7:6). Orthodox Christians could consider this difference to be a function of what changed (along with divorce laws) with the arrival of the Messiah. See Matthew 19:3–4.

[3]By a secular fundamentalist state, I mean a state that in ways analogous to a religious fundamentalist state imposes on the public space, public institutions, and public professions a particular normative, secular, post-religious view of proper action and discourse, including laicist norms for deportment and speech, which will conflict with the first three understandings of medical professionalism (Engelhardt 2010c, 2010d).

[4]In the Eastern rites of the Orthodox Church, the prayers during the prothesis, that is, during the proskomedia, mention is made of six of the Holy Unmercenary Physicians. The liturgical term *prothesis* identifies both the rite of preparation before the Liturgy, as well as the table or side altar north of the main altar. It is at the side altar that the prothesis or

proskomedia takes place, during which the bread is prepared for the Liturgy. "Proskomedia" is derived from the Greek for oblation. The bread used is leavened bread, for it is clear from the text of the New Testament that at the Last Supper when Christ celebrated "the festival of unleavened bread" (azymes) He did not use unleavened bread, but a loaf of leavened bread (*artos*) (Matthew 26:26; Mark 14:22; Luke 22:19; I Corinthians 11:23). Jesus changes the very sense of the Passover. As the Christ, as the Messiah, He has brought Redemption so that the character of the Passover is transformed. From that point on, unleavened bread is not to be used. In taking out the seventh particle from the bread that will be consecrated during Liturgy, the priest prays, "[in honor and memory] of the holy, glorious and wonder-working unmerce-naries Cosmas and Damian [It is related of Sts. Cosmas and Damian of Rome, whose feast day is the 1st of July and who were martyred in the year A.D. 284, that "The standard fee that they requested from their patients—that is, those among the race of men whom they healed—was singular: believe in Jesus Christ through Whom they wrought cures" (*Great Synaxaristes July* 2008, p. 1).], Cyrus and John [Sts. Cyrus and John (a non-physician companion of St. Cyrus) of Rome, who were martyred in A.D. 292, and whose feast day is the 31st of January, directed their patients to prayer and repentance. "In this manner, [St. Cyrus] converted the pagans to the knowledge of God, and further strengthened the faithful" (*Great Synaxaristes January* 2003, p. 1169).], Panteleimon and Hermolaos "and of all the holy unmercenary healers" (*Liturgikon* 1989, p. 249). [St. Hermolaos, who was not a physician, baptized St. Panteleimon, whose feast day is July 27th, the day in A.D. 304 on which he was martyred. St. Panteleimon, who is invoked during the prayers of the Blessing of the Waters and the Mystery of Holy Unction, both treated and baptized patients. "The only recompense he sought for the cures was that his patients acknowledge and confess the true Physician, Jesus Christ" (*Great Synax-aristes July* 2008, p. 1209).] The six named, who practiced medicine (or assisted those in the practice of medicine) without charging for the care they gave, were also martyrs not just for being Christians. They were killed for being Christians who, in the face of a pagan empire, made it clear to their patients that the only real cure for sickness and death is Christ. They understood that the surrounding pagan culture could seduce Christians, but that it could not violate their conscience (only they themselves could do that). Despite a hostile dominant culture and its requirements, the holy unmercenaries were totally unembarrassed about being fully committed, proselytizing Christians. The holy unmercenary physicians realized that because physicians accompany their patients in the face of suffering and the threat of death, Christian physicians have a special obligation to teach all how to prepare to face the dread judgment seat of Christ. The holy unmercenaries were martyred for their determination to provide health care as Christians should, namely, proclaiming in their practice the good news of the Kingdom.

[5]One should note that some traditional Christian health care professionals continue to recognize the importance of praying for and with their patients, so that acting as a Christian remains integral to their sense of medical professionalism. See, for example, Strang 2011.

[6]Vattimo is of the view that the contemporary secular moral culture's demoralization of traditional moral choices into life-style or aesthetic choices is integral to an eschewal of vio-lence and a pursuit of peace. His view is that if people abandoned absolute moral commitments

and commitments to a transcendent reality, they would have little about which to fight. Obviously, he has forgotten about the *Iliad* or wars for control of oil fields.

It seems clear that the reconciliation of peace and liberty in the postmodern or late-modern world will be attained only on condition that esthetics prevails over objective truth. The variety of lifestyles and the diversity of ethical codes will be able to coexist without bloody clashes only if they are considered, like the artistic styles within an art collection (Vattimo 2004, p. 58).

Vattimo's point is that the contemporary secular search for world peace has come to involve the rejection of metaphysics in the sense of any reference to an unconditioned reality or perspective.

References

Bunch, C. 1990. Women's rights as human rights: Toward a re-vision of human rights, *Human Rights Quarterly* 12.4: 486–498.

Cantor, Julie D. 2009. Conscientious objection gone awry—restoring selfless professionalism in medicine, *New England Journal of Medicine* 360 (April 9): 1484–1485.

Engelhardt, H. T., Jr. 2010a. Kant, Hegel, and Habermas: Reflections on 'Glauben und Wissen,' *The Review of Metaphysics* 63.4: 871–903.

Engelhardt, H. T., Jr. 2010b. Moral obligation after the death of God: Critical reflections on concerns from Immanuel Kant, G. W. F. Hegel, and Elizabeth Anscombe, *Social Philosophy & Policy* 27.2: 317–340.

Engelhardt, H. T., Jr. 2010c. Religion, bioethics, and the secular state: Beyond religious and secular fundamentalism, *Notizie di Politeia* 26.97: 59–79.

Engelhardt, H. T., Jr. 2010d. Political authority in the face of moral pluralism: Further reflections on the non-fundamentalist state, *Notizie di Politeia* 26.97: 91–99.

Great Synaxaristes of the Orthodox Church, January. 2003. Buena Vista, CO: Holy Apostles Convent.

Great Synaxaristes of the Orthodox Church, July. 2008. Buena Vista, CO: Holy Apostles Convent.

Kant, Immanuel. 1964. *Immanuel Kant's Critique of Pure Reason*, trans. Norman Kemp Smith. New York: Macmillan.

Kant, Immanuel. 1959. *Foundations of the Metaphysics of Morals*, trans. Lewis White Beck. Indianapolis: Bobbs-Merrill.

Kant, Immanuel. 1956. *Critique of Practical Reason*, trans. Lewis White Beck. Indianapolis: Bobbs-Merrill.

Liturgikon. 1989. Englewood, NJ: Antakya Press.

Margolin, T. 2008. Abortion as a human right, *Women's Rights Law Reporter* 29.2–3: 77–97.

Meyers, Christopher & Robert D. Woods. 1996. An obligation to provide abortion services: What happens when physicians refuse? *Journal of Medical Ethics* 22: 115–120.

Oholoth. 1989. *Babylonian Talmud*, ed. I. Epstein, trans. H. Bornstein. London: Soncino Press.

Pellegrino, Edmund & David Thomasma. 1988. *A Philosophical Basis of Medical Practice.* New York: Oxford University Press.

Pellegrino, Edmund & David Thomasma. 1981. *For the Patient's Good.* New York: Oxford University Press.

Rawls, John. 1971. *A Theory of Justice.* Cambridge, MA: Belknap Press.

Savulescu, Julian. 2006. Conscientious objection in medicine, *British Medical Journal* 332: 294–297.

Strang, Cecily Weller. 2011. Is intercessory prayer a valid nursing intervention? *Journal of Christian Nursing* 28.3 (April): 92–95.

Vattimo, Gianni. 2004. *Nihilism and Emancipation*, ed. Santiago Zabala, trans. William McCuaig. New York: Columbia University Press.

Zampas, C. & J. Gher. 2008. Abortion as a human right—International and regional standards, *Human Rights Law Review* 8.2: 249–294.

CHAPTER SIX

Clinical Ethics Radically Reconsidered: Bioethics, Common Morality, and the Law[1]

I. Bioethics without Foundations

As far as the foundations of secular bioethics, there are none.[2] There is no canonical secular morality; there is no canonical secular bioethics. There is an intractable plurality of moralities and bioethics. There are no foundations , there is no sound rational argument that can secure any one particular secular morality or bioethics as canonical. There is no way out of this difficulty through an appeal to social contracts, which are plural (Bishop 2011), and whose authority is in question, once foundations are lost, once one has gone beyond the minimal state. The history of bioethics discloses persistent disagreement (Koch 2012). There are multiple incompatible clusters of intuitions supported by disparate narratives, such that each account or narrative is freestanding within the horizon of the finite and the immanent. Some, such as those from Singapore and China, which affirm a one-party capitalist state (Fan 2010 and 2011; Fan et al. 2012; Lim 2012; Li & Wang 2012), as well as from the Philippines (Alora 2001), collide strongly with the supposed common morality and bioethics of Beauchamp and Childress (Beauchamp & Childress 2012). Some moralities and bioethics are social-democratic (Daniels 1985; Buchanan 2009). Others are embedded in libertarian understandings of various sorts (Engelhardt 1986, 1996, 1991; Kukathas 2007). Secular moralities and bioethics are diverse (Hoshino 1997).

What ought one to make of secular morality and secular bioethics and secular clinical ethics, since their longed-for justification through sound rational argument fails? How is one to think of them in a culture after God? Because there is no canonical, secular, sound rational argument to establish the liberal, social-democratic moral vision or the political authority of a liberal, social-democratic constitution and the governments such constitutions authorize, how should one understand the fields of secular bioethics and secular clinical ethics with their liberal, social-democratic content? Beyond constituting quasi-political movements, how should one understand these fields? Or is there, as Tom Koch argues, a self-deception that dominates contemporary bioethics and that involves *inter alia* an affirmation of a neoliberal economics of scarcity (Koch 2012, p. 250)? Do bioethicists self-deceive themselves due to the psychological challenge of reconsidering their self-identity (i.e., some may actually imagine themselves to be moral experts or "morally" successful ethicists who draw comfort and self-esteem from their supposed expertise)? Are large segments of the public mistaken about the significance and roles of bioethics, especially clinical ethics? What can or ought the future of bioethics and clinical ethics to be, given that there is no canonical, secular, common, or universal morality? Why despite all these puzzles do health care ethics consultants succeed so well (Engelhardt 2011, 2009, 2003)?

It is, after all, the success of clinical bioethics that, by accident of association, has made academic bioethics appear successful, which of course it is not, if success lies in establishing a conclusive rational warrant for the morality and ethics forwarded. The aspirations of academic secular bioethics have not succeeded in establishing a canonical bioethics. The academy has failed to justify a canonical morality, because, as we saw in chapter two, this is impossible. At best, one can conclude that moral philosophy and academic bioethics have failed to appreciate sufficiently their situation as after God and after morality. Nevertheless, secular bioethics has succeeded politically and functions in triumph as a political movement whose political agenda is widely passed off as a moral conclusion. Bioethicists have emerged with a remarkable self-identity. Bioethicists appear to be the intellectuals who have succeeded in being relevant to society through doing something that "really" matters. One can be proud to be a bioethicist or clinical ethicist.

Tom Beauchamp and James Childress, with the aid of Eunice and Sargent Shriver, as well as the Kennedy Foundation through the Kennedy Institute, helped establish bioethics, even though Beauchamp and Childress eschewed the term "bioethics," giving preference to "biomedical ethics." The Center for Bioethics of the Kennedy Institute, with its total-immersion courses, ordained cadres of a new order of secular chaplains who transformed the ethos of health care practice, the oversight of research, and the functioning of advisory panels of various genres. They made bioethics the moral and intellectual master of medical ethics (Engelhardt 2002).[3] These courses at the Kennedy Institute, along with the *Principles of Biomedical Ethics* (1979, 1983, 1989, 1994, 2001, 2009, 2012), abetted the development and flourishing of bioethics. As it was, it was still too risqué for some former Christian theologians and scholars wholeheartedly to accept all of the secular bioethics that were becoming dominant (e.g., that secular bioethics had no conclusive arguments against infanticide). Nevertheless, despite whatever their initial relative conservatism may have been on some matters, Beauchamp and Childress embraced without hesitation a strong social-democratic, political agenda and took the first steps to a post-Christian morality and bioethics, the full force of which is still just beginning to be appreciated. It is enough in this chapter to acknowledge some of the implications for secular bioethics, both academic and clinical, of being beyond foundations, of being in a culture after God.

II. Living with Moral Pluralism

Against the background of the loss of foundations for secular morality and bioethics, one can better appreciate that there is no conclusive rational basis for taking any particular secular morality or bioethics to be canonical. Theory is understandably not just in disarray but brought into question. It cannot establish what one ought to do, once a God's-eye perspective is lost. In this light, one can also better understand Tom Beauchamp's observation that secular bioethics can proceed without attention to theory. Beauchamp even reminds us that it is best not to pay attention to and/or be embarrassed by the failure of theory. After all, theory cannot vindicate the dominant secular morality and culture, much less Beauchamp and Childress's common or "universal" morality.[4] As Beauchamp puts it, quite understandably, "this [moral] theory part of the landscape of bioethics . . . [will] vanish soon, because it is serving no useful purpose" (Beauchamp 2004, p. 210). Since it is impossible, given deep disagreements regarding basic moral premises and rules of evidence, to establish any particular concrete morality or bioethics as canonical, theory fails to aid in securing a particular canonical secular morality or bioethics. Without the possibility of establishing a particular canonical morality by sound rational argument, one cannot identify, much less ground, a canonical, common, or "universal" morality or bioethics. Without such a warrant for morality or bioethics, why take bioethics and its practitioners seriously? Is this state of affairs disastrous both for those that seek counsel from clinical bioethicists and for such bioethicists themselves? Are such bioethicists like "Those who stay on the job [and] become like old prison lags, the long-time prisoners who mop the floor and proclaim the institution fine because the floor is clean" (Koch 2012, p. 253)?

Where, then, do we find ourselves? Theory can offer analyses, exegeses, comparisons, and defenses of alternative secular moralities and bioethics. Theory can lay out the content and the character of the various claims of particular or regional moralities, including the dominant secular morality of our society, drawing out the implications in specific areas or regarding specific cases. Theory can lay out alternative geographies of morality and bioethics. But theory cannot establish which particular morality should serve as *the* canonical, common, or "universal" morality, so as to provide a secular canonical ethics for bioethics to apply. As Beauchamp admits,

> The reasons for the demotion of ethical theory are the lack of distinctive authority behind any one framework or methodology, the unappealing and formidable character of many theories, the indeterminate nature of general norms of all sorts, the turn in bioethics to more practical issues, and most importantly, the stumbling and confusing manner in which philosophers have attempted to link theory to practice (Beauchamp 2004, p. 216).

Three points are crucial. First, there is "the indeterminate nature of general norms of all sorts" (Beauchamp 2004, p. 216); second, there is "the stumbling and confusing manner in which philosophers have attempted to link theory to practice" (Beauchamp 2004, p. 216). Finally, as already underscored, no particular secular morality or bioethics can by sound rational argument be established as canonical. What is one then to make of bioethics under these circumstances?

Beauchamp appears to accept something like a biopolitical view of this state of affairs. He is willing to live with core ambiguities regarding key terms and principles in morality and bioethics, including his cardinal principle of autonomy, as long as the agenda of his biopolitics is advanced. One should note that a strategic ambiguity is often rhetorically useful in building political coalitions, in that a certain amount of ambiguity serves the force of political persuasion by appealing in different ways to different audiences. Clear definitions exclude particular bases of support, while strategically ambiguous definitions can help to build political coalitions. Politics is not an area that encourages analytic precision or clear sound rational argument. Instead, politics in its practice is marked by the art of persuasion, sophistry in the classical sense of the term. One need not be Foucaultian in order to recognize that statecraft is the exercise of persuasion and power.

Consider the ambiguities of autonomy, the focus of Beauchamp and Childress's first principle. The meaning of autonomy is multiple. The term autonomy, as well as the principle of autonomy, is plural, compassing different principles of autonomy with different intensions and extensions. For instance, one can identify at least four different understandings of autonomy (and therefore four different principles of autonomy), each with a distinctly different meaning.

1. Autonomy as a source of authority—When persons meet who do not agree regarding God's commands, regarding what moral rationality requires, or regarding what common customs dictate (if there be any), they can always draw authority from the consent or permission of those who decide to collaborate peaceably (Engelhardt 1996). Autonomy in the sense of the conveyance of authority through permission for common collaboration is at the root of the authority of contracts, the market, and the minimal state, but not of the more-than-minimal state. No value and/or no virtue is imputed to the practice of gaining common authority for peaceable collaboration. It is simply the case that if one enters into this practice of gaining authority from permission, one can, together with others who also explicitly enter the practice, share the authority of common permission, the authority of consent that is derived from the collaborators. The

source of this authority is nothing other than the consent or permission given by those who collaborate.

2. Autonomy as a value or goal—Autonomy can also be valued as an end in itself or as an overriding good. Various philosophies and ideologies have valued persons choosing on their own, setting their own goals as autonomous agents, rather than submitting to the authority of others. When persons freely submit to the authority of others, they do not violate the principle of autonomy as permission, but they reject giving an overriding value to autonomy. Thus, when one sells oneself into temporary slavery (i.e., allowing another to compel one's services rather than being allowed to pay damages for the failure to provide promised services), such as when joining the military, one values other goods more highly than the good(s) of autonomy. During the Enlightenment and following the French Revolution, views regarding autonomy as an overriding value became salient, often construing freedom or liberty as a good in itself. The value of autonomy is cardinal to many contemporary accounts of bioethics.

3. Autonomy as *the* rational choice—The existence of a canonical, content-full moral choice is at the core of a rational "Kantian" way of life and as such is held by Kant to be obligatory for all rational beings. This sense of autonomy does not affirm one's choosing as one wants (*Willkür*), but only as one rationally *should* will (*Wille*). For example, according to Kant, to act autonomously one must rationally choose in conformity with what the moral law requires as the choices of rational agents *qua* rational agents. Here Hegel notes in his critique of Kant in the "Moralität" section of *Elements of the Philosophy of Right* that Kant either imports content without sufficient argument or leaves crucial terms underdefined so that a thick or ambiguous set of moral commitments is imported without due notice into Kant's notion of moral rationality.

4. Autonomy as union with God—Through freedom from sin and distorting passions, one can be granted union with God. This is the traditional Christian account of freedom, which is expressed in "You shall know

the truth and the truth shall set you free" (Jn 8:32). This account of freedom realizes that the good, the right, and the virtuous are such only
when they are aimed at the Holy, the Persons of the Trinity. One can
aim properly through purification of the soul and submission to God's
commandments, so that free from improper attachments one can come
into union with God. In this case, truth is not propositional but refers to
the Persons of the Trinity. Christ, after saying "you shall know the truth
and the truth shall set you free," explains Who the Truth is: "I am the
way, the truth, and the life: no man cometh unto the Father but by Me"
(Jn 14:6). One only becomes truly free by becoming a god by grace (i.e.,
through the uncreated energies of God [St. Athanasius, *De incarnatione
verbi dei* §54.3]).

These four senses of autonomy are in many ways incompatible. They at most
show or possess some family resemblances. There is no obvious way to parse
the meaning of autonomy in the principle of autonomy, because autonomy is
multiple in its meanings.

The first sense, autonomy as permission, can be affirmed in the face of
skepticism regarding Kant's claims about what rational agents should choose.
Moreover, autonomy as permission, in contrast with the second account, simply
identifies a source of authority (i.e., permission) that can serve as the basis for
peaceable collaboration among moral strangers. It is not a rationally required,
independent, right-making condition (i.e., apart from its standing within the
practice of permission-giving itself), nor is it a claim made about the value of
freedom or about acting peaceably, nor is it claimed that autonomy has a particular content. Indeed, in terms of the first meaning of autonomy, no claim is
even made about the moral importance of this practice of gaining authority,
but only that this practice exists as a possibility that can bind peaceable moral
strangers, should they wish to enter into it. The meaning of autonomy is, in
short, plural.

Given this state of affairs, what can one then say about the principle of autonomy? What precise meaning for Beauchamp's account of bioethics does autonomy have, if any? In particular, it should be clear that there is no one canonical
view about the importance or meaning of autonomy or of the significance of the

principle of autonomy. Beauchamp appears without any concern in recognizing and conceding this state of affairs with its deep ambiguities.

> What it is about autonomy that we are to respect remains unclear, and it remains obscure what "respect" means. Most obscure of all is how practice is affected by a theory of autonomy. The contemporary literature in bioethics contains no theory of autonomy that spells out its nature, its moral implications, its limits, how respect for autonomy differs from respect for persons (if it does), and the like (Beauchamp 2004, p. 214).

Autonomy is not taken by Beauchamp to identify a particular interpretation or meaning of autonomy. At best, for Beauchamp and Childress (1979) the principle of autonomy functions as a guiding heuristic to identify a diverse cluster of moral concerns associated with the character of choice, self-determination, and collaboration with others. That is, autonomy as a principle draws attention to a complex and heterogeneous cluster of moral intuitions and concerns bearing on choice and self-determination that, within the dominant secular moral narrative, have some family resemblances. The result is that an appeal to autonomy can in different contexts identify different moral and bioethical concerns, to which it may be important to attend. However, secular morality cannot establish any particular content-full sense of autonomy as canonical. There is, after all, a plurality of moral concerns associated with choice, self-determination, freedom, and liberation, which are nested within disparate moral frameworks.

Again, Beauchamp appears to be at peace with the central ambiguities of autonomy. Once more, a plausible interpretation of this state of affairs is that Beauchamp's agenda is at bottom political, so that his contentions should be understood as a form of political rhetoric. To put this state of affairs in Hegelian terms, the political is the higher truth of the moral in Beauchamp and Childress's bioethics. Like Richard Rorty, and like the later Rawls, Beauchamp can be understood as having taken a political turn so that the dominant secular morality he affirms reflects his support for the social-democratic positions in law and in public policy that he embraces. Given such an interpretation, Beauchamp would, and indeed should, tolerate a broad range of theoretical positions and different construals of autonomy. Their unity would not be conceptual but political, not that of a uniting idea, but of a political coalition: the support that the various notions of autonomy afford is that of advancing a social-democratic policy agenda. From this perspective, Beauchamp would want to reassure bioethicists that "there is no need to embrace only one of the [moral] frameworks that have seemed in intractable conflict. One can, without inconsistency, embrace principles, rules, virtues, rights, narratives, case analysis, and reflective equilibrium" (Beauchamp 2004, p. 210). One can use whatever works, whatever has rhetorical success.

Given this political interpretation of Beauchamp's position, the morality and bioethics of the dominant secular culture, by being established at law and in public policy, become the common secular morality and bioethics. Moral philosophy and bioethics provide clusters of rhetorical strategies that can through their very ambiguity prove politically useful in advancing political or public-policy agendas, such as a liberal, social-democratic movement to refashion society in general, and health care policy in particular. Once one recognizes the dominant secular morality and its bioethics as constituting dimensions of strategies integral to a socio-political movement, if one is part of that movement, one can choose among moral and bioethical arguments on the basis of which best helps rhetorically to advance one's political or public policy agendas. There appears to be no obvious political gain from openly and honestly admitting to this state of affairs, in fact to the contrary. The higher truth of secular bioethics becomes secular biopolitics.

Given this state of affairs, bioethics consultants or clinical ethics consultants (i.e., most academic bioethicists) earn a living by advancing a particular health care policy or by expositing a particular bioethical perspective that has become established at law. In the case of clinical ethics or clinical ethics consultation, one can offer the service of expositing a particular established law and public policy bearing on decisions regarding health care and the biomedical sciences. Following Karl Marx (1818–1883) and Friedrich Engels (1820–1895), one can recognize that there is no independent basis for one's morality and bioethics. One need only recognize morality and bioethics as part of "the ruling ideas of the epoch," as concretely realized in a particular jurisdiction (Marx & Engels 1967, p. 39). One can then sell one's services as a "conceptive ideologist," as a defender and/or expositor of "the ruling ideas" established at law and in public policy in a particular jurisdiction or jurisdictions. As a step toward securing status and approved market constraints to support their profession, clinical ethicists can seek to become recognized and/or approved "conceptive ideologists" through some form of certification, licensing, or official recognition.[5] In this circumstance, moral and bioethical theories play various roles as political rhetoric and/or marketing devices. In a culture after God, bioethics is biopolitics.

III. A Common Morality? A Common Bioethics?

A critical re-interpretation of secular bioethics is thus in order. Among other things, this involves deciding how to understand Beauchamp and Childress's claims regarding a common morality, in the face of the circumstance that there is no common morality or secular canonical morality. Beauchamp and Childress in *Principles of Biomedical Ethics* (Beauchamp & Childress 1979) assert that there is a common morality. Crucially, they proceed as if, given this common morality, appeals to the principles of autonomy, beneficence, non-maleficence, and justice can give concrete guidance for moral and bioethical decision-making,[6] despite the prevailing moral pluralism, and despite Beauchamp's recent acknowledgement of core ambiguities in the principles. In the first edition of their *Principles of Biomedical Ethics*, Beauchamp and Childress simply remark regarding the existence of a common morality: "Most of the principles and rules that we will consider are accepted by most deontological theories and can also be discovered in the 'common morality'" (Beauchamp & Childress 1979, p. 34). They repeat this claim verbatim in the second edition (1983, p. 33). In the third edition, Beauchamp and Childress state, "Most of the principles and rules adopted in this book are accepted by most deontological theories and can also be discovered in the 'common moral consciousness'" (Beauchamp & Childress 1989, p. 37).

By the fourth edition, which appeared in 1994, they finally provide an account of what they hold common morality to be.

> In its broadest and most familiar sense, the *common morality* comprises socially approved norms of human conduct. For example, it recognizes many legitimate and illegitimate forms of conduct that we capture by using the language of "human rights." The common morality is a social institution with a code of learnable norms. Like languages and political constitutions, the common morality exists before we are instructed in its relevant rules and

regulations. As we develop beyond infancy, we learn moral rules along with other social rules, such as laws. Later in life, we learn to distinguish general social rules held in common by members of society from particular social rules fashioned for and binding on the members of special groups, such as the members of a profession (Beauchamp & Childress 1994, p. 6).

This account of common morality with its reference to "social approval," "social rules," and a "social institution" seems open to, if not to underscore, a political interpretation so that the common morality would be the morality established at law and in public policy, the particular regnant ethos. However, their account at this point does not make it clear whether each society has its own common morality (like, for example, Hegel's *Sittlichkeiten*) or whether Beauchamp and Childress are asserting that all humans share one common, universal morality. One is not helped by Beauchamp and Childress to see which society, or part thereof, gets to approve "the norms of social conduct." Is this determined by a democratic procedure, and if so, guided by what "constitutional" constraints?

It is only in the fifth edition (2001) that Beauchamp and Childress more clearly, but nonetheless somewhat rhetorically, advance the claim that there is one common human morality in the sense of one universal morality shared by all "morally serious" persons. Beauchamp and Childress, by employing the rhetorically weighted term "morally serious," invite agreement with their position. Who, after all, would want to deny being "morally serious"?

All persons who are serious about living a moral life already grasp the core dimensions of morality. They know not to lie, not to steal property, to keep promises, to respect the rights of others, not to kill or cause harm to innocent persons, and the like. All persons serious about morality are comfortable with these rules and do not doubt their relevance and importance. They know that to violate these norms without having a morally good and sufficient reason is immoral and should lead to feelings of remorse. Because we are already convinced about such matters, the literature of ethics does not debate them. Such debate would be a waste of time.

We will refer to the set of norms that all morally serious persons share as *the common morality*. The common morality contains moral norms that bind all persons in all places; no norms are more basic in the moral life. In recent years, the favored category to represent this universal core of morality in public discourse has been human rights, but moral obligation and moral virtue are no less vital parts of the common morality (2001, p. 3).

The difficulty is that people do in fact disagree as to when it is morally licit, forbidden, or obligatory to take property, break promises, honor rights claims advanced by others, and kill other humans. "Morally serious" persons disagree about when it is appropriate to lie or to tell the truth. For example, the norms of civilized society involve dissimulating one's true feelings, with the norms for truth-telling varying remarkably across cultures. As has already been mentioned in chapter four, the Christianity of the first centuries and Orthodox Christianity differ from Western Christianity in recognizing an obligation at times to lie.[7] Beauchamp and Childress do recognize that there are a number of moral accounts of a common morality, and in their reflections they give special attention to William Frankena (1908–1994) and W. D. Ross (1877–1971). What is at stake beyond a rhetorical and strategically vague but powerful appeal to being "morally serious" is unclear.

In the fifth edition, Beauchamp and Childress also hold that their common morality will allow some customary moralities to be criticized as deficient in not meeting the moral standards set by their "common morality." To do this, they invoke a "coherence model of justification" that at best begs the question as to which morality (i.e., their common morality or the customary morality) is canonical and why. If by a coherence model of justification they mean to engage a wide reflective equilibrium, the problem is that Beauchamp has expressed skepticism as to what this could mean. "I am asserting that it has never been made clear how the method [a wide reflective equilibrium] connects to practical problems, how one would know whether it has been followed, and how it might be used by others in bioethics. . . . It continues to be unclear whether anyone in bioethics has followed the reflective-equilibrium model (I include myself), despite its standing as the most widely mentioned model" (Beauchamp 2004, p. 213). In any event, in the fifth edition they state: "This strategy [distinguishing and comparing common morality and customary morality] allows us to rely on the authority of the principles in the common morality, while incorporating tools to refine and correct unclarities and to allow for additional specification of the principles" (Beauchamp & Childress 2001, p. 403). At this point, it would seem that they wish to identify their common morality with a supposed universally binding morality, which is in reality a common political agenda.

This concern with common morality has been associated with an increased invocation of human dignity and human rights. The appeal to human rights is presumed to strengthen Beauchamp and Childress's position. But claims of human rights are notoriously rhetorical through being politically powerful albeit conceptually unclear. To quote from Kozinski:

> The post-World-War II overlapping consensus on moral goods that was to serve as the political foundation of the democratic charter, then, was an illusion. Though citizens may have shared a common lexicon of "human rights" and "democratic values," in reality, it was a house built on sand with a sinking foundation of disparate understandings of that lexicon and radically disparate traditions of practical rationality: Thomist, Lockean, Humean, Kantian, Rousseauian, Nietzchean, Deweyean—or an eclectic and incoherent mix of these or other less systematic ways of thought and practice (Kozinski 2010, p. 175).

The supporters of human rights, Beauchamp and Childress included, have embraced a political agenda. Nevertheless, Beauchamp and Childress in the sixth edition (2009) state that their common morality is a universal morality. The language they engage suggests that this may be an empirical claim. However, they provide no supporting studies that convincingly show

> that the common morality is a product of human experience and history and is a universally shared product. The origin of the norms of the common morality is no different in principle from the origin of the norms of a particular morality in that both are learned and transmitted in communities. The primary difference is that the common morality is found in all cultures (Beauchamp & Childress 2009, pp. 3–4).

Indeed, they claim that "Our hypothesis is simply that all persons *committed to morality* adhere to the standards that we are calling the common morality" (Beauchamp & Childress 2009, p. 4).

Of course, everything turns on the notion that "all persons committed to morality" accept *their* common morality. Their view appears to assume a background canonical morality that allows one to identify who these persons are, as well as the canonical morality that persons should and do hold. That they assume a particular morality to be the common morality is also clear in the 2012 edition of *The Principles of Biomedical Ethics* (Beauchamp & Childress 2012). Here they state that "We have defined the *common morality* in terms of 'the set of norms shared by all persons committed to morality'" (Beauchamp & Childress 2012, p. 417). The issue is which is the morality to which all should be or are implicitly committed. As with Beauchamp and Childress's reference to those who are "morally serious" and to "those who are committed to morality," there is rhetorical power but insufficient conceptual specificity or detailed argument. How does one determine what that morality is or who morally serious persons are?

Beauchamp and Childress appear to have finally come to the view that whether a common morality exists is an empirical question that can be addressed through anthropological study, such that

> [s]hould it turn out that the persons studied do not share the norms that we hypothesize to have their roots in the common morality (we claim to present only norms pertinent for biomedical ethics), then the research would have shown that there is no common morality of the sort we have envisioned, and our hypothesis would be falsified (Beauchamp & Childress 2012, p. 418).

Their thesis of a common morality in this account would not turn on a conceptual criterion for being "morally serious," but rather empirically on whether a particular morality is common. If this interpretation is correct, how many of which people (e.g., professors of moral philosophy, educated persons, persons generally, persons never convicted of a felony, etc.) need to hold what norms to make them the common morality? How does one go about the anthropological, sociological project of determining this state of affairs? Can it really be that Beauchamp and Childress do not in fact see that the moral project has already been falsified and that morality has collapsed into a plurality of competing moralities, while they all along continue to assert that there is a common, indeed universal, morality?

The cardinal difficulty is that Beauchamp and Childress do not give an adequate justification of their claim that there is a common morality despite the circumstance that there is wide and pronounced disagreement as to when it is obligatory, licit, or forbidden to have sex, reproduce, transfer property, tell the truth, or kill humans. It may be that all humans in being incarnate beings have concerns about sex, reproduction, pleasure, possessions, suffering, and death, but their moral views regarding these matters are manifestly diverse. There is no one morality or bioethics regarding these matters. One encounters radically different moral life-worlds (e.g., that of the secular social-democrat from Cambridge, Massachusetts, that of the Confucian familist from Singapore, or that of the pious Muslim from Tehran). If there is no sound rational argument that can identify one among the many different conflicting moralities and bioethics as canonical, then in what sense can there be a common morality? Nevertheless, Beauchamp and Childress assert that there is a common morality, and that it is the universally binding morality. They imply that those who do not agree with them are not morally serious. Yet, they give no basis for establishing what counts as moral seriousness.

Despite their claims about the existence of a common morality as a universally binding morality, a political interpretation of Beauchamp and Childress's position still appears most plausible, especially if one holds that within the sphere of the immanent, the political is the higher truth of secular morality. The political account is particularly plausible, given Beauchamp's pessimism regarding theory, indeed even regarding the impossibility of an appeal to a reflective equilibrium that could establish what counts as the content of a common morality. Appeals to balancing moral claims and/or moral concerns will not help either unless one can identify a canonical balance by which definitively to balance moral claims and concerns. As a moral project, the search for a common morality appears to be a self-deception. However, matters change if "common morality" points to the morality that Beauchamp and Childress's political agenda is aimed at establishing. That is, the common morality can be read as that morality that, given Beauchamp and Childress's political agenda, they seek globally to enact through law and public policy.

It may be the case that both Beauchamp and Childress recognize that one morality is indeed common, but only in the sense of being the morality that *they* hold should be globally regnant, that they hold should be universally established at law and public policy. If so, Beauchamp and Childress would be taking a position similar to that of Hegel and Rorty, namely, that a particular morality exists concretely only in being the morality established at law and public policy, or as that morality that some particular group aspires to impose by law. Politics then provides the standpoint from which to identify a common morality and its bioethics, in that the state establishes a morality as common in the sense that it is realized through law and public policy. The political turn also allows one to identify the morality that one wishes to establish through one's political movement as common in anticipation of future political success. The result is that with Rorty politics is "[t]he right way of reading these [moral] slogans [about common humanity, natural human rights, and the philosophical foundations for democratic politics, in that it] lets one think of philosophy as *in the service* of democratic politics, as a contribution to the attempt to achieve what Rawls calls 'reflective equilibrium' between our instinctive reactions to contemporary problems and the general principles on which we have been reared" (Rorty 1989, p. 196). Crucially at stake is a "shift from epistemology to politics" (Rorty 1989, p. 68). After the failure of the universalistic aspirations of secular morality and bioethics, one is left with morality as politics.

In the case of *The Principles of Biomedical Ethics*, secular bioethics and its common morality are realized in the realm of the social-democratic political agenda that Beauchamp and Childress endorse and seek to advance. If one's goal is political, one will be at peace with philosophy and bioethics' failure to provide foundations and with the ambiguity of key concepts such as autonomy and reflective equilibrium, while nevertheless speaking of a common morality that turns out to be a discourse that anticipates the establishment of one's favored morality, one's political agenda at law and in public policy. Common morality is common in anticipation of the coming realization of a political agenda. Beauchamp and Childress can thus identify those moralities that do not accord with their political agenda as "deficient" customary moralities. Or to put the matter a bit differently, the common secular morality is the customary morality that accords with the favored political agenda. Beauchamp and Childress can thus anchor the communality and universality of their morality in the future, in the realization of their political agenda. For them, all turns on their political commitments.

For Hegel, these considerations would be beyond the scope of his reflections, because they would require philosophical prophecy, or at least an anticipation of the future, and Hegel warns that philosophy cannot look to the future: "the owl of Minerva begins its flight only with the onset of dusk" (Hegel 1991, p. 23). But Beauchamp and Childress, given their political agendas, are oriented to the future, to a moral view that they seek to establish at law and in public policy. From this future perspective, they can then speak of a common morality. Such a perspective would allow Beauchamp and Childress to speak of their "universal" common morality, while the truth of their claims is in the end a promissory note based on the hoped-for success of their political agenda. Their political agenda is their morality, so they may assume that their "common" or "universal" morality is common and "universal," albeit it is currently neither universal nor common.

IV. Why, Despite Moral Pluralism, Secular Health Care Ethics Consultants Succeed so Well

The political construal of secular morality and bioethics allows one better to appreciate the success of clinical ethics, despite intractable moral pluralism, despite intractable moral disagreements. Clinical bioethics succeeds by making reference not to a canonical morality or to a political agenda, but to that ethics currently established at law and in public policy. The success of clinical bioethics lies in the circumstance that the ethics about which secular clinical ethicists are experts is that ethics *actually* established in a polity through law and public policy. Despite intractable moral pluralism, clinical ethicists can nevertheless be experts about those mores and/or norms established at law and in public policy. Clinical ethicists are not anthropological or sociological experts able to establish which norms are widely held, nor are they able to show, were they to know those norms, what would morally follow from such an anthropological or sociological fact of the matter of the norms being widely held. Clinical ethicists would need canonical, secular, sound rational arguments that do not exist. It is about these norms that there are disputes in most large-scale societies, which lie at the roots of political controversies.

Clinical ethicists are not experts as to which professional norms or ethics should be followed apart from that which is established at law and in public policy. For example, there are states in the United States that establish norms for the practice of medicine, which do not include those norms established by the Code of Ethics of the American Medical Association, to which association the overwhelming majority of physicians in the United States do not belong. In any jurisdiction, apart from such an establishment at law and/or policy of particular professional norms, as for example through state licensing authorities, clinical ethicists are not authorities able to give guidance as to which professional norms or norms of medical ethics should govern. In the United States, unlike in countries where the norms of the local medical profession are imposed with the color of law on all physicians, American medical ethicists (who are conceptually different from clinical ethicists) can at best lay out disparate codes for the practice of medicine and particular specialties, as well as how they constrain members of particular associations of physicians.

The roles of health care ethics consultants as a result have strong family resemblances with the roles of lawyers. Lawyers do not directly give advice regarding "widely-held social norms," nor do attorneys give guidance about professional norms beyond those norms established at law and in public policy. Similarly, health care ethics consultants give what is tantamount to legal advice in functioning as experts about the norms and/or morality established at law and in public policy (including those bearing on tort law). They can give answers to questions, for example, as to who in a particular jurisdiction is in authority to make medical decisions for incompetent patients and with respect to the circumstances under which an advance directive is valid. To repeat once more, health care ethics consultants function by giving quasi-legal advice regarding that morality established at law and public policy (Engelhardt 2012, 2011, 2009, 2003). One thus sees why, despite the moral pluralism that would appear at first blush to be a cardinal impediment, health care ethics consultants, clinical ethicists, or clinical bioethicists, however one styles the profession, have succeeded so well in advancing their trade. Health care ethics consultants can function successfully despite intractable moral and bioethical disputes, because they do not in fact function as moral or ethics experts. Instead, they usually help families, physicians, nurses, and others to understand the implications for clinical decisions of established law and public policy bearing on health care and the biomedical sciences.

Like lawyers, clinical ethicists can identify and characterize grey zones and then make suggestions about how to act with the least moral (read legal and public policy) risk. In addition, by means of consultations and through entering notes into the patients' charts regarding controverted cases, clinical ethicists can help show that due diligence has been taken in reaching a decision. Establishing that due diligence has been taken tends to serve as a protection against malpractice suits and other legal adversities. Health care ethics consultants thereby support effective risk management. Last but not least, clinical ethicists while noting the constraints of law and public policy can function, as do lawyers, as expert mediators among disputing parties. When they function well, they function as talented, legally cognizant mediators. In none of this is there any need for an agreement regarding a canonical morality or canonical bioethics. There is no need for ethics expertise as traditional morality had once conceived of it (i.e., knowing what is the really right thing to do). Clinical ethicists do not know better than others what people should do, apart from law and public policy. Instead, secular clinical ethicists by appealing to that ethics enshrined in law and established health care policy can bypass the problems of moral and bioethical pluralism. They need only know the norms of the morality and bioethics established at law and in health care policy in their particular jurisdiction. Health care ethics consultants can therefore function well and even flourish in the face of moral pluralism, in a secular society whose established morality and bioethics are without foundations and where in addition robust moral pluralism prevails.

The result of this state of affairs is that there is not just an American clinical bioethics and a European clinical bioethics, but also a German clinical bioethics, an Italian clinical bioethics, a Chinese clinical bioethics, a Japanese clinical bioethics, a Texan clinical bioethics, and a Californian clinical bioethics, not to mention a Norwegian clinical bioethics. In each jurisdiction, given its own law and public policy bearing on health care and the biomedical sciences, the ethics of clinical ethics consultation (however one wishes to style the field) will be different. This is the case in that a clinical ethicist must know local law and established policy in order to practice clinical bioethics. Again, in this matter clinical ethicists have a great similarity to lawyers. Clinical ethics is jurisdiction-specific, although, as with some lawyers, a clinical ethicist may be able to practice competently in different jurisdictions. In general, some talents (e.g., for mediating disputes) may be presumed for competent practice in nearly every jurisdiction.

The matter is different for bioethicists who have expertise regarding a particular morality and its bioethics, which morality and bioethics are not only held to have a force apart from law and public policy, but which are also applied within particular institutions. This involves circumstances such as when a morality or bioethics is established in an institution nested within a non-geographically-based moral community. For example, a Roman Catholic clinical ethicist in a Roman Catholic hospital does function as a moral expert about a morality that is recognized by a particular community as having force apart from secular law and public policy, as being in fact grounded in the will of God. In addition, for such Roman Catholic health care ethics consultants, ecclesiastical law also plays a role, and it is understandable that Roman Catholic health care ethics consultants be subject to Roman Catholic canon law and require the approval of the local bishop. Relevant knowledge concerning Roman Catholic canon law (e.g., excommunication for performing an abortion) will therefore be important. In short, here there can be a morality about which a bioethicist can and should be a moral expert, where a morality and a bioethics qua particular morality and/or bioethics are held to have force. Such moralities and bioethics have been neither demoralized nor deflated. In this circumstance, Christian bioethics has a concrete and sectarian meaning. It is different in content and character, depending on whether it is an Episcopalian or Orthodox Christian bioethics. These Christian bioethics differ in terms of their content, as well as with respect to who are recognized as authorities and/or as being in authority (e.g., bishops) to settle disputes. There are also different relevant literatures. The whole sense of appropriate religious bioethics, including clinical bioethics, differs from religion to religion. One might consider, for example, the special role of rabbinic authorities in providing clinical ethical guidance in Orthodox Jewish hospitals.

In summary, despite moral pluralism and in the absence of foundations, secular clinical ethicists possess a very useful expertise, even though there is no canonical secular morality or bioethics about which such health care ethics consultants can be experts. Secular clinical experts are experts regarding the morality and ethics established at law and public policy within their polity, especially about how to apply that established morality and bioethics in particular situations. The practice of clinical ethics is like the practice of law (in fact, the public recognition of clinical ethics has allowed its practitioners to practice law without being admitted to the bar), which also does not require moral or ethical expertise. One does not need to have studied philosophical theories and other accounts of the law in order to practice law successfully. The successful practice of the law does not require that there be a canonical account of the foundations or moral significance of the law. One does not need a philosophy of law to practice law. There is, after all, no canonical secular account of the authority of secular law and public policy beyond its being imposed by a particular *modus vivendi*. Instead, there is an intractable plurality of accounts of secular morality and of the law, not to mention a large number of conflicting codes of law.[8]

V. Beyond Self-Deception: Bioethics and Clinical Ethics Reconsidered

In order to appreciate the success of secular clinical ethicists, one must radically revise one's assumptions about what is required to count as an expert clinical ethicist. If the appeal by health care ethics consultants explicitly or implicitly is to that ethics established at law and public policy, there is no need for, and there are good reasons against, secular clinical ethicists ever holding themselves to be normative ethicists or to be experts about what *ceteris paribus* one should do morally. After all, given moral and bioethical pluralism, the secular normative issue of what would be right, good, virtuous, or just to do is a matter of persistent disagreement. However, which morality is established at law and in public policy is a fact of the matter. Again, the success of health care ethics consultants is best explained by the circumstance that secular clinical ethicists give quasi-legal advice while rarely if ever providing straightforward moral or bioethical advice. Health care ethics consultants can function well in the contemporary dominant secular culture, despite intractable moral pluralism, as well as in the face of the demoralization and deflation of the secular morality and bioethics of the West. Clinical ethics is after morality.

If this account of bioethics and clinical ethics is justified, why do not all bioethicists and clinical ethicists recognize its truth? Of course, if one is a conceptive ideologist earning one's living as a bioethics expert, it may not help one's career to be too frank about the foundationless character of secular morality and bioethics. It may not be a good marketing strategy to underscore the actual character of clinical ethics. Also, if one has a political agenda, there may be no good reasons for, and there may be good reasons against, acknowledging publicly and clearly that one's moral concerns are really a political agenda. One may simply wish to establish the clinical ethics one favors. One's candor will be limited by political considerations. There will be significant conflicts of interest between earning one's living as a conceptive ideologist (e.g., a secular bioethics or ethics expert) and committing oneself to forthrightness. There have always been tensions between personal political agendas and full forthrightness about the policies one is advancing. The ethos of consultancy and of the political life is not one necessarily marked by frankness concerning the service one is selling or concerning one's political agenda, if such forthrightness is likely to undermine one's marketability or political agenda.

Let me underscore that this state of affairs does not impeach my view of those who act guided by career or political expediency. What else would one expect? Moreover, all surely do not act out of expediency. Some clinical ethicists also are undoubtedly honestly misled by their success in working through to resolutions of bioethical and clinical ethical quandaries so that they are brought to think of themselves as moral or bioethical experts. But of course, such "working through" is what good lawyers do in their practice of the law without being moral experts. Nevertheless, some clinical ethicists may derive an important dimension of their self-identity and self-esteem from their ungrounded view of themselves as moral experts. They may see themselves as clinical ethical experts apart from and beyond what they know about the morality and norms established at law and in public policy, and beyond their talents as mediators and in selling themselves as consultants. This is all personally understandable, but it does not count against the foundational reconsideration of bioethics and clinical ethics advanced by this chapter. Secular bioethics and clinical ethics are not what many thought the field to be.

In that secular bioethics and secular clinical ethics will reflect secular law and secular political agendas at odds with traditional Christian belief, believing patients, their families, and health care providers will find themselves in a micro culture war. They will be obliged, as chapter five shows, to remain true to their obligations to God. To say the very least, this will not meet with approval from secular institutions or from secular law and health care policy. Traditional Christians will thus come face to face with the profoundly secular, post-Christian character of the bioethics that emerged out of the cultural and religious chaos of the 1960s and 1970s. They will find themselves as moral strangers within the secular, post-Christian culture, indeed as its moral enemies.

Notes

[1]This chapter is drawn in part from a lecture, "Bioethics after Foundations: Feeling the Full Force of Secularization," delivered at the Centro Evangelico di Cultura "Arturo Pascal" and the Consulta di Bioetica ONLUS, Turin, Italy, January 31, 2012. An ancestral version of this chapter appears as Engelhardt 2013.

[2]I must admit to having since my youth been disappointed by the claims of moral philosophy regarding sound rational argument. When I was still a Roman Catholic, I had tried to my utmost to use philosophy to secure its natural law, natural theological, and other rationalist claims. I was shocked by my failure. I found that the moral-philosophical and -theological arguments of Roman Catholicism required the concession of crucial and controverted initial premises and rules of inference. Then I discovered that the same difficulty lies at the basis of any secular moral-philosophical viewpoint, morality, or bioethics. This chapter is a special gloss on this difficulty in bioethics.

[3]*Confiteor quia peccavi nimis.* From the early 1970s, I was culpable in part for the development and success of the dominant secular bioethics. I helped teach the Kennedy Institute summer courses and myself directed courses in bioethics supported by the National Endowment for the Humanities Seminars for Medical and Health Care Teachers between 1974 and 1980. Also, from 1977 through 1982 as the Rosemary Kennedy Professor of the Philosophy of Medicine at Georgetown University, I made my modest contribution to the development of the field. I am as guilty as any for what naively took place in the 1970s and early 1980s.

[4]Let me be quite clear that my reflections concerning Beauchamp and Childress's bioethics are not advanced in criticism of them. Personally, I am deeply indebted to them both and consider them to be my friends and colleagues. Moreover, I acknowledge them as likely the two most important figures for the emergence of bioethics in the latter part of the 20th century. Their *Principles of Biomedical Ethics* gave the new field the substance and direction it felt that it needed. My critical repositioning of their work recognizes their importance. I have

approached their work in an Hegelian spirit (caveat lector: I have taught Hegel for decades, but I am not a Hegelian). My goal is to lay out the higher truth of their work.

[5]For an overview of the drive in the United States on the part of clinical ethics consultants to establish themselves as a profession, see Kodish & Fins 2013.

[6] *Mea culpa*. I must confess my involvement in the emergence of the so-called four principles. Beauchamp and Childress's four principles grew out of the success of the National Commission's three principles of respect for persons, beneficence, and justice in guiding the commissioners in the articulation of regulations for research involving human subjects (National Commission 1978, pp. 4–10). The three principles of the *Belmont Report* themselves were in part developed out of principles suggested in a background paper I had authored.

A. One should respect human subjects as free agents out of a duty to such subjects to acknowledge their right to respect as free agents.

B. One should foster the best interests of individual human subjects.

C. One should have concern to maximize the benefits accruable to society from research involving human subjects, taking into particular regard interest in values such as (1) the amelioration of the human condition through advances in the biomedical and behavioral sciences and technologies; (2) preservation of human autonomy as a general value; (3) increase in knowledge apart from any consideration of its application to the amelioration of human condition; (4) the personal satisfaction of human subjects derived from their feeling of having contributed to the common good or to the advancement of human knowledge by participation in research (Engelhardt 1978, pp. 8–5, 8–6).

The first two principles were recast under the rubrics of a principle supporting respect for persons and a principle of beneficence (Jonsen 1998, p. 103). The third principle was substantially recast as a principle of justice.

Albert Jonsen in his history of the emergence of bioethics gives an account of the emergence of the focus on principles of bioethics. He states that, in the development of the Belmont principles, his fellow commissioner, Joseph V. Brady,

professed that he was attracted to three principles only: beneficence, freedom, and justice. I seconded Brady's point because these three principles seemed to do what ethical principles should do—namely, serve as rational justification for decisions and policies. We also had in our dossier of philosophical essays H. Tristram Engelhardt's paper which had suggested three basic principles: "respect for persons as free moral agents, concern to support the best interests of human subjects in research, intent in assuring that the use of human subjects of experimentation will on the sum redound to the benefit of society." Tom Beauchamp had also contributed a paper entitled "Distributive justice and morally relevant differences." After much discussion, the commissioners took Engelhardt's first two principles and Beauchamp's principle of distributive justice and crafted "crisp" principles: respect for persons, beneficence, and justice. Stephen Toulmin was directed to redraft the report for presentation at the March meeting. . . . [These] principles found their way into the general literature of the field, and, in the process, grew from the principles underlying the conduct of research into the basic principles of bioethics (Jonsen 1998, pp. 103, 104).

The final outcome was a broad public appeal to principles.

[7]St. John Chrysostom (344–407) emphasizes the obligation at times to deceive others. "The straightforward man does great harm to those he will not deceive" (Chrysostom 1984, p. 51).

[8]There is a significant demand for clinical ethicists, given the post-traditional character of Western society. In the face of the loss of the authority of traditional authority figures (e.g., physicians), the weakening of intermediate structures, and the fracturing as well as increasing infrequency of intact traditional families, clinical ethicists can, do, and will play an important default role. Moreover, they are relatively easy to train as well as (generally) relatively inexpensive. Using clinical ethicists instead of lawyers who have specialized in health law has advantages analogous to using nurse practitioners instead of physicians. Nevertheless, lawyers and physicians have more social prestige, which invites clinical ethicists to attempt to secure for themselves a prominent status in their own right.

References

Alora, Angeles Tan & Josephine M. Lumitao (eds.). 2001. *Beyond a Western Bioethics: Voices from the Developing World*. Washington, DC: Georgetown University Press.

Beauchamp, T. L. 2004. Does ethical theory have a future in bioethics? *Journal of Law, Medicine, and Ethics* 32: 209–217.

Beauchamp, T. L. & J. Childress. 1979. *The Principles of Biomedical Ethics*. New York: Oxford.

Beauchamp, T. L. & J. Childress. 1983. *The Principles of Biomedical Ethics*, 2nd ed. New York: Oxford.

Beauchamp, T. L. & J. Childress. 1989. *The Principles of Biomedical Ethics*, 3rd ed. New York: Oxford.

Beauchamp, T. L. & J. Childress. 1994. *The Principles of Biomedical Ethics*, 4th ed. New York: Oxford.

Beauchamp, T. L. & J. Childress. 2001. *The Principles of Biomedical Ethics*, 5th ed. New York: Oxford.

Beauchamp, T. L. & J. Childress. 2009. *The Principles of Biomedical Ethics*, 6th ed. New York: Oxford.

Beauchamp, T. L. & J. Childress. 2012. *The Principles of Biomedical Ethics*, 7th ed. New York: Oxford.

Bishop, Jeffrey. 2011. *The Anticipatory Corpse*. Notre Dame, IN: University of Notre Dame Press.

Buchanan, Allen. 2009. *Justice & Health Care*. New York: Oxford University Press.

Chrysostom, St. John. 1984. *Six Books on the Priesthood*, trans. Graham Neville. Crestwood, NY: St. Vladimir's Seminary Press.

Daniels, Norman. 1985. *Just Health Care*. New York: Cambridge University Press.

Engelhardt, H. T., Jr. 2013. Bioethics and moral pluralism, *Notizie di Politeia* 105 (June): 7–21.

Engelhardt, H. T., Jr. 2012. Bioethics critically reconsidered: Living after foundations, *Theoretical Medicine and Bioethics* 33.1: 97–105.

Engelhardt, H. T., Jr. 2011. Core competencies for health care ethics consultants: In search of professional status in a post-modern world, *HealthCare Ethics Committee [HEC] Forum* 23.3 (September): 129–145.

Engelhardt, H. T., Jr. 2009. Credentialing strategically ambiguous and heterogeneous social skills: The emperor without clothes, *Hospital Ethics Committees [HEC] Forum* 21.3 (September): 293–306.

Engelhardt, H. T., Jr. 2003. The bioethics consultant: Giving moral advice in the midst of moral controversy, *HealthCare Ethics Committee [HEC] Forum* 15.4 (December): 362–382.

Engelhardt, H. T., Jr. 2002. The ordination of bioethicists as secular moral experts, *Social Philosophy & Policy* 19.2: 59–82.

Engelhardt, H. T., Jr. 1996. *The Foundations of Bioethics*, 2nd ed. New York: Oxford University Press; 1st edition, 1986.

Engelhardt, H. T., Jr. 1991. *Bioethics and Secular Humanism*. Philadelphia: Trinity Press International.

Engelhardt, H. T., Jr. 1978. Basic ethical principles in the conduct of biomedical and behavioral research involving human subjects, *The Belmont Report*, Appendix vol. 1, sec. 8, pp. 1–45. Washington, DC: Department of Health, Education, and Welfare, publication # (12) 78–0013.

Fan, Ruiping (ed.). 2011. *The Renaissance of Confucianism in Contemporary China*. Dordrecht: Springer.

Fan, Ruiping. 2010. *Reconstructionist Confucianism*. Dordrecht: Springer.

Fan, Ruiping, Xiaoyang Chen, & Yongfu Cao. 2012. Family-oriented health savings accounts: Facing the challenges of health care allocation, *Journal of Medicine and Philosophy* 37.6: 507–512.

Hegel, G. W. F. 1991. *Elements of the Philosophy of Right*, ed. Allen W. Wood, trans. H. B. Nisbet. New York: Cambridge University Press.

Hoshino, Kazumasa (ed.). 1997. *Japanese and Western Bioethics*. Dordrecht: Kluwer/Springer.

Jonsen, Albert. 1998. *The Birth of Bioethics*. New York: Oxford University Press.

Kukathas, Chandran. 2007. *The Liberal Archipelago*. New York: Oxford University Press.

Koch, Tom. 2012. *Thieves of Virtue: When Bioethics Stole Medicine*. Cambridge, MA: MIT Press.

Kodish, Eric & Joseph J. Fins. 2013. Quality attestation for clinical ethics consultants, *Hastings Center Report* 43.5 (Sept.–Oct.): 26–36.

Kozinski, Thaddeus J. 2010. *The Political Problem of Religious Pluralism*. Lanham, MD: Rowman & Littlefield.

Li, Jun & Jue Wang. 2012. Individuals are inadequate: Recognizing the family-centeredness of Chinese bioethics and Chinese health system, *Journal of Medicine and Philosophy* 37.6: 568–582.

Lim, Meng-Kin. 2012. Values and health care: The Confucian dimension in health care reform, *Journal of Medicine and Philosophy* 37.6: 545–555.

Marx, Karl & Friedrich Engels. 1967. *The German Ideology*. New York: International Publishers.

Rorty, Richard. 1989. *Contingency, Irony, and Solidarity*. New York: Cambridge University Press.

CHAPTER SEVEN

Common Ground as Battleground: Seeking an Anchor in God[1]

I. Morality, Bioethics, the Culture Wars, and Western Christianity: Assessing the Current Terrain

There is no cultural peace. We are in a culture war defined by disagreements. Salient among the disagreements are bioethical battles about abortion, human embryo stem-cell research, therapy for sexual dysfunction in homosexual couples, artificial insemination of unmarried women, reproduction in marriage with the use of donor gametes, health care allocation, physician-assisted suicide, and euthanasia, to name only a few issues. In great part, these disputes exist because of the collision of traditional Christian morality and bioethics with the morality and bioethics of the dominant secular culture. Most salient is traditional Christianity's rejection of the demoralization of morality and bioethics, as well as of the aggressive secularization of the public space (Hunter 1991). The cultural geography of these profound disagreements frames the public discourse of bioethics and health care policy. The character of this public discourse is crucially tied to the secularization and the de-Christianization of the West. Contemporary bioethics itself arose within the collapse of mainline Christianity.

This chapter shows how the emergence of contemporary secular bioethics was closely associated with ecclesial and theological changes in Roman Catholicism, the largest of the Christian denominations, which changes led to the abandonment of its previous paradigm of medical ethics and the emergence of secular bioethics. Contemporary secular bioethics under the term *bioethics* as it developed at Georgetown University, a Jesuit university, in the 1970s was intimately tied to conditions within post-Vatican II Roman Catholicism. Contemporary secular bioethics has important roots in the disputes characterizing Roman Catholicism in the late 1960s and early 1970s. To appreciate the place of Christian bioethics in the contemporary debates, this chapter examines as well the role of Roman Catholic thinkers in attempting to bring peace to the culture wars by denying as well as obscuring difference. It is traditional and/or conservative Christians who are prominent belligerents in the culture wars. The contemporary bioethical culture wars also importantly reflect consequences of the post-Vatican II (1962–1965) changes in Roman Catholicism, which have left it ever less monolithic in its opposition to the secularity that shapes the morality and bioethics of the dominant culture. The contemporary culture wars are located within this complex territory of conflicting social forces. The cardinal question then arises: Given the disarray of Western Christianity, will the moral and bioethical battles in the culture wars continue?

This is not an easy question to answer, especially given the continuing secularization and disorientation of much of Western Christianity. What resources remain to sustain Christianity's counter-cultural character along with its responses to the secular transformation of morality, bioethics, and health care policy? Is Western Christianity not itself about to be thoroughly demoralized and in the mode of Paul Tillich (1886–1965) deflated? Can Western Christianity continue to supply recruits for the culture wars? This serious issue regarding the future of the culture wars and the future context for the disputes about morality, bioethics, and health care policy is a central focus of this chapter. Will the cultural belligerencies concerning morality and bioethics continue? There are grounds for doubting the staying power of Western Christianity. The secularization of Western Christianity, along with false perceptions regarding the character of the disputes resulting especially from a continued commitment to the moral-philosophical project, raise the possibility that even many Christians will no longer fully appreciate what is at stake: the collision between a secular moral vision with its bioethics, and the moral vision grounded not in philosophy but in an experience of God. What is offered in this chapter is a geography of the contemporary Western Christian theological terrain, along with its differences from Orthodox Christianity. The chapter closes with examining what it is to have a theology along with moral and bioethical norms grounded in God.

II. Making Way for a New Paradigm for Medical Moral Reflection

As the last chapter has shown, secular academic bioethics is an arena of interminable disputes, for which theoretical reflections can at best provide a geography of a contentious intellectual territory, but not a way out. Health care ethics
consultation, for its part, has successfully taken possession of a domain of the
practice of law, so that it offers what amounts to legal advice. However, the ethics established at law and in public policy is often strongly in tension with the
obligations of Christian health care professionals. This complex phenomenon
of secular bioethics occasions the culture wars because, if nothing else unites
secular bioethics, it is united by an understanding of itself as after Christianity. Chapter four addresses this point by showing why traditional Christians
find themselves in positions in which they are unable to compromise with the
demands of law and public policy established by secular fundamentalist states
where a particular secular ideology plays a role analogous to the role religion
plays in a religious fundamentalist state (Engelhardt 2010a and 2010b). But who
are those who remain in opposition to the secular state's violation of their consciences? What is the character of their opposition? Answering such questions
is core to understanding the culture wars and the place of morality and bioethics
therein. This chapter focuses primarily, but not exclusively, on the role played by
Roman Catholicism, in that it is the largest and by far the most organized of the
Christianities. Moreover, it is the origin of secular bioethics.

The belligerence of the culture wars depends on the vigor of the disputing
parties. The party of the secular is generally quite dedicated. Therefore, the character and strength of the battles depend on the strength of the response of those
committed to traditional Christian moral and bioethical positions, primarily
traditional Christians who reject the secular demoralization and deflation of
morality and bioethics. As a consequence, these conflicts have a different character in different polities, depending chiefly on the strength of the religious groups
within their jurisdictions. Often, the response of the locally dominant Christianities will be mild at best. Foreshadowing recent changes in Roman Catholicism, the mainline Protestant Christian churches from the mid-18th and early
19th century abetted secularization and desacralization as they themselves were
transformed.[2] A powerful early and continuing influence on the secularization

of Protestantism was Immanuel Kant's project of reducing religion to its moral significance, so that it did not matter to which religion one belonged, as long as one lived a "moral" life. Doctrinal substance became irrelevant and a "rational" ethos could be affirmed.

> We have good reason to say ... that "the kingdom of God is come unto us" once the principle of the gradual transition of ecclesiastical faith to the universal religion of reason, and so to a (divine) ethical state on earth, has become general and has also gained somewhere a *public* foothold, even though the actual establishment of this state is still infinitely removed from us (Kant 1960, p. 113, AK VI 114).

Kant endorsed a moral and social gospel. Faith in such a universal religion of reason was sufficiently widespread among intellectuals at the beginning of the 19th century that some liberal Jews, admittedly for a complex set of reasons,[3] considered entering into some form of congregational union with liberal Protestants of equally sparse confessional commitments (Hess 2002, esp. pp. 176–182).

Before the mid-20th century, the results of secularization were already widespread in central Europe. In Germany in particular by the late 19th century, mainline Protestantism was largely moribund.[4] As Eduard von Hartmann (1842–1906) noted, "Liberal Protestantism has necessarily become an irreligious phenomenon of history, because Protestantism has taken the interest of modern culture to be the criterion" (von Hartmann 1874, p. 87). Mainline Protestantism was effecting its own *Selbstzersetzung*, its own self-destruction. This secularization was described in various ways and promoted by Friedrich Schleiermacher (1763–1834), Arthur Schopenhauer (1788–1860), Ludwig Feuerbach (1804–1872), and David Strauss (1808–1874). There was a widespread *Verweltlichung* (secularization) of Protestant Christianity (Overbeck 1919, p. 245). By the early 20th century in Germany, the transformation had been thoroughgoing. As Émile Durkheim (1858–1917) puts it, "the old gods are growing old or already dead, and others are not yet born" (Durkheim 1947, p. 427). An analogous secularization and deflation of dogma marked Protestantism in many areas of the northern United States, especially in New England.[5] It was in reaction against liberal Protestantism that fundamentalist Christianity developed its identity at the end of the 19th and the beginning of the 20th century.[6]

Finally, a Protestantism emerged that was *sotto voce* after God, a liberal Protestantism that realized itself in a social gospel and moral commitments without a metaphysics of transcendence. Some of these Protestants were influenced by and were intellectual descendants of Hegel. As Charles Taylor puts it,

> Thus while Hegel is not in the main line of descent of liberal Protestantism, he is the point of origin of another important movement towards a demythologized, one might say, 'de-theologized' Christianity. Contemporary theologies of 'the death of God' are his spiritual grandchildren. The filiation is either direct, as with Paul Tillich who very much influenced the theologians of this school, or through the young Hegelian Ludwig Feuerbach (Taylor 1975, p. 495).

One must therefore wonder about the meaning of the gloss by Emil Fackenheim on Karl Barth regarding Hegel: "We may rely on Karl Barth's apt formulation that Hegel seeks to do for the modern Protestant world what St. Thomas Aquinas has done for the Catholic Middle Ages" (Fackenheim 1967, p. 10). An Orthodox Christian would take this to be a subtle way of also criticizing Aquinas's effect on Western Christianity. In any event, by the late 20th century, one had with figures such as Paul Tillich (1886–1965) Christian theologians without belief in the God of the Christians. As Richard Rorty remarked,

> when people asked why [Tillich] didn't stop pretending to be a Christian theologian and instead bill himself as a Heideggerian philosopher . . . [h]e would say in effect that it was precisely the job of a Christian theologian these days to find a way of making it possible for Christians to continue using the term 'Christ' even after they had given up supernaturalism (as he hoped they eventually would)" (Rorty 1991, p. 70).

A post-Christian Christianity had emerged.

Contrary to the assertion of Edward S. Shapiro, in the dominant secular culture it is not the case that "If a Christian is secularized and becomes an atheist or an agnostic, he ceases being a Christian" (Shapiro 2014, p. 42), as the counterexamples of G. W. F. Hegel and Paul Tillich ably attest. Christians, like Jews, can remain Christians within the contemporary culture even when they are atheists

or at least agnostics.[7] Thomas Luckmann appreciates this deflation or immanentization of the transcendent (an old theme articulated by Hegel in 1802).

> The span of transcendence is shrinking. Modern religious themes such
> as "self-realization," personal autonomy, and self-expression have become
> dominant. More recently, they have fused either with the newly emerg-
> ing mix of pseudo-science and magic or with certain rearticulations of the
> intermediate and great transcendences in the ecological components of the
> "New Age." The shrinking of transcendence thus does not mean a loss of
> the "sacred." The dominant themes in the modern sacred cosmos bestow
> something like a sacred status upon the individual himself by articulating
> his autonomy. As the transcendent social order and the great transcendences
> cease to be generally significant, matters that are important to the privatized,
> partly egoistic and hedonistic, partly ecological, symbolically altruistic indi-
> vidual become sacralized (Luckmann 1990, p. 138).

The only question is whether Jews and Christians can resist these powerful
forces in the dominant secular culture. Will they become Jews and Christians
after God?

A fate similar to mainline Protestantism and Reform Judaism was initially
resisted by Roman Catholicism. It vigorously responded to threats of secularization through Pope Pius IX's (1792–1878, elected 1846) *Syllabus of Errors* (December 8, 1864) and other condemnations of modernism, the complex movement
that devalued supernatural commitments and sought accommodation to the
secular culture. There was as well the condemnation by Pope Leo XIII (1810–
1903, elected 1878) of Americanism, which was considered a heresy for supporting *inter alia* the separation of church and state. Americanism was addressed,
for example, in a letter by Pope Leo XIII to Cardinal Gibbons of Baltimore of 22
January 1899 (Denzinger 1965, pp. 656–658, novus numerus textum 3340–3346;
vetus numerus 1967–1976).[8] Rome was able to bring order by acting from the
top down. This included having all seminarians under oath reject modernism
(September 1, 1910). Save with regard to the Roman Catholic intellectual class,
these measures were largely successful, such that generally parishes were for
the most part flourishing, pious, and engaged in charitable outreach. Although
these measures were repressive, they fit into an ecclesial culture that was itself

generally repressive and had forbidden, among other things, vernacular translations of the Mass (placing them on the *Index of Forbidden Books*) until the late 19th century.[9] Despite all of these difficulties, there was a high rate of adult conversions.[10] Tendentious histories depict the pre-Vatican II church as ineffective and shallow,[11] notwithstanding the fact that pre-Vatican II Roman Catholicism was marked by high devotion reflected in real "social justice" achieved through hospitals and parochial schools manned by nuns and brothers. Liturgical life in the Roman Catholic church before Vatican II was surely often distorted, as pious Roman Catholics said the rosary while priests read the Mass in Latin at amazing speeds. Nevertheless, there is objective evidence of success before and then collapse after Vatican II (1962–1965). A sense of the sacred was nurtured along with high levels of Mass attendance. Pre-Vatican II Catholicism was generally functional, and the Catholicism of Vatican II, with that of Popes John XXIII (1881–1963, elected 1958), Paul VI (1897–1978, elected 1963), and John Paul II (1920–2005, elected 1978) was generally dysfunctional, secularized, and indeed desacralized.

It must be noted that two features of pre-Vatican II Roman Catholicism made it ripe for a revolution that generated liturgical as well as doctrinal transformation and confusion, if not chaos (Hull 2010). The first was a liturgical movement that had been developing throughout the early 20th century bent on radically recasting the traditional Tridentine Mass. As an example, one might consider the work of Fr. Gerald Ellard, S.J., and his *The Mass of the Future* (Ellard 1948). An overview of the roots and character of the sweeping changes is offered by one of their most important advocates and agents of the changes, Archbishop Annibale Bugnini (1990), as well as by critics of those changes (Wiltgen 1967). Many of these 20th-century liturgical movements that led to Paul VI's Novus Ordo Mass had roots in the Jansenist liturgical agenda of the 18th century. Before Vatican II there were clear signs of movements that would create a rupture in the ritual habits that had given Roman Catholicism continuity and coherence. The second feature was a view of papal authority that became widespread with Pope Pius IX, which held that the pope had the authority in a fundamental fashion to alter and set aside liturgical tradition. As a result of this view of papal authority, the majority of Roman Catholics accepted the radical liturgical changes instituted by Pope Paul VI. This would have been impossible prior to the further accretion of papal authority subsequent to the Council of Trent (1545–1563), Pius IX (1792–1878, elected 1846), and Vatican I (1869–1870), before which the pope's authority was held to be more limited.[12]

This is not to say that dispute and dissent did not accompany the changes introduced during and after Vatican II. There was a significant minority of Roman Catholics who to various degrees did not agree with the changes and at times reacted in fear regarding their likely consequences. This minority regarded the changes as revolutionary, as with respect to the Council's declaration regarding the authority of the College of Bishops, the affirmation of which Yves Congar (1904–1995) characterized as an October Revolution.[13] These individuals tended still to have a commitment to the traditional Roman Catholic approaches to morality and medical ethics. They realized that a major disorienting transformation of Roman Catholicism had been initiated. Archbishop Annibale Bugnini himself admits:

> The path of liturgical reform has been marked not only by experimentation
> and adaptation but also by opposition. While some indulged in uncontrolled
> experimentation, to the detriment of the faith and the sacredness of worship
> of the Lord, others took a hard stand on the past and launched a systematic
> attack on the reform (Bugnini 1990, p. 277).

In an attempt to limit the negative reaction that was already salient, the preparation of the new calendar for the Novus Ordo Mass proceeded in secrecy (Bugnini 1990, p. 315). A gulf opened between the reformers and the defenders of the old Mass. The controversies that resulted were strident and were associated with significant demographic changes.

The hemorrhage of clerics and congregants that had begun during Vatican II provoked a warning on September 25, 1969, from Alfredo Cardinal Ottaviani and Antonio Cardinal Bacci (Ottaviani & Bacci n.d.) that the changes were undermining Roman Catholicism. The difficulties accelerated after the *de jure* establishment among Roman Catholics of the Novus Ordo Mass in November 1969. Roman Catholicism was marked by a dramatic loss of priests, religious brothers and sisters, and laity. There was in particular a loss of vocations. In the United States, the number of diocesan seminarians fell from 6.3 per ten thousand Roman Catholics in 1965 to 0.51 per ten thousand in 2002 (Jones 2003, p.

29), while the number of religious seminarians fell from 4.87 per ten thousand in 1965 to 0.21 per ten thousand in 2002 (Jones 2003, p. 30). In the seven years following the replacement of the Tridentine Mass by the Novus Ordo Mass in 1970, the number of priests in the world declined from about 410,000 to about 245,000. The period was also characterized by a major loss of communicants. For example, in the period from 1965 to 1974, weekly church attendance among Canadian Protestants dropped 19%, but among Canadian Catholics 29% (*Index* 1980). As has been observed, "the ritual chaos within Roman Catholicism surely made a contribution to destabilizing a major social institution in Western culture" (Solomon et al. 2012, p. 12). Dietrich von Hildebrand (1889–1977) in describing those who forwarded the new liturgy noted: "They seem to be unaware of the elementary importance of sacredness in religion" (Hildebrand 1969, p. 135).

What followed was a dramatic implosion of Roman Catholicism, marked by a one-shot decline in church practice in the sixties and the early seventies (Greeley 1990).

By 1990 Roman Catholicism was qualitatively different from Roman Catholicism as it had existed in 1962 at the beginning of Vatican II. A substantial and dramatic change in its ecclesial paradigm had occurred. The result was that Roman Catholicism came to be experienced by most Roman Catholics within a fundamentally different lifeworld. Major demographic and structural changes were under way. Its hospitals lacked the presence of sufficient religious (i.e., nuns and brothers) to staff them, its parishes were in need of priests, and its parish-based schools, which no longer possessed the financial advantages of their teachers being primarily nuns, were closing. The institutions that remained in the 1970s were deeply different from what had existed in 1962. It is not just that Roman Catholicism's public face in its hospitals, churches, and parochial schools has been altered, but in addition what it means to experience Roman Catholicism as an ecclesial body has changed. As China began its Cultural Revolution in 1966 and as student unrest began in America and Western Europe, Roman Catholicism went through a revolution of its own. In the process, the lived character of Roman Catholicism was dramatically transformed. All of this occurred against the background of profound disagreements and significant tensions within Roman Catholicism about its future. It was not just that Roman

Catholics now ate meat on Fridays, but the very structure and experience of Roman Catholic piety had been altered.

There were disputes regarding many of the cardinal dogmas and disciplines of Roman Catholicism, which in the 1960s became politically incorrect (e.g., not approving homosexual acts). More significantly, there were disagreements about how to live as a Roman Catholic. Roman Catholics faced a dramatic cleft between alternative lifeworlds: traditional versus post-traditional. What had been experienced as a united lifeworld had abruptly been shattered into hostile enclaves.

> After the papal decision against artificial contraception in 1968, the debate becomes increasingly acrimonious, and a yawning gap began to appear between the church's central administration and a large majority of Catholics, including pastoral leaders and theologians. Since the election of John Paul II in 1978, that gap has grown and hardened, turning into a power struggle about a whole series of issues and concerns, such as mandatory celibacy for priests, the exclusion of women from the ordained ministry, doctrinal uniformity and academic freedom, the morality of homosexual acts, divorce and remarriage, abortion. The result of this prolonged and increasingly angry power struggle has been a growing religious cynicism, grounded in a sense that the church that speaks justice to the world refuses to practice justice within the church itself. Today's young adults have grown up in an increasingly polarized and often cynical church, where they've heard mostly criticism about Catholicism and little of what is positive and constructive (Ludwig 2000, p. 3).

Mainline Roman Catholicism was transformed from a functional and very successful religious community making converts and producing vocations with a common understanding of tradition of what it is to be a Christian into a significantly dysfunctional body that had become a battlefield in the culture wars against tradition. Roman Catholicism became a denomination from which congregants and clergy were rapidly exiting. These conflicts were world-wide (Bouyer 1970).

What emerged was an ecclesial environment that was deeply in contrast with the Orthodoxy that Roman Catholicism had left behind a millennium before.

If today the entire liturgy has become the playground of private "creativity," which can romp at will just as long as the words of consecration are kept in place, at work is the same reduction of vision whose origin lies in an erroneous development typical of the West but quite unthinkable in the Eastern Church (Ratzinger 1995, p. 112).

The vast changes in piety, belief, and liturgical attitude over the millennium of separation, especially following Vatican II, produced substantively different religious communities (i.e., not just Roman Catholic versus Orthodox, but traditional versus post-traditional Roman Catholicism) separated by their attitudes, their understandings and ecclesial ways of life, and therefore by their experience of what it means to live the Christian faith.

Both in doctrine and in liturgy, what really matters is lost when one feels obliged to distill a juristical minimum, beyond which everything is left subject to arbitrariness. Here too we would do well to learn to look once more beyond the fence of Western thinking and to make the attempt to understand anew the original vision which has remained largely intact in the East (Ratzinger 1995, p. 112).

Roman Catholicism was substantively altered as a result of changes in how it was lived and practiced. A new mind and experience of ecclesial community emerged over against what had predominated in the past. The new Roman Catholicism was contrasted strongly with various traditional groups (e.g., the Society of St. Pius X) that were attempting to re-orient themselves as most of Roman Catholicism entered a dramatically different liturgical space. Western Christianity has become essentially different, although committed hold-outs persist and flourish. As a consequence, there has been a significant closing of churches due to the decline in the number of both parishioners and priests (Weidemann 1989).

The impact was not just demographic but affected the very character of its scholarship. Roman Catholicism fell into widespread theological chaos. As Richard McCormick observed,

The Second Vatican Council, after speaking of the renewal of theological disciplines through livelier contact with the mystery of Christ and the history of salvation, remarked simply: special attention needs to be given to the devel-opment of moral theology. During the past six or seven years moral theology has experienced this special attention so unremittingly, some would say, that the Christianity has been crushed right out of it (McCormick 1981, p. 423).

Roman Catholicism was qualitatively transformed, along with its theological, philosophical, and medical moral assumptions. The style of scholarship had changed through abandoning its Scholastic character, but it was still unclear what kind of theological scholarship should replace it. It was also unclear how it should approach the field of medical ethics. Roman Catholicism had experienced a truly astonishing rupture from its pre-Vatican II past, leading to a recasting of the self-identity of the world's largest Christian denomination. There had been a wide-ranging paradigm change. Many Roman Catholics were astonished by the speed, drama, and depth of the changes, not to mention their consequences for the integrity of Roman Catholicism. One might think of a 1971 somewhat polemical volume by John Eppstein, *Has the Catholic Church Gone Mad?* (Epp-stein 1971), which was published with a *nihil obstat* and an *imprimatur*, no less. The way in which ordinary Roman Catholic life, and in particular the life of priests and religious, was experienced, was radically changed. One had entered into a new and unfamiliar life-world. There had been a secularization and a recasting of moorings whose implications were at the time largely unclear.

Rapid changes in norms of Christian piety, liturgy, spirituality, demography, and the nature of scholarship in the 19th and 20th centuries led in Western Christianity to an equally dramatic salience of widespread foundational theo-logical uncertainties, producing pervasive religious identity crises and changes in the dominant Christian ethos, which had been integral to the dominant Western ethos before its secularization. The dominant Western culture, which had been Christian, became robustly post-Christian. This transformation was largely unanticipated, dramatic, and often divisive. In part, these changes were reflected in the mid-20th-century radical death-of-God theology to which we will return in chapter 8. As William Hamilton described the texture of the changes in theology:

The death of God radical theologians, recently given far more visibility than they either desired or deserved, are men without God who do not anticipate his return. But it is not a simple not-having, for there is an experience of loss. Painful for some, not so for others, it is loss nonetheless. The loss is not of the idols, or of the God of theism, but of the God of the Christian tradition. And this group persists, in the face of both bewilderment and fury, in calling itself Christian. It persists in making use of the phrase "death of God," in spite of its rhetorical color, partly because it is a phrase that cannot be adapted to traditional use by the theologians today (Hamilton 1966, p. 6).

The post-Vatican II world framed a dominant culture that defined itself as after tradition. It was integral to a cult of the new that was emerging with strength. In the dominant culture, the framework of theological experience had changed fundamentally so that old points of certainty were substantively undermined and obscured. As Altizer and Hamilton gloss this state of affairs, the changes that underlay the death of God in the dominant culture radically altered what 20th-century Christianity came to mean in the public space. The culture was profoundly altered.

There once was a God to whom adoration, praise and trust were appropriate, possible, and even necessary, but that now there is no such God. This is the position of the death of God or radical theology. It is an atheist position, but with a difference. If there was a God, and if there now isn't it should be possible to indicate why this change took place, when it took place, and who was responsible for it (Altizer & Hamilton 1966, p. x).

For many, this fundamental change seems oxymoronic, in that God had been recognized as the one necessarily existing being. Now God is absent. More than anyone, it was the Western theologians who had killed Him in the culture. They had cut away the old moorings. A new context for orientation, or for that matter for disorientation, became regnant.

These changes brought often dramatic institutional transformations, which recast the character of most Christian universities and colleges (Gleason 1995; Hauerwas & Westerhoff 1992; Marsden & Longfield 1995; Sloan 1973). For example, Roman Catholic education, after having largely maintained its religious and cultural integrity from the Middle Ages into the mid-20th century, was radically transformed. It became post-Christian. As Burtchaell observes,

The Catholic establishment thus fended off both Modernism and Americanism until the destabilizing 1960s, when lay autonomy, an embarrassment about scholarly mediocrity, and the drive for recognition by the then secular American academy and the acceptance of its liberal dogma abruptly destroyed the Catholic self-assuredness of an intellectual advantage (Burtchaell 1998, p. ix).

The result was that a new academic orthodoxy, a zealous heterodoxy secular in character, emerged that "excluded Christian belief as unworthy of study in the new orthodoxy of secularism" (Burtchaell 1998, p. ix). The mention of God as a ground for morality had become a conversation stopper (Rorty 1999). In the dominant culture after God, the mention of God could lead nowhere. The foundational roots and points of orientation for the dominant culture had changed. As a result, "God-talk" took on a saliently problematic valence, even in many Christian universities and colleges.

In Roman Catholicism, very powerful, destructive, anti-traditional emotions were unleashed within a cultural environment that had become hostile to tradition, leading to a convulsion of painful transformations.

> Catholics were displeased with their hymns; their saints, their curia; their liturgy; their concordats; their journalism; their ethnic parishes; their architecture; their aloofness from Masons, cremation, and Baptist prayers at high school graduations; their fish on Friday; their Thomism and their Bible translations; their sisters in heavy serge habits and headgear; their clericalism; their sacred art; their church histories; their reproductive rate; their seminaries; their maladaptive missionary style . . . and their parochial schools and colleges. The sense of shame was stronger still among the higher education leaders, for they were smart enough to have gone to Stanford, the Sorbonne, MIT, and Oxford (Burtchaell 1998, p. 707).

There was an emotionally valenced rejection of what Roman Catholicism had for centuries been. This rejection occasioned culture wars marked by passion, even if not by blood. In this context, Roman Catholic leaders, "especially the educators, were in the onset of their pietist phase and enjoying the flush of self-hatred" (Burtchaell 1998, p. 708). A wide-ranging iconoclasm with strong family resemblances to the 16th-century Protestant iconoclasm broke in on the Roman Catholicism of the mid-1960s. The past was to be erased or at least to be recast under a strongly adverse valence. An entire lifeworld was being negatively re-evaluated and then, if not obliterated, substantively transformed. In the ruins of what only a few years previously had been a unified, powerful, and self-confident Roman Catholicism, there was both confusion and strife. As an epiphany of this iconoclasm, in the zeal to recast the character of their churches, often exquisite old altars were torn out of churches. The very feel and life of the churches changed. A new ecclesial lifeworld was established, replacing what had been. The religious, academic, and intellectual world of Roman Catholicism was in free fall. A thoroughgoing cultural revolution had occurred, producing a new ecclesial cultural framework.

The result was a second Reformation that often brought with it a commitment to a destruction of the past.

> And so it went. "The less Catholic it is," declared the vice president of Chicago's Mundelein College (which would disappear), "the better the Catholic college will be." A faculty draft report on academic freedom at the University of Dayton, run by the Marianist Fathers, was more blunt. The purpose of a Catholic university, it claimed, was "to become secularized; for to be secularized means to come of age" (Woodward 2013, p. 29).

The changes have been rapid, dramatic, and thoroughgoing. A great leap forward into an abyss of disbelief or at least a recasting of the meaning of belief has taken place. Something quite novel has emerged. In place of the tradition that had been rejected, Roman Catholic schools of higher education and scholarly associations were fundamentally reshaped, at times collapsing in the process. "Catholic schools at all levels were adversely affected by the widespread tendency to repudiate older forms of institutionalized Catholic activity in favor of more direct forms of Christian service such as the civil rights movement, the peace movement, or 'inner city work'" (Gleason 1995, p. 319). The changes were broadly encompassing and perversely transformative. The changes involved a wide-ranging disengagement from the certainties and the ethos of the Christian tradition, which changes were tied to an attempt to see and live everything anew.

Religious uncertainties became central to the lifeworld of the Roman Catholic academy.

> "Who Are We?" was the title chosen by Ernan McMullin for his 1967 presidential address to the American Catholic Philosophical Association. In it he took note of the "massive failure of confidence" occasioned by the collapse of Neoscholasticism and suggested that the ACPA consider designating itself by the "perhaps more philosophically relevant title, 'Christian.'" McMullin's counterpart of the Catholic Theological Society of America, Walter J. Burghardt, S.J., put the issue in harsher terms. Asking whether the CTSA could, "in hard-nose reality, justify...[its] relatively unproductive existence," he answered his own question with a flat No! A newer group, the Catholic psychologists, had been publishing a learned journal for only five years when it carried an article calling for the dissolution of the society because it represented "a divisive, sectarian, ghetto mentality." The American Catholic Sociological Society, which had been formed to pure "Catholic sociology," threw off its last remaining confessional link in 1970 by changing its name to Association for the Sociology of Religion. In so doing, according to a recent student, it exchanged a putative "tunnel of privileged vision" for broader access to "the human chorus we call religion" (Gleason 1995, pp. 319-320).

The alterations were made not only with great zeal, but in the shadow of the loss of a common paradigm of what constituted Christian theology, so that there were often strident disagreements about what should be embraced by Roman Catholic theology.

As a consequence, a common vision of the importance of maintaining continuity with the Christian past and of affirming the tradition no longer predominated in the West, but rather the very opposite. For many, what had been self-evident became incomprehensible or indeed self-evidently to be repudiated. Nothing less than a revolution was seen to be required. For example,

> although *Worship* was the title of the leading Catholic liturgical journal, the lay executive director of the Liturgical Conference declared that it was precisely the idea of "worship" that had to be eliminated from religion. The Sister Formation Conference, whose autonomy had already been trimmed,

effectively disappeared in the postconciliar turmoil, and so did the Jesuit Educational Association (Gleason 1995, p. 320).

As Gleason clearly recognized, foundational confusion and conflict defined the day. It was a period of rapid alteration in which disorientation was itself embraced. Many lost the sense of where to look for orientation: "the crisis is not that Catholic educators do not want their institutions to remain Catholic, but that they are no longer sure what remaining Catholic means" (Gleason 1995, p. 320). Indeed, there were bitter disputes as to what "Catholic" should mean. As with the priests in the Novus Ordo Mass, there was mass disorientation (the double pun intended). There was a loss of a shared understanding of the goals of Roman Catholic education, not to mention of worship and piety. The dominant culture had become so profoundly after traditional Christianity and after traditional worship that points of orientation had for many disappeared. The traditional ritual fabric of Roman Catholicism was obliterated and a substantively new fabric established, which redefined ritual space and ritual propriety. As a consequence, when the dust settled, so much had been lost that nothing less than a radically new vision and experience of Christianity had emerged.

This was a period, as in Protestantism in the 19th century, during which Bible texts were recast in their meaning through being subjected to a hermeneutic of disbelief grounded in a project of reinterpreting biblical texts from a perspective that, among other things, did not recognize Jesus as God. Everything took on a new meaning as Scripture was now read from the perspective of a secular hermeneutic of suspicion. Regarded from a perspective of disbelief, the texts naturally appeared quite differently, because what they at their core said was brought into question. What counted as information and what counted as noise changed dramatically. Although many who went to the seminary may have initially hoped to become traditional Roman Catholic priests, they were told this was impossible. Seminarians found their course of study marked by attacks on traditional Christian commitments that had for many undermined their original sense of vocation. Their seminary experience became a disorienting induction into a framework of disbelief, an experience that in the case of Roman Catholic seminaries also involved a deeply troubling encounter with homosexuality (Rose 2002; Engel 2006). As Thomas Sheehan observed,

In Roman Catholic seminaries, for example, it is common teaching that
Jesus of Nazareth did not assert any of the divine or messianic claims the
Gospels attribute to him and that he died without believing he was Christ
or the Son of God, not to mention the founder of a new religion....[T]he
Gospel accounts of the claims Jesus supposedly made to be Christ and God
did not come from his own mouth but were interpretations his followers
created in the decades after his death (Sheehan 1984, pp. 35, 37).

The meaning and message of the Scriptures were in this context subject to an
alien matrix of re-interpretation so that all was substantively re-articulated. It
was an age defined by its breaking away from Christian society (Paz 1974, p. 27).
Attending a seminary became a road to disorientation and disbelief.

Within a decade after Vatican II, Roman Catholicism had a substantially
different character. The chaos of a Reformation was this time internal to Roman
Catholicism and self-inflicted.

In 1971, *Newsweek* again polled American Catholics for a cover story—
"Has the Church Lost Its Soul?"—that, with copious charts, went on for
seven pages. What we found was a once apparently cohesive community
in disarray: As one liberal monsignor bluntly told us, "The Church is one
god-damned mess." Nearly as many American Catholics, for instance, said
they now looked for spiritual guidance to evangelist Billy Graham as did
those who still looked to the pope. By "soul" I meant "an integral Catholic
subculture with its own distinctive blend of rituals and rules, mystery and
manners" which, as I saw it then, "has vanished from the American scene"
(Woodward 2013, p. 31).

The result was a loss of structure, focus, and mission. Most harmed were orders
of nuns.

[T]he Sisters of the Immaculate Heart of Mary splintered into traditional
and reformed factions, and the latter eventually disappeared. So did a lot of
the other communities of nuns. By the end of the sixties, women's religious
orders were reporting defections of up to six thousand a year, plus a precipi-
tous drop in new novices. The vocation crisis, at least in the United States,
became a steady state of relentless attrition (Woodward 2013, p. 28).

The widespread and salient presence of Roman Catholicism in health care delivery, which once bore the clear stamp of its medical ethics, abruptly went into decline as Roman Catholicism was no longer able to staff its hospitals with religious sisters and brothers. It was a self-wrought secularization on the scale of the Secularization in central Europe in 1803. A different and weaker Roman Catholicism emerged, and emerged quickly.

It was a time in which the novelty of disorientation itself had not only a crushing effect on many but also for many offered a titillating, seductive appeal. A radical revolution was under way. A whole new, post-Christian life seemed appropriate. A crusade on behalf of disbelief, on behalf of a culture after God, was launched. For those who embraced this alienation from the past and from the tradition, there was a giddy sense of a new age dawning and an anti-traditionalist joy and freedom of tearing apart and down what had for centuries been embraced. Moreover, what was so confusing for many devout Roman Catholic faithful was that the scholars who were deconstructing Jesus as Messiah and God, thus undercutting traditional belief, were quite often "Roman Catholic exegetes and theologians, most of them priests, faithfully ensconced at the heart of their infallible Church" (Sheehan 1984, p. 35). An impassioned self-destruction of Roman Catholicism was occurring, drawing from the passions of the "faithful" as well as abetted by the very heart of radically recast ecclesial institutions. A robust contradiction was embraced, which filled the institutions of Roman Catholicism with forces at odds with the traditional Christianity that had previously flourished. What was a simple Roman Catholic seminarian to make of this state of affairs?

Of course, there is another quite different and much more complete story to be told which critically highlights how both Scripture and tradition have been "critically" recast in their significance and meaning by post-traditional exegetes. Martin Hengel (1926–2009), for example, has pointed out that, contrary to and opposed to the critical textual account and its attempted revision of the significance of the New Testament, a different account is much better sustained by the actual history of biblical texts. A traditional view of the Scriptures was in fact much more plausible than that which the revisionary view advanced. For example, Hengel, contrary to the secular project of textual deconstruction, writes on behalf of a tradition-sustaining argument with regard to the Gospel of St. John and his letters. "Furthermore, it seems to me to [be] unmistakeable that the Gospel and the letters are not the expression of a community with many voices, but above all the voice of a towering theologian, the founder and head of the Johannine school" (Hengel 1989, p. ix). Hengel's contention is that an ideologically driven failure carefully to inspect and determine the history of the biblical texts has led to radically false conclusions that do not recognize that history vindicates St. John as both the witness and the author of the reports regarding the events found in his Gospel and letters. The result of Hengel's findings is that the "critical" approach, which has been engaged to deconstruct the traditional appreciation of the New Testament, turns out to be a basis for misleading conjectures. The attempt to undermine the scriptural foundations of traditional Christian belief fails. This attempt is in need of a critical rejection. "The more critical it makes itself out to be, the more 'creative' it becomes: what is said by the texts which have come down to us is all too often replaced by more or less free conjecture in the face of text and 'context'" (Hengel 1989, p. xi). This is a harsh but justified riposte to those who would wish to deflate the traditional significance of the Scriptures. A false paradigm has been driving the radical re-reading of biblical texts. The result is that the so-called critical approach to biblical texts is shown to be foundationally misguided, creating its facts to fit its expectations. "'Once upon a time,' as we must say now, David Friedrich Strauss (1808–1874), the founder of radical gospel criticism in the nineteenth century, compared the Fourth Gospel to 'Christ's seamless robe.' Nowadays, even a conservative theologian would no longer dare to say anything like that. 'Christ's seamless robe' has long become a patchwork 'coat of many colours'" (Hengel 1989, p. 1). In the light of a careful examination of the evidence, Hengel's historical research brings the critical revision of St. John's Gospel radically into question and defends the tradition. One is forced to take a critical stand against the attempted critical deflation of the significance of the New Testament. "The time is past when Protestant hypercriticism could put the Fourth Gospel in the middle of the second century. P^{52} makes it improbable that it was written after 110. In other words, the *terminus ad quem* is really the time of Trajan" (Hengel 1989, p. 3). The Gospel of St. John had in short been falsely re-interpreted by those who sought to deflate its traditional meaning, and in the process it was misperceived within a quite secular interpretive framework.

The realization was that a secular framework had distorted the appreciation of the Scriptures. This radical misinterpretation was already well known long before Martin Hengel's work. For example, as E. L. Mascall (1905–1993) argued in 1965,

> Enough has, I think, nevertheless been said to show that the impoverished secularized versions of Christianity which are being urged upon us for our acceptance today rest not upon the rigid application of the methods of scientific scholarship nor upon a serious intuitive appreciation of the Gospels as a whole in their natural context, but upon a radical distaste for the supernatural. Even scholars whose own religious practice implies the acceptance of the supernatural are frequently so imbued with this prejudice that in their study of the New Testament they take it as a matter of course that the supernatural element is, if not to be totally denied, at least to be consistently minimised (Mascall 1966, p. 282).

Despite the actual history, a post-traditional project still asserts itself deceptively and vigorously with its agenda in hand. The traditional Christian encounter with and affirmation of Jesus as Christ and the Son of God is rejected by a culture that seeks to be fully after God. "[T]he radical Christian wagers upon the Christ who is totally profane" (Altizer 1966, p. 157). Nevertheless, a traditional vision and experience remain and appear best warranted by the actual history, not to mention the continued miraculous presence of God. It should be added in emphasis that a defense of traditional belief similar to Hengel's can be given of the five books of Moses and their current textual character (Halivni 1997).

The dramatic cultural shift following Vatican II involved a foundational desacralization of core elements of Western culture that were transformed both by the absence of once substantive bonds with the past and by the presence of a new, post-traditional Roman Catholicism. An important sense of holiness disappeared. For example, there was no longer the asperges of the congregation with holy water that prior to Vatican II and its changes had preceded High Mass on Sunday in many parishes. Age-old pieties ranging from fish on Friday, remnants of the Lenten fast, and Masses in Latin, to the priest facing east disappeared, creating a significant cultural vacuum. The result was that the life-world of Roman Catholicism was starkly altered, a life-world that had maintained many important connections with the religious life of the Middle Ages and even elements from the first millennium. The Reformation had finally come to Roman Catholicism. In addition, the desacralization of the largest Christian denomination in the West constituted a new post-traditional presence in substitution for what had been a sustaining force. The culture was thus affected by both the removal of important historical connections and the emergence of a significantly different religious body.

The changes after Vatican II, especially after the imposition of the novel Pauline liturgy (i.e., the Novus Ordo Mass), were so widespread and disruptive that Pope Paul VI (1963–1978), who had fashioned them and imposed them, recoiled in horror at what was happening. As early as 1968, Pope Paul VI

> marked the end of the 1967–1968 "Year of Faith" with a profession called the *"Credo of the People of God"* (June 30, 1968). In the preface to this Credo, he speaks of the "disquiet which agitates certain modern quarters with regard to the Faith" and says: "We see even Catholics allowing themselves to be seized by a kind of passion for change and novelty" (Fastiggi 2012, p. 62).

On the 29th of June, 1972, Pope Paul VI made the following candid but nevertheless astonishing statement: "It was believed that after the Council there would be a day of sunshine in the history of the Church. There came instead a day of clouds, storm and darkness, of search and uncertainty. Through some fissure the smoke of Satan has entered the Temple of God."[14] Vatican II and Pope Paul VI had succeeded in letting loose forces that for centuries had been building up in Roman Catholicism (Hull 2010, p. 216–229). Vatican II and the new Pauline Mass acted as a catalyst that set off a chain reaction. "'Auto-demolition' was Pope Paul VI's description of the suicidal movement ravaging the Roman Church in the 1970s" (Hull 2010, p. 188). On July 31, 1975, Pope Paul VI abruptly removed Bugnini from his authority over liturgical reform.[15] Paradoxically, although Popes Paul VI, John Paul II, and Benedict XVI recognized individual problems associated with Vatican II and its aftermath, they lacked the courage forthrightly to acknowledge that Vatican II had radically undermined Roman Catholicism. However, it must be acknowledged that then-Cardinal Ratzinger saw the connection between the change in the Liturgy and the crisis in Roman Catholicism: "I am convinced that the crisis in the Church that we are experiencing is to a large extent due to the disintegration of the liturgy" (Ratzinger 1998, p. 148). The result was a revolutionary transformation of the life of Roman Catholics that reached from a radically new Mass to the abandonment of old pieties such as fish on Fridays (i.e., abstinence from meat on Fridays). The life of Roman Catholicism began to die out. What had been a vigorous ecclesial body was in ruins as churches, church schools, and hospitals began to close. The consequences for bioethics were also dramatic, in that these changes in Roman Catholicism sent into desuetude a 300-year-old literature in medical morality and engendered the circumstances that supported the birth of contemporary bioethics at Georgetown University, a Roman Catholic institution.

A desacralization of the public space has nevertheless been accomplished not only by the actions and revolt of new-age Christians who stepped away from tradition and who articulated a Christian culture that is after God, but by Jews as well. Jews faced not just the recognition of the complex textual character of the Torah, especially as it is seen in a secular culture, but also the shock and challenge of the Holocaust. In this context, many reform and conservative Jews invoked the Holocaust as an excuse for a new, post-theistic, theological discourse, while re-reading Scripture within a hermeneutic of disbelief so as to serve their secular purposes. For instance, Rubenstein (1924–) argues that:

> Religious Jews have been compelled either to retreat to a fideistic dogmatism which ignores modern scholarship, or to seek a new rationale for their theological commitments. For many, the problem of finding a new rationale has been aggravated by the death of their personal God. After Auschwitz many Jews did not need Nietzsche to tell them that the old God of Jewish patriarchal monotheism was dead beyond all hope of resurrection (Rubenstein 1966, p. 227).

Rather than sternly and critically responding to such secular criticism aimed at undermining traditional belief, many gave in to the temptations to conform and then felt the floor underneath them collapse. As a consequence, once-observant faith on the part of many in the enduring power and presence of God was lost; Christianity and Judaism were exposed to being recast.

What then of Judaism? It is the way we Jews share our lives in an unfeeling
and silent cosmos. It is the flickering candle we have lighted in the dark to
enlighten and to warm us. Somehow it will continue for a very long time
because there will always be some men who will accept and affirm what they
were born to be. Ultimately, as with all things, it will pass away, for omnipotent Nothingness is Lord of All Creation (Rubenstein 1966, p. 225).

Such a revision of Judaism and Jewishness re-interpreted what had been the
tradition so that it became a transformed tradition that was located after God.
All became relocated in terms of the absurd. After Auschwitz, the traditional
God of many Jews had become dead, so that for them "the Father-God is a dead
God. Even the existentialist leap of faith cannot resurrect this dead God after
Auschwitz. Nevertheless, after the death of the Father-God, God remains the
central reality against which all partial realities can be measured" (Rubenstein
1966, p. 238).

The result is that, in the shadow of the undermining force of a secular critical
re-interpretation of faith, an eclipse of God occurred, a loss of the experience
of God. For many Jews and Christians, especially for those who accept the supposed implications of attempted attacks on the tradition, the very character
and meaning of religion had been brought into question. The conclusion has
been embraced that "Our prayers can no longer be attempts at dialogue with a
personal God. . . . [I]n the time of the death of God a mystical paganism which
utilizes the historic forms of Jewish religion offers the most promising approach
to religion in our times" (Rubenstein 1966, p. 240). Due to this turn from traditional belief, a culturally traumatizing rupture followed: the presence of God
was obscured by a thick and complex fabric of passions for the new and post-
traditional, as well as for self-indulgence, that has uprooted many from the traditional nexus of faith and the experience of God. A novel lifeworld that deformed
the religious life of many gained a misleading prominence. This change became
publicly manifest, driven by a fabric of post-traditional agendas. A new, indeed
an old, pre-Christian world once more claimed prominence. "For the first time
in two thousand years the nude body has appeared upon the shores of the Medi-
terranean. These men and women know only the pleasures of the flesh; there
is nothing banished by this pagan race" (Rubenstein 1966, pp. 256–257). This

re-emergence of a pagan lifeworld occurred as the significance of traditional Judaism and Christianity were for many dramatically deconstructed. What has happened for Reform and Conservative Jews has taken place for mainline Christians as well: traditional belief and traditional observance have collapsed. Here Rubenstein correctly observes: "What remains of Judaism and Christianity in contemporary America is largely pagan" (Rubenstein 1966, p. 259). Rituals, for example, marriage and funerals, remain, but they are cut off from a recognition of the transcendent God Who properly locates and defines their meaning, so that the rituals can now only serve and affirm needs that can be recognized within the horizon of the affirmatively immanent. Rubenstein grants the cardinal role of ritual, but sets the meaning of ritual apart from the intrusive prophetic voice of God and from a dialogue in prayer with the Creator God. In this context, a resurgent paganism becomes "a wise intuition of man's place in the order of things" (Rubenstein 1966, p. 259). There is a persistence of ritual (Solomon et al. 2012), but cut off from the transcendent in a context in which "The death of God is a cultural fact" (Rubenstein 1966, p. 246). The texture and life of non-orthodox Judaism has been altered as radically as has been the lifeworld of mainline Christianity.

All of this was already manifest in the late 19th century in what Nietzsche appreciated as following from the secular culture's killing of the recognition of God and the subsequent loss of any point of ultimate orientation. An overwhelming disorientation characterized the context in which people found themselves. After having lived in terms of a point of ultimate reference, one was left no final point of orientation. All this is underscored in Nietzsche's parable of the mad man.

> 'Whither is God?' he cried: 'I will tell you. *We have killed him*—you and I. All of us are his murderers. But how did we do this? How could we drink up the sea? Who gave us the sponge to wipe away the entire horizon? What were we doing when we unchained this earth from its sun? Whither is it moving now? Whither are we moving? Away from all suns? Is there still any up or down? Are we not wandering as through an infinite nothing? Do we not feel the breath of empty space? Has it not become colder? Is not night continually closing in on us? Do we not hear nothing as yet of the noise of the gravediggers

who are burying God? Do we smell nothing as yet of the divine decomposition? Gods, too, decompose. God is dead, God remains dead. And we have killed him (Nietzsche 1974, p. 181).

The dominant culture has become a culture after God. Among the consequences of this vast cultural transformation is that final points of reference can no longer be discerned in a culture after God. One is left without any hint of ultimate moorings. Everything is ultimately unhinged. This transformation of the very experience of reality within the dominant culture of the West into a place after God was largely completed by the early 1960s. With these cultural changes came a loss of taken-for-granted points of enduring meaning. All became transient and provisional. Mark Taylor has summarized some of these complex and often bewildering developments.

> Individuals appear to be unsure of where they have come from and where they are going. Thus they are not certain where they are. Furthermore, the "texts" that have guided and grounded previous generations often appear illegible in the modern and postmodern worlds. Instead of expressing a single story or coherent plot, human lives tend to be inscribed in multiple and often contradictory texts (Taylor 1984, p. 3).

The transcendent has for many been reduced to the immanent so that "God came to be regarded as the creation of human beings" (Taylor 1984, p. 4).

Against the backdrop of these profound cultural transformations, a deep animus against tradition has taken root. For Roman Catholicism, as already observed, this animus drove immense changes in norms of piety, conduct, and liturgy. The very character of religious devotion was altered. A whole new lifeworld of being a Christian emerged that would have been unimaginable for many in the early 20th century, a lifeworld at odds with the lifeworld of the ancient Church. A post-traditional form of Christianity became the rule in the latter part of the 20th century that would have been generally unforeseeable at the beginning of the 20th century. An appreciation of traditional Christianity nearly disappeared, and its collapse is still under way. A transvaluation of values occurred so that the dominant culture has come to regard traditional Christians and Jews as bigots. For example, they appear as people who malign homosexuals and those who cohabit and reproduce without marriage. A rapid disengagement from organized religion has become salient and is still under way. "In this country alone [the USA] . . . about 7.5 million more Americans are no longer active in religion since 2012, according to the 2014 General Social Survey" (Erlandson et al. 2015, p. 19). The point is that a substantively different and radically deflated framework for Christianity, Christian experience, and Christian morality has become dominant not only in contemporary culture, but also at the center of Western Christianity itself. Something new and, from the perspective of traditional Christianity, heretical and even frightening has emerged. In this culture, children now grow up apart from and defended against a recognition of the God Who lives. They are nurtured in a social fabric that is structured so as to avoid a recognition of, much less an encounter with, God. Nevertheless, despite Auschwitz, Vatican II, and the secular recasting of the public culture of the West, a traditional Christianity has endured, even though its morality and bioethics have become ever more strongly counter-cultural. The source of this traditional Christian otherness over against the surrounding post-theistic culture lies in the origins of Christianity itself, in the Christianity of the Apostles and the Fathers, namely, in Orthodox Christianity. Against the tenor of the times, disregarding the animus to set traditional Christianity aside, and despite heretics prominent within its fold, Orthodox Christianity remains a light in a world after God. The ancient Christianity of the first centuries remains alive and well.

III. From a Scholastic Medical Ethics to Contemporary Secular Bioethics

It is only against the background of these wide-ranging ecclesial and theological changes that one can appreciate why the robust medical-moral literature that existed in Roman Catholicism before and into Vatican II disappeared overnight. This considerable body of medical-moral manuals had taken shape within the manualist tradition that first developed in the early 17th century, growing out of post-Tridentine Roman Catholicism and the Counter-Reformation. It was a literature to which even Roman Catholic saints such as Alphonsus Maria de Liguori (1696–1787) contributed (Liguori 1862). The manuals were meant to serve as easily accessible resources for Roman Catholic clerics and others, so as uniformly to guide them and to aid them in facing intellectual and moral challenges. These manuals became integral to the intellectual and moral framework of Roman Catholicism. By the end of the 19th and the early 20th century, the manualist project had produced a significant focus on medical-ethical issues, including a large number of medical-moral manuals in English.[16] It was an influential body of scholarship.[17]

This tradition of medical-moral reflection was characterized by a strong faith in reason. In fact, those who engaged in this enterprise saw themselves not as Roman Catholic or Christian moralists, but as "scientific" moralists *simpliciter*. They were convinced that they belonged to a moral-scientific tradition that could lay out for all people—atheists, Christians, Jews, and Muslims alike—the norms that should guide the proper conduct of medicine. A striking example of this view is a statement by Fr. Gerald Kelly, S.J., in 1958.

> But the [Roman] Catholic moralists do have a just claim to special competence in the *science of ethics*, the science of moral right and wrong, the science of applying the moral law to the problems of human living. They are highly trained and experienced men in this particular field. Their preparation for this professional capacity is intensive and comprehensive; they usually teach the science of morality over a number of years; and they are constantly dealing with practical applications of this science. Aside from any question of religion, the [Roman] Catholic moralists represent by far the world's largest group of specialists in the science of ethics. And they have a tradition of scientific study that extends over centuries (Kelly 1958, p. 34).

This confidence in reason was mirrored in most examples of this literature. For another instance, consider the claim that Fr. John Kenny, O.P., makes in introducing his book.

> Moral principles are not the heritage of any particular religion; they belong to the whole human race, and should be known and practiced by every human being. The application of these principles to the many and varied problems of medical practice constitutes the subject matter of medical ethics. . . . It must first be noted that ethics holds to a few postulates which are derived from other fields of philosophy (Kenny 1962, p. 1).

These books in Roman Catholic medical-moral theology were regarded as works in medical ethics, not in medical-moral theology. Because of its commitment to the univocity of moral rationality, the medical ethics of pre-Vatican II Roman Catholicism saw itself to be the same as proper secular medical ethics.

In the United States, medical-moral manuals were tied to a parallel tradition of writing codes for Roman Catholic physicians and hospitals. These codes developed out of a movement begun in June 1915 (a year after the inception of the Catholic Hospital Association) by Charles B. Moulinier, S.J., which led to Michael P. Bourke overseeing the creation of a code of ethics in 1920 for the Diocese of Detroit. In 1921, a surgical code was adopted by what at the time was styled The Catholic Hospital Association (now called Catholic Health Association). After the Second World War and as progress in medicine accelerated, interest increased in having, as well as giving, direction for the practice of medicine. Out of this background of producing codes of ethics, a document emerged titled "Code of Ethics—1948," first published in 1949.[18] This was followed by one of the most influential of the manuals, the one by Gerald Kelly already quoted above, which functioned as a quasi-companion to the Code. Kelly's book was first published as a series of pamphlets (Kelly 1949, 1950, 1951, 1953, 1954) before its first appearance as a book in 1958 (Kelly 1958).

These and a multitude of other works in this genre were a part of a coherent scholarly tradition recognized within the Roman Catholic academy. It produced a large literature that was approved by the hierarchy and that informed Roman Catholic physicians, health care workers, chaplains, and educated laity. It shared a common vision both of the tradition's goals and of its scholarly requirements. It was an established Roman Catholic research program guided by a well-accepted paradigm. The result was that the intellectual footprint of Roman Catholic reflections on medical morality was large. Although this medical ethics tradition was sectarian in depending on a particular sense of the morally rational, those who worked within it were fully unaware of its parochial character. This medical-moral literature exceeded not only anything produced by Protestants, but even the secular literature of the time.

After Vatican II, the entire project of producing medical-moral manuals collapsed; it abruptly disappeared. As Paul Ramsey succinctly observed, "The day is past when one could write a manual on medical ethics" (Ramsey 1970, p. xvi).

With Vatican II, the previous paradigm of Roman Catholic medical ethics was abandoned, along with Roman Catholicism's overarching Scholastic commitments of which it was a part, not because the medical-moral literature had been explicitly rejected, but because the overarching intellectual and moral framework of Roman Catholicism had changed. The Second Vatican Council was supposed to lead to a focus on personalism and biblical study. Although there were publications in bioethics that did style themselves as personalist (Sgreccia 2012), what followed was a crisis of intellectual orientation within which it was unclear as to what scholarly paradigm should guide. Everything had changed. As Paul Ramsey observed, "Due to the uncertainties in Roman Catholic moral theology since Vatican Council II, even the traditional medical ethics courses in schools under Catholic auspices are undergoing vast changes, abandonment, or severe crisis" (Ramsey, 1970, p. xvi).

The abandonment of the centuries-old Scholastic, manualist paradigm was associated with rejection of the old background and overarching paradigms of piety and liturgy in favor of new paradigms of piety and liturgy. Moved by ecumenical concerns, there was an approximation of a reformed Protestant mindset, as Archbishop Bugnini acknowledged: everything was removed from the new liturgy "that could constitute the slightest risk of a stumbling block or a source of displeasure for our Separated Brethren, that is, for the Protestants."[19] There was in addition an attempt made to remove from the Mass "texts that smacked of a negative spirituality inherited from the Middle Ages" (Bugnini 1990, p. 773). The ethos and life-style of Roman Catholicism were transformed. As a consequence, the previous theological and moral paradigm went into crisis, because the traditional encompassing paradigm for liturgy and piety that had determined the mindset of Roman Catholicism had been abandoned. *Lex orandi, lex credendi est*; the law of prayer is the law of belief. Not only was the Latin Mass replaced by a Mass in the vernacular, but the character of the Mass had changed. It was not just that Roman Catholics no longer abstained from meat on Friday or during Lent (with the exceptions of Ash Wednesday and Good Friday), or that Latin was no longer the language of seminaries. The very way of life that had framed Roman Catholicism had changed. Ritual shapes the life-world so that radical changes in ritual lead to radical changes in the Roman Catholic way of life (Solomon et al. 2012). With a new liturgy, prayer, approaches to piety, and the abolition of traditional roles of fast and abstinence, a new life-world with a new form of belief was taking shape, although it was unclear what its full character would be. The consequences of Vatican II are still underway. In this new life-world, the old medical ethics tradition was too much a part of the past to seem plausible any longer. However, it was quite unclear as one entered the 1970s what would replace the medical ethics of the manualist tradition for Roman Catholicism.

What followed was a secular bioethics. As John Collins Harvey's (a for-mer member of the Roman Catholic International Study Group in Bioethics) account of the development of bioethics has shown, there was a direct connec-tion between post-Vatican II Roman Catholicism and the emergence of secular bioethics (Harvey 2011). As Harvey argues, a crucial role was played by Roman Catholic intellectuals such as André Hellegers (1926–1979), the first director of the Kennedy Institute of Georgetown University, and Sargent Shriver (1915–2011), who with the support of the Kennedy family and the Kennedy Foundation was its moral and financial backer. They had generally embraced the revolution in piety and liturgy following Vatican II. They were also convinced that a new medical morality was needed and that this moral philosophy could elaborate and justify the bioethics and health care policy they wanted to embrace politi-cally. They were confident that this new moral vision could re-direct Roman Catholicism's appreciation of medicine and the biomedical sciences. The result was the creation of the first academic center for the new field: the Center for Bioethics of the Kennedy Institute of Ethics at Georgetown University. A cadre of intellectuals was assembled who through publications and "total immersion" courses engendered, if they did not singlehandedly create, the new field of bio-ethics.[20]

Hellegers affirmed Vatican II, although he considered himself a liberal dis-senter from elements of the magisterium of the post-conciliar church. Being a dissenter, one should note, had become a badge of honor at the Kennedy Insti-tute, as is clear from LeRoy Walters' (the first director of the Center for Bioethics within the Kennedy Institute) praise of Hellegers.

In André's own life and work, there are several striking examples of his cour-age and willingness to protect dissent. The first two Catholic theologians whom André invited to the Kennedy Institute were Warren Reich and Charles Curran. Both had been active in the attempt to reform Catholic moral theology in the late 1960s, and Warren Reich had been a visible and active supporter of Charles Curran when Catholic University and the Vatican had tried to set limits on the scope of his theological inquiries. Warren was the first long-term Catholic scholar at the Institute, and Charles Curran our first visiting scholar. In 1974 and 1975, André invited Bernard Häring, another burr under the Vatican's saddle, to join us as a visiting scholar (Walters 2003, p. 228).

Hellegers was convinced that philosophy and empirical research could and should refashion Roman Catholic medical ethics. For Hellegers, the first point at issue was the Roman Catholic prohibition of artificial contraception, regarding which in particular Hellegers supported change. Hellegers had served on the Roman Catholic commission considering the acceptability of artificial contraception (McClory 1995). In reaction to Pope Paul VI's condemnation of contraception in *Humanae Vitae* (1968), Hellegers argued:

> Had the encyclical stated that the data, advanced by the commission, were wrong or irrelevant, or were insufficient to warrant a change in teaching, that would have been one thing. It is quite another thing to imply that agreement with past conclusions is the *sine qua non* for acceptance of a study. Such wording pronounced the scientific method of inquiry irrelevant to Roman Catholic theology (Hellegers 1969, p. 217).

Hellegers rejected the theological understanding underlying *Humanae Vitae* and in its stead proposed a new theological approach. Hellegers had faith in the role that his sense of theological rationality should play in refashioning and developing doctrine.

Hellegers used the Kennedy Institute to bring other dissenters to join in building the nascent field of bioethics. He was confident that this new field of bioethics would support his moral and dogmatic vision. Those who joined Hellegers had the sense that a new and soon-to-be-influential paradigm for medical ethics was emerging. And, of course, they were right. As Warren Reich recalls,

Thus, when I came to Georgetown as a "dissenter," I felt radically disconnected from my past academic pursuits and had no clear vision of my
professional or intellectual future. Furthermore, after the 1960s I felt that
I, together with countless others throughout the world, was experiencing
the decisive end of one cultural, moral, and social era and the beginning of
another, the contours of which were not yet defined. Thirty-one years later,
I see that my serendipitous situation of being suspended between cultures
in 1971 was precisely the requisite spiritual and intellectual condition for the
task of trying to absorb and articulate the contours, meanings, and normative issues of a new social, intellectual, and political reality that was rapidly
taking shape before our very eyes, the future of which we did not know
(Reich, 2003, p. 166).

A new paradigm of bioethics took shape, and with it a new field of scholarship
was established. Within seven years Warren Reich would publish the first edition of *The Encyclopedia of Bioethics* (1978), aided in part by other persons with
theological backgrounds (Warren Reich is a former priest) such as Tom Beauchamp and James F. Childress. There was a hunger for change. Hellegers was
able within a Roman Catholic university to frame a paradigm for a new field,
bioethics, which filled the void left by the disappearance of manualist medical
ethics. The collapse of the old paradigm, as well as the genesis of the new field
of bioethics with its new paradigm of morality and scholarship, can only be
appreciated against the background of Vatican II, along with the ecclesial and
intellectual crises it engendered, leading to a change in the paradigm for the
discipline of medical ethics.

As John Collins Harvey (2013) and Paul Schotsmans (Schotsmans 2005)
have shown, the post-Vatican II Roman Catholic influence on the emergence of
secular bioethics was exerted not just directly through the Kennedy Institute,
but indirectly through Francesc Abel, S.J. Abel was at the Kennedy Institute from
the year of its inception (1971) until he returned to Barcelona in 1975 where he
played a crucial role in establishing the Institut Borja de Bioethica (Barcelona),
as well as the International Study Group in Bioethics of the International Federation of Catholic Universities (one might recall my role beginning in the mid-
1980s with the Study Group as mentioned in chapter one). The result was the

genesis out of Roman Catholicism of a secular bioethics movement that came to shape moral reflection on medicine and the biomedical sciences in Western Europe. As Schotsmans summarizes,

> Describing bioethics in Europe is impossible without honoring the found-
> ing fathers of bioethics. Several eminent bio-ethicists have to be mentioned,
> like Edouard Bone, S.J. (Brussels, Belgium), Maurice de Wachter (Montreal,
> Canada, and Maastricht, Netherlands), Richard Nicholson (London, UK),
> Nicole Lery (Lyon, France), Patrick Verspieren (Paris, France) and—even
> more than all the others—Francesc Abel (Barcelona, Spain) (Schotsmans
> 2005, p. 38, quoting Abel 1999, pp. 17–18).

One might note the names of prominent Roman Catholic bioethics scholars such as Bone, de Wachter, and Vespieren. Reviewing the history, Schotsmans concludes that it

> makes clear that bioethics in Europe started mainly in the South [i.e., among
> Roman Catholic thinkers]. . . . The creation of Barcelona's Institut Borja de
> Bioethica is certainly one of the earliest developments in European bioeth-
> ics. At the same time, fortunately enough, the European dimension of the
> bioethical debate was stimulated by the creation of the European Associa-
> tion of Centers of Medical Ethics (EACME). F. Abel played an eminent role
> in this organization. The Barcelona Institute (with F. Abel) developed an
> international research and communication network (Schotsmans 2005,
> p. 38 ff).

Bioethics in Western Europe, like bioethics in the United States, grew out of a change in moral-philosophical focus within Roman Catholicism.

The bioethics born of Roman Catholicism was grounded in fully secular moral commitments and premises. The modern secular phenomenon of bio-ethics, while still drawing on a faith in reason from Roman Catholicism, recast its sense of moral rationality in order to adapt and to fill the scholarly ecologi-cal niche in Roman Catholicism that had once been filled by the medical-eth-ics manualist tradition. The medical ethics of the manualist tradition thought of itself as equivalent to good secular medical ethics, although it carried with it very particular moral understandings rooted in Roman Catholicism (e.g., the natural-law conviction that artificial contraception is forbidden). The new bioethics also carried with it very particular moral premises (e.g., about the capacities of moral philosophy and the existence of human rights), but now after Vatican II and *aggiornamento* the premises were drawn from the dominant secular culture, not from Roman Catholic tradition. This bioethics of the 1970s, because it was really a secular bioethics, came to thrive beyond the borders of Roman Catholicism and indeed beyond Christianity. It became the dominant approach to secular bioethics. Now a new crisis threatens in which Roman Catholicism is again playing an important role. Secular bioethics is discovering that the philosophical assumptions it embraced in the 1970s cannot supply a canonical anchor in being or in reason. The bioethics of the 1970s is confronted with post-modernity.

IV. They Never Knew What Hit Them: Aggiornamento Transforms the Cultural Context for Bioethics

Pope John Paul II, who followed Pope Paul VI after the brief papacy of Pope John Paul I (26 August–28 September 1978), never adequately appreciated the radical character of the post-Vatican II transformation of Roman Catholicism. In the face of a dramatic loss of congregants and clergy, there continued to be praise for the fruits of liturgical renewal and Vatican II (Mt 7:17–20). Nor did John Paul II rectify the chaos, along with the loss of vocations and congregants that followed Vatican II. If anything, under the papacy of John Paul II the chaos and controversies grew worse because what was taking place, a crisis due to the loss of old paradigms without an acceptance of a new productive paradigm, was not adequately understood. The disarray among Roman Catholics proved contagious and affected Protestants as well. As Kenneth Woodward reports, much of what was to happen to Roman Catholicism was already clear at Vatican II and shortly afterwards.

> Presbyterian theologian Robert McAfee Brown told me[:] "I concluded that if Catholicism was not going to be the same, then Protestantism is not going to be the same either." . . . What struck me most, apart from the headline-making results on sex-related issues, was the sheer confusion revealed in the pollsters' personal interviews. The sudden change in traditional dos and

don'ts, like abstaining from meat on Fridays, left many Catholics feeling boundary-less. Reading their responses, I remembered what sociologist Peter Berger had said of the curial officials who had warned of chaos if the Council's liberalizing reformers got their way (Woodward 2013, p. 27).

The outcome for mainline Western Christianity has been wide-ranging, involving among other things a demoralization of moral theology, along with a deflation of the force of dogma.[21] The religion that emerged was not a serious alternative to the secular culture. People simply lost interest in the Western Christianities.

With Pope John Paul II and Benedict XVI, there were attempts to engage the dominant culture and reach out to those, especially the youth, alienated from a church that had insisted on traditional doctrinal commitments, including a traditional Christian sexual morality that restrained the life-styles of young and old alike. The strategy of outreach that was adopted has not proven successful in restoring numbers of the faithful. As Edward Leigh observes,

> It is clear that, over the last 40 years, none of the attempts to woo the young with folk Masses, 'raves in the nave,' and so on have [sic] had a significant positive effect on the decline in church-going. Trying to attract converts by making their experience of church-going more like that of their ordinary lives and leisure activities, and by soft-pedalling on 'hard sayings,' has clearly failed (Leigh 2009, p. 19).

Another way to put the matter is that the new Pauline liturgy created a new religious space within which traditional morality and dogma did not fit. The loss of congregants and vocations with and after Vatican II was a function of a change of life-world, an abandonment of a paradigm for life that left many Roman Catholics without a bond to the new Roman Catholicism. The rupture has been deep and abrupt. The post-Vatican II recasting of the life-world of Roman Catholicism did not produce a new Pentecost, as had been promised. The reforms satisfied the personal emotional and intellectual needs of the reformers, but not that of enough of the ordinary congregants, leading to a profound disconnection, which was followed by a loss of laity and vocations. According to any objective criteria, the post-Vatican II changes were highly counter-productive. The demographic decline has been dramatic (Jones 2003). With this collapse of Roman

Catholicism, the public space of the West has been redefined. Within this secular public space, as we have seen, secular bioethics has been demoralized and deflated, leading to the question of what this will mean for Roman Catholic and more specific Western Christian bioethics. Will Roman Catholic bioethics also be demoralized and thus set within a "weak" moral theology?

Gianni Vattimo has in particular critically addressed one of the consequences of these developments: the "resecularized religiosity" (Vattimo 2007, p. 94) introduced by John Paul II and continued by Benedict XVI. This "secularized religiosity" has supported the continuing secular transformation of public spaces, further opening up the cultural niche within which the new secular bioethics flourishes. Vattimo addressed these cultural changes in an interview published in 2007 in which he spoke to the discordance between the goals of John Paul II and Benedict XVI and what was actually produced by their attempts at evangelization.

> One of my favorite examples of this comes from the Roman Catholic Church's celebration of the Year of the Jubilee in 2000. Many young people came to Rome to see and hear from the pope. This was perceived by many as an example of the rise in religiosity among today's youth. But, after they had left and when it came time to clean up the area where the youth had spent the night, they found three hundred thousand condoms (Caputo & Vattimo 2007, p. 96).

Vattimo's interviewer then responded, "The number I heard was actually twenty thousand." Vattimo's riposte was, "No, there were more. Of course, there is difficulty in the counting" (Caputo & Vattimo 2007, p. 96). Vattimo's point is that the "primitive religiosity" engaged by John Paul II and Benedict XVI (Caputo & Vattimo 2007, p. 96) through media Masses and youth assemblies has not strengthened, but if anything has further weakened, Roman Catholicism. John Paul II and Benedict XVI's media Catholicism has failed substantively to integrate piety, dogma, and ritual into a new and compelling paradigm. "The threat is that, with the means of the mythologies created by television, we reconstruct a sort of primitive religiosity, a form of superstition—a religious show [is produced] in contrast to devotion" (Caputo & Vattimo 2007, p. 96). Crowds have been taken to be an index of success.

Vattimo appreciates that in a desperate need to re-attract its lost flock, a media Catholicism has been produced that is only further severed from the substance of Christianity. That is, there has been an attempt to draw large crowds grounded in

> a decision the Vatican has taken in order to begin to attract all those people who left the Church because of the dogmatic preaching of Pope John Paul II. And although I still haven't heard about the number of condoms left after World Youth Day in Cologne [2005], I did read about a controversy that arose over plans for police to distribute condoms at World Youth Day. The church tried to halt plans to distribute them, according to the spokeswoman of the German police unions (the union commonly distributes them at large public gatherings to protect the public) (Caputo & Vattimo 2007, pp. 96–97).

The commitment to reconnect with the youth and others alienated from Western Christianity has occurred without acknowledging the constraints set by traditional moral norms, leading to the bizarre outcomes that Vattimo notes. The attempts of John Paul II and Benedict XVI may have only further abetted secularization and encouraged the enlargement of the cultural space within which a demoralized bioethics can flourish. Once again, Roman Catholicism turns out to be changing the cultural geography so that morality and bioethics will be further refashioned, this time as a morality and bioethics after modernity.

In contrast, traditionalist Christians have for many reasons held their own. In part, this may be because the majority of them, especially fundamentalist Protestants, are not embedded within the moral-philosophical assumptions that tied much of mainline Western Christianity, first and foremost Roman Catholicism, to the conceits of secular moral philosophy and thus to secular culture. Mainline Christians have more consanguinity with the philosophy-oriented, so-called *via antiqua*. After all, mainline Western Christianity is a close sibling of the contemporary, dominant, secular culture, as a result of mainline Christianity's commitment to the prevailing secular morality and moral philosophy. The mainline Christian churches of the West have also supported the secularization of the West through rendering Christian concerns for the transcendent into immanent concerns for a social gospel, and for social justice, that are to be articulable and justifiable without reference to God, much less to Christ. As with Pope Francis, as will shortly be shown, there was a move from a focus on the morality and bioethics of sexuality, reproduction, and end-of-life decision-making to a focus on social justice and the allocation of health care resources.

This has occurred in the shadow of a hyper-ecumenism that has sought to reach out even to atheists. One might recall Friedrich Hayek's observation that when Christian clerics talk of social justice rather than of obligations to charity, it is an indication of an immanent displacement of a once transcendent moral-metaphysical view and its concerns. They have likely lost their faith.

> [Social justice] seems in particular to have been embraced by a large section of the clergy of all Christian denominations, who, while increasingly losing their faith in a supernatural revelation, appear to have sought a refuge and consolation in a new "social" religion which substitutes a temporal for a celestial promise of justice, and who hope that they can thus continue their striving to do good. The Roman Catholic church especially has made the aim of "social justice" part of its official doctrine; but the ministers of most Christian denominations appear to vie with each other with such offers of more mundane aims—which also seem to provide the chief foundation for renewed ecumenical efforts (Hayek 1976, p. 66).

Talking about social justice allowed the mainline Christian churches to disengage from traditional belief and yet still seem to be Christian. One should recall that Christianity in the first three centuries did not preach social justice to the Roman Empire, but instead charity. The Church of the first centuries did not trust that a pagan government would rightly tend to the needs of the poor. To the contrary, Christians were sure that the empire's social justice would be a pagan social justice hostile to Christian commitments. Second, and more importantly, the obligation to feed the poor fell on Christians themselves who are required personally to turn to the poor in need. Social justice is not a concept with roots in the Apostles and the Fathers. There is instead in Christianity a radical demand to turn personally to meet the needs of the poor. In contrast, post-traditional Christianity has socialized charity and in the process reshaped the cultural context, along with bioethics and health care policy, within which law and public policy are appreciated by the Western Christianities (Francis 2013).

V. Is Peter Singer an Anonymous Christian?

Despite the increasing moral and metaphysical gulf separating traditional Christianity and its bioethics from the dominant secular culture, Roman Catholicism's faith in reason has led its theologians to attempt through philosophical reflection to deny this gulf. They argue that the seemingly deep gulf separating Christian theology from secular unbelieving moral philosophy and its bioethics is an illusion. After all, both Christians and atheists can be committed to feeding the poor and criticizing an individualistic consumerism. A paradigm example is provided by *Peter Singer and Christian Ethics* (Camosy 2012). Charles Camosy, a Roman Catholic theologian, argues that there is a common ground uniting Peter Singer's concern for the poor and the moral vision of Roman Catholicism. This Camosy holds to be the case, although Peter Singer is widely known for a morality and bioethics radically at odds with the commitments of traditional Christianity (Singer 2011). Camosy states, for example, "If those who take Singer's approach are united in the spirit of intellectual solidarity with the Church, and *vice versa*, both will see that we have a fundamental trajectory in common" (Camosy 2012, p. 251). Camosy envisages the followers of Peter Singer and of Jesus Christ being able together to overcome what Camosy takes to be the guiding vision of the contemporary West, namely, the normativity of a "consuming, private, supposedly autonomous individual" (Camosy 2012, p. 251). The assumption is that materially equivalent goals or trajectories (e.g., to feed the poor) are actually common goals or trajectories. This assumption leads to the further claim of a basic harmony between the Roman Catholic mission and the commitments of Peter Singer. This is an understandable assumption, given the Roman Catholic commitment to the dialectic of faith and reason, *fides et ratio*.

Materially equivalent behavior can constitute essentially different acts with fundamentally different meanings. Thus, if both Peter Singer and a Christian under similar circumstances give equal amounts of their resources to feed the poor, the acts have a different significance, in that the Christian's love of the poor is anchored beyond the horizon of the finite and the immanent in love and obedience to God. Although both may act from love for the poor, only Christians will also have acted first and foremost out of love and submission to God.[22] Peter Singer's feeding of the poor will not be an act of love for the poor.

Or at least, the love of the poor will have a different meaning. A love anchored in obedience to God is a love anchored in the very meaning of the universe and therefore quite distinct from a love anchored only in one's own will, immanent concerns, and philosophical arguments regarded apart from God. As Moses Maimonides recognizes, doing what one should because God commands it is quite different from the same behavior done on the basis of a philosophical argument. The latter, because it does not acknowledge God's commands, does not merit salvation.[23] The same behavior (i.e., feeding the poor) when set within different life-worlds (that of the traditional Christian versus that of the utilitarian agnostic) will be quite distinct acts with quite different trajectories or goals.[24] Also, it is quite different to redistribute resources to the poor through taxation versus giving the same amount of resources to the poor out of love of God and neighbor. Traditionally, Christians recognize that the former cannot substitute for the latter. The Christian act of charity is a personal act that binds the giver to the recipient and the recipient to the giver in grateful prayer, and both to God, a matter Roman Catholicism discovered as its charity hospitals died for want of vocations to support their staffs with religious brothers and sisters.

Peter Singer's rejection of contemporary individualistic consumerism is articulated in a life-world distant from the Christian rejection of the individualism of contemporary consumerism. Again, for Singer, a solidarity among persons grounded in a set of utilitarian considerations articulated apart from God contrasts with a traditional Christian rejection of consumer individualism because of a focus on love of God and love of neighbor. The differences lie not merely in differences of philosophical-moral accounts or in a secular sense of solidarity, but in the foundational truth that Christianity's bond with others is anchored in God, which in the case of right-believing and right-worshipping Christians is nurtured in the reality of Christ embodied in the liturgical community of the Church (Eph 1:22–23). The central Christian criticism of individualistic consumerism is Eucharistic. It underscores a union through and in the Body and Blood of Christ. In the Liturgy of St. Basil the Great, the priest prays after the epiclesis, "And as for us, partakers of the one bread and of the cup, do thou unite all to one another unto communion of the one Holy Spirit" (*Liturgikon* 1994, p. 292). Christians recognize that, because of God, humans are not isolated individuals. Consumerism is to be condemned because it disunites

Christians from love of God and each other as Christians, and of others from being united in the image of God. Between Singer and traditional Christians, there is no agreement about the nature of reality, morality, the nature of humans, the meaning of being a person, or the wrongness of consumerism.[25]

Charles Camosy's attempt to bridge the gulf between Christianity and atheism is highly significant: it is a symptom of a Roman Catholic and more broadly a mainline Christian attempt to discount the difference between Christianity and the secular world. This is as one would expect if one holds that a single moral rationality underlies both Christian and secular moral understandings. It reflects Roman Catholic theology's having embraced the rationalist horn of Euthyphro's dilemma: the demands of the holy are to be fully understood in terms of a secular rational account of the right, the good, and the virtuous. The person who embraces secularity and who lives after God sees everything within a life-world at odds with traditional Christianity. The two are moral strangers to each other.

The depth of the differences separating traditional Christianity and its bioethics from the dominant secular culture and its bioethics can only be adequately appreciated with reference to the theocentric character of traditional Christianity, which recognizes that the right, the good, and the virtuous can only be understood in terms of the holy. Traditional Christians know that the gulf between Christians and the secular world is constituted through the difference between aiming one's life at the transcendent personal Creator, versus having an ultimate concern only for creation, including one's fellowmen, insofar as this can be understood apart from God. In the first chapter of the Letter to the Romans, St. Paul condemns the pagan Greek culture's affirmation of that which appears to be fully and truly human, understood apart from a recognition of God (Rom 1:18–32). The Greek pantheon celebrated the full range of human passions, engagements, and concerns portrayed as incarnate in a plastic art of idols that in great beauty affirmed the immanent realization of human life, insofar as this can be celebrated apart from the transcendent God. Because of a failure to orient to the transcendent God, St. Paul recognizes that this refined, indeed sophisticated, pagan Greek culture with its focus on the creature, on that which is most truly human considered apart from God, was profoundly perverse. Its beauty and sense of temperance, *sōphrosynē*, were in fact distorted in being disconnected from God.

Against this background, we can appreciate the traditional Christian view that any orientation towards creatures, apart from a proper recognition of the transcendent, will harmfully fall short of the mark. To return to Singer and Camosy, any attempt to aid the poor or articulate a bioethics apart from an appropriate orientation to God will cause harm. As a painful instance, one might recall (as already mentioned in chapter three) how the welfare programs of President Lyndon Johnson, while attempting to aid the poor, destroyed poor families, especially black families. The result included very serious, albeit unintended, enduring, adverse consequences (Moynihan 1965). Wrongly focused love harms and destroys. There is a gulf between authentic Christianity and the world after God. However, it is a gulf that post-Vatican II Roman Catholic moral theology with its continued faith in reason augmented by commitments to ecumenism and dialogue wishes to bridge.

The gulf separating the immanent with its bioethics from traditional Christian bioethics with its recognition of the transcendent divides traditional Christian bioethicists from those "Christian" bioethicists who have developed their bioethics without any necessary reliance on particular Christian norms for behavior. Such culturally Christian bioethicists may drop the name of Jesus or invoke Christian images; their views have no necessary dependence on Christianity. Here, one might recall Stanley Hauerwas's criticism of Paul Ramsey (1913–1988) as having "insufficient resources to show how Christian practice might make a difference for understanding or forming the practice of medicine" (Hauerwas 1995, p. 16). As a result, Ramsey's work was marked by "the irony . . . that it is unclear you need Jesus' preaching of the kingdom for such an ethic" (Hauerwas 1995, p. 24). Hauerwas argued that this disconnection of Ramsey's work from concrete views and norms of Christians

> helps us understand why Ramsey, in spite of his strong declarations to be working as a Christian ethicist, prepared the way for the developments that Gustafson laments—that is, the subordination of theological ethics to medical ethics. If the social gospel prepared the way for the Christian social ethicist to become a social scientist with a difference; in many ways the more

orthodox Ramsey prepared the way for the Christian ethicist to become a medical ethicist with a difference, the difference being the vague theological presumptions that do no serious intellectual work other than explaining, perhaps, the motivations of the ethicist (Hauerwas 1995, pp. 25–26).

It was in response to such a Christian bioethics without Christian substance that Hauerwas in 1979 in a paper for the Ethics Advisory Board of the Department of Health, Education, and Welfare underscored:

[B]y speaking from a theological perspective I do not pretend to speak from principles that are or should be shared by everyone in our society. You should also know that my own methodological presuppositions in this respect are not widely shared among those that work in theological ethics. Rather the assumption is that theological ethics must develop arguments that should compel consent from all rational subjects irrespective of their religious convictions or lack of religious convictions. Of course, that results in the somewhat ironical state of affairs that committees such as this one invite representatives of religious communities to show how their communities' particular convictions throw light on an issue only to be told that Christian views on the subject are not necessarily related to their religious convictions. Christian ethicists therefore say what any right thinking moral philosopher or person would say. Well I simply do not believe that. It will be the heart of my argument that theological beliefs do make a difference for how *in vitro* fertilization is understood. But since my own views are correlative to my theological convictions it raises the issue of how seriously the committee can take them for consideration of public policy (Hauerwas 1979, pp. 2–3).

The predominant ethics and bioethics of the mainline Western Christianities are in contrast with traditional Christianity in being embedded in the norms of the general culture, not in the particular norms of Christianity.

The differences are stark that separate the life-worlds of those who live their lives aimed at the transcendent God incarnate in history, and those who live within the horizon of the finite and the immanent, eschewing all ultimate meaning, indeed denying all meaning beyond that horizon. The meanings that structure these life-worlds are framed by different histories and by different commitments. The differences are even more strident when God is recognized as the God of the Christians with a history anchored in an Incarnation and Resurrection of that God, along with thick norms regarding abortion, sexual conduct, and suicide. The two frameworks of meaning are embedded, nested, supported, and carried within different moral communities whose conflicts drive the contemporary culture wars. As a consequence, traditional, non-secularized Christians, whether Roman Catholic or Protestant, look odd. Such is surely the case with regard to Orthodox Christianity. Rather than being the norm, "they have become a 'peculiar people', anomalous in their primary beliefs, assumptions, values and norms" (Gilbert 1980, p. ix).

Given the role of the social gospel and of moral philosophy, the border between the secular culture and much of mainline Western Christianity is often unclear. As a consequence, many mainline Christians do not appreciate the full force of contemporary cultural conflicts, even though the differences between the secular culture and traditional Christianity are stark. Roman Catholicism and a good proportion of Protestants remain tied to moral philosophy as it was understood before the recognition of the failure of moral philosophy to secure foundations for its claims. The result is that mainline Christians are promised a connection with the general secular culture through philosophical rationality. Roman Catholicism, in particular, cannot easily lose its faith in reason, as did the general Western culture when it became post-modern, because faith in philosophy lies at the very core of Roman Catholicism, though, as we will shortly see, Pope Francis is attempting to recast this faith. It was through embracing the rationalist horn of Euthyphro's dilemma as much as through any of its new doctrines that Roman Catholicism emerged as a separate religious denomination.[26] The result is that, despite the depth of the gulf, Roman Catholicism remains convinced that the differences that separate Roman Catholicism from the secular culture can be overcome by better philosophical arguments, or at least by the mysterious process of dialogue.

In Roman Catholic moral theology and bioethics, the denial of any gulf between Roman Catholic moral reflection and secular moral reflection is striking. Josef Fuchs (1912–2005), for example, asserts, "If, therefore, our church and other human communities do not always reach the same conclusions, this is not due to the fact that there exists a different morality for Christians from that for non-Christians" (Fuchs 1980, p. 11). In a similar fashion, Charles Curran holds that

> Obviously a personal acknowledgement of Jesus as Lord affects at least the consciousness of the individual and his thematic reflection on his consciousness, but the Christian and the explicitly non-Christian can and do arrive at the same ethical conclusions and can and do share the same general ethical attitudes, dispositions and goals. . . . The explicitly Christian consciousness does affect the judgment of the Christian and the way in which he makes his ethical judgments, but non-Christians can and do arrive at the same ethical conclusions and also embrace and treasure even the loftiest of proximate motives, virtues, and goals which Christians in the past have wrongly claimed only for themselves. This is the precise sense in which I deny the existence of a distinctively Christian ethic; namely, non-Christians can and do arrive at the same ethical conclusions and prize the same proximate dispositions, goals and attitudes as Christians (Curran 1976, p. 20).

This identification of moral theology and Christian bioethics with secular moral rationality means that such a moral theology and Christian bioethics will be thrown into crisis; the failure of philosophical rationality is now widely acknowledged. Roman Catholicism remains confident that philosophy, or at least right reason, can reclaim for Christianity a secularized Western culture, but this faith in reason is unfounded.

VI. The Wrong Diagnosis, the Wrong Treatment

Roman Catholicism still possesses an amazing faith in philosophy. This faith both gave birth to the bioethics of the 1970s and shaped Roman Catholicism's understanding of the proper engagement in the bioethical battles of the culture wars. The engagement is to be philosophical. Consider (1) John Paul II's characterization of the secularization of Europe in terms of a failure of philosophy, as well as (2) his philosopher's appeal to philosophers to repair the damage: "I appeal also to *philosophers*, and to all *teachers of philosophy*, asking them to have the courage to recover, in the flow of an enduringly valid philosophical tradition, the range of authentic wisdom and truth—metaphysical truth included—which is proper to philosophical enquiry" (John Paul II 1993, §106, p. 151). For John Paul II, the secularization of the West reflects as much a philosophical failure as a failure of Western Christianity to preserve traditional Christian life.

> It should also be borne in mind that the role of philosophy itself has changed in modern culture. From universal wisdom and learning, it has been gradually reduced to one of the many fields of human knowing; indeed in some ways it has been consigned to a wholly marginal role. . . . In the wake of these cultural shifts, some philosophers have abandoned the search for truth in itself and made their sole aim the attainment of a subjective certainty or a pragmatic sense of utility. This in turn has obscured the true dignity of reason, which is no longer equipped to know the truth and to seek the absolute (John Paul II 1998, §47, pp. 71–73).

Faith in the moral-philosophical project of the Greeks, reborn in the High Middle Ages, still remains so strong that, in response to the de-Christianization of Western Europe, rather than enjoining a return to the spiritual disciplines of the Christianity of the first millennium in order to renew Christian culture, Pope John Paul II instead affirms a hope for salvation from the Greeks, from philosophers.[27] Faced with the decline of Western Christianity, John Paul II concluded that the spiritual and moral secularization of Western Europe is in significant measure due to bad or timorous philosophers, philosophers not willing to do real metaphysics and therefore supposedly unable adequately to ground moral philosophy so as to secure the norms of Christian life. According to this account, the de-Christianization of Western Europe can be understood in terms of a failure adequately to embrace the inheritance from Athens, rather than that from Jerusalem. This approach implicitly endorses the rational-philosophical foundation of secular bioethics.

John Paul II's response was striking. He recognized the decline, if not collapse, of mainline Western Christianity. He experienced at first hand the deep and wide-ranging secularization of Europe. He saw that "[d]echristianization, which weighs heavily upon entire peoples and communities once rich in faith and Christian life, involves not only the loss of faith or in any event its becoming irrelevant for everyday life, but also, and of necessity, *a decline or obscuring of the moral sense"* (John Paul II 1993, §106, p. 158). Yet, confronted with this major crisis in Christian belief in general and in Roman Catholicism in particular expressed in a major decline of vocations, a shrinking number of congregants, the collapse of Roman Catholicism's ministry of social justice through charitable hospitals, and an increasing theological chaos, John Paul II's response was *not* to call people back to the mind of the Fathers through the traditional Christian ascetic life. He asked for better philosophers to correct philosophical error. In particular, he *did not ask* for the re-establishment of the traditional Christian fasts, along with a commitment to traditional personal prayer, almsgiving, and vigils. Instead, he issued a call for philosophy to regain full faith in its own capacities and to assert its traditional central role in Western culture and Roman Catholicism. John Paul II's call was for a renewal of faith in reason and philosophical reflection. For him, to restore Christian culture and Christian faith one had to renew and reinvigorate Roman Catholicism's medieval intellectual synthesis of faith and reason. It is as if the king of Nineveh in the book of Jonah had proclaimed intensive philosophical seminars instead of a strict fast and repentance in order to hold back God's wrath.[28] John Paul II made the wrong diagnosis and offered the wrong therapy. He failed to stem the loss of congregants.

This faith in reason, in philosophy, and the view that philosophy is central to the restoration and maintenance of a Christian culture emboldens many Roman Catholics with the expectation that through more and better moral-philosophical argument, and through better philosophical argument more generally, Roman Catholicism can close the gulf dividing the dominant secular culture from authentic Christianity. Philosophy in general, and moral philosophy in particular, remain for Roman Catholicism the prime weapons in the culture wars. Consider, for example, Joseph Cardinal Ratzinger's faith in reason.

> [U]ltimately the only weapon is the soundness of the arguments set forth in the political arena and in the struggle to shape public opinion. This is why it is so crucial to develop a philosophical ethics that, while being in harmony with the ethic of faith, must however have its own space and its own logical rigor. The rationality of the arguments should close the gap between secular ethics and religious ethics and found an ethics of reason that goes beyond such distinctions (Ratzinger & Pera 2006, pp. 130–31).

Ratzinger, not yet Pope Benedict XVI, held that the gulf between Christianity and the dominant secular culture could be closed not by converting others to Christianity from that culture, but by arguing with that culture to correct moral conclusions. One is almost moved to wonder whether this approach of Ratzinger (Pope Benedict XVI) reflects a faith in Jesus Christ as the Son of God, or instead in Christianity as a philosophical tradition. Nevertheless, Ratzinger recognized

> The fact that the university became the new seat of research and of the teaching of theology without a doubt enervated its ecclesial dynamism and furthermore severed theology from vital contact with spiritual experiences. Yet another important consequence comes into view: the intensity of the change which had taken place distanced Christian thought drastically from the pattern of the first millennium and from Oriental and Greek culture. "Scientific theology soon found itself Western and Latin, far beyond its conscious choice." All these dangers are in large measure present even today. A theology wholly bent on being academic and "scientific" according to the standards of the modern university, cuts itself off from its great historical matrices and renders itself sterile for the Church (Ratzinger 1995, p. 116).

Many difficulties lie in the way of such an undertaking succeeding. First and foremost, the two sides, the secular culture and the authentically Christian, articulate their arguments and their intellectual concerns within fundamentally different frameworks or paradigms. It is like an argument between homeopaths and those physicians who practice the now-dominant scientific medical paradigm. Although the same terms may be used by both parties (e.g., "congestive heart failure"), they have different meanings, different extensions and intensions when they refer to disease and proper treatment (Engelhardt 2011). Those in the dominant secular culture engage a moral discourse without foundations, which is demoralized and deflated. In contrast, traditional Christians live in the presence of the transcendent God in terms of Whom they understand the content and significance of their behavioral norms to be anchored. As a result, traditional Christians and secular moralists at dispute about any moral issue will argue past each other, a point made by Agrippa and confirmed by ordinary experience. However, given Roman Catholicism's commitment to philosophical rationality, it is unclear whether they will stand out as different, as do traditional Christians. Unlike the Roman Catholics of the Incarnate Word Hospital of the 1930s in San Antonio where my mother worked as a nurse, giving the greeting of "Praised be the Incarnate Word" to every patient, family member, and staff member, post-Vatican II Roman Catholic hospitals are now marked by politically correct, quasi-consumerist commitments. Such a greeting would be too divisive. A *Selbstzersetzung* of Roman Catholicism similar to that by which von Hartmann characterized the liberal Christians of the 19th century will likely continue (von Hartmann 1874).

Second, Roman Catholic moral-theological reflection through its commitments both to philosophical rationality and to ecumenism may remove any moral commitments that cannot be articulated in the most general terms. Apart from the challenge to this undertaking from the failure of the moral-philosophical project, there is the loss of an appreciation of any difference that could set the discourse of Roman Catholic bioethical reflection apart and distinguish it from the language of secular bioethics. A Christian bioethics in this mode will be Christian only in quoting Christian bioethicists who quote other Christian bioethicists who nevertheless attempt to argue as philosophers and philosophically minded bioethicists (see, for example, Cahill 2005). Roman Catholicism lies not just at the origins of contemporary secular bioethics, but eschews any foundational anchorage in the peculiarities of Christianity.

Given that Roman Catholicism as a distinct denomination was created in great measure by a fusion of Aristotelian, Platonic, Stoic, and Christian commitments, the failure to secure philosophical foundations brings cardinal elements of Roman Catholicism into question, including its affirmation of the purported ability of its moral philosophy to serve as a moral theology that can secure a canonical grounding for its moral-theological claims, especially those claims supposedly rooted in natural law. The failure of the philosophical project may even work as a *modus tollens*, raising doubts about what has become the Western Christian moral-theological project as a whole (Buckley 1987). This future will at the very least bring into question not only the rationalist framework of contemporary secular bioethics, but that bioethics embraced by Roman Catholicism. The secularization of the West and the failure of well-crafted philosophical argument to remedy the loss of foundations do not bode well for mainline Western

Christianity and especially for Roman Catholicism, given its rationalist defense of its morality and bioethics.

VII. Scrying the Future: The Impact of Pope Francis

What does all of this mean for Roman Catholicism and its future engagements with and contributions to morality and bioethics? How will Roman Catholicism be able to speak to medical law and health care policy? What impact will changes in Roman Catholicism, Christianity's largest denomination, have on how morality and bioethics are understood and on the character of the moral and bioethical battles in the culture wars? In almost all plausible futures, because of the faith in reason at its roots, Roman Catholicism will likely enter into a deeper crisis (i.e., a further loss of congregants, as well as greater unclarity regarding Roman Catholicism's dogmatic commitments, along with questions becoming more salient concerning its connection with the Church of the Apostles and the Fathers). This faith in reason has up to now not only sustained Roman Catholicism's belief in its key claims regarding natural law being knowable apart from a recognition of God, but also supported its attempts through philosophical reflection to engage the larger culture.[29] Because of Roman Catholicism's embrace of philosophy as its guide, it will be drawn ever more to internalize post-modern moral philosophical accounts as these become prominent in philosophy, thus accommodating further to the secular culture.

By a "post-modern turn" is meant a recognition of, and acquiescence in, moral pluralism: an acceptance that different persons with different moral views, with different moral assumptions, and with differently formed consciences will properly choose differently. They will properly make different life-style choices. This acquiescence in moral pluralism is tightly connected to the demoralization of morality and bioethics (i.e., an intractable moral and bioethical pluralism that is not regarded as in itself radically defective, as lamentably reflecting man's fallen state in a culture after God). In short, there is the possibility that Roman Catholicism itself will support a broad embrace of a morality and a bioethics after God.

If this journey to becoming a post-traditional Christian denomination continues, Roman Catholicism will become ever more like the mainline Christianities.

Roman Catholicism will give greater accent to secular moral assertions from social justice to human dignity and human rights, while also effecting major accommodations with the secular culture on issues ranging from the ordination of priestesses to the acceptance of active homosexuality. In the culture wars, Roman Catholicism will be ever less a critic of secular bioethics. It will, like mainline Christianity, reflect the culture at large. This among other things will support the demoralization of morality and bioethics. This in great measure may happen because Pope Francis is committed to restoring Roman Catholicism to a major social role. This will require stepping back from politically incorrect bioethical positions (e.g., the condemnation of abortion, the artificial insemination of lesbians, and euthanasia) that place Roman Catholicism in a social and political ghetto reserved for religious fundamentalists. Instead, Roman Catholicism will turn to more socially acceptable, indeed populist, issues, such as criticizing the market and capitalism, thereby gaining a major role in cultural and political debates. To make such a change, Roman Catholicism will need to develop a rationale or perspective that can justify ceasing to underscore its politically incorrect moral and bioethical positions. A "weak" post-modern turn by Roman Catholicism that would support this change would come with dramatic implications for Roman Catholic morality and bioethics. Attempting to "fit in" to the contemporary culture will speed the general demoralization of morality and bioethics.

That a post-modern turn is underway in Roman Catholicism is supported by the pope's recent statements and interviews, as well as by his Apostolic Exhortation of November 24, 2013 (Francis 2013). In the reflections that follow, Pope Francis is interpreted not as a bumbling or incautious speaker, or as an uninformed author. As his successful ecclesiastical career demonstrates, Pope Francis is an experienced and intelligent man who has an agenda developed over a lifetime. In this essay, he is interpreted as speaking and writing to support a considered set of goals that has wide-ranging implications for morality, bioethics, and health care policy. There is no reason to assume that he is making things up on the spot. In this chapter, Pope Francis is approached as a person who knows what he is doing. Like Popes John Paul II and Benedict XVI, he is committed to a media papacy, although with an Argentine populist overlay. He seeks to proceed in a pastoral mode, but without dogmatic emphasis on the constraints of the traditional morality and bioethics regarding sexuality, reproduction, and end-of-life decision-making. This pastoral turn through which no doctrine is officially set aside or changed, but through which some doctrines are ignored and then forgotten, will re-frame the geography of Roman Catholic moral theological commitments (e.g., allowing Roman Catholics to receive communion after divorce and remarriage, but without the necessary annulment).

From what he has said and written, Pope Francis, with his friend the late Carlo Cardinal Martini, appears to be committed to bringing Roman Catholicism to set aside its alienation from the dominant culture (Martini & Sporschill 2012). Having for centuries been the dominant cultural force in large parts of Europe, Roman Catholicism has chafed in its current role as an adversarial religion in the culture wars. Cardinal Martini wanted, and Pope Francis wishes, to overcome this cultural and social marginalization. Roman Catholicism aspires again to be mainstream, as the mainstream Christianities had once been mainstream in the United States (Dorrien 2013). Pope Francis gauges accurately the general dissatisfaction in the dominant secular culture with Roman Catholicism's defending the traditional Christian morality and bioethics of sexuality, reproduction, and end-of-life decision-making. As a recent *Time* magazine article (December 23, 2013) celebrating Pope Francis as "Person of the Year" noted, "People [are] weary of the endless parsing of sexual ethics" (Chua-Eoan & Dias 2013, p. 53). Many have rejected "the doctrinal police work so important to [Pope Francis's] recent predecessors" (Chua-Eoan & Dias 2013, p. 53). Pope Francis began at once to step away from doctrinal stridency. Pope Francis generally avoids speaking to traditional moral issues such as sexuality (e.g., the treatment of the sexual dysfunction of homosexuals and transsexual surgery), reproduction (e.g., reproduction outside of marriage, artificial insemination of lesbians, *in vitro* fertilization with embryo wastage, and abortion), and end-of-life issues (e.g., stopping hydration and nutrition for the permanently comatose, physician-assisted suicide, and euthanasia). Pope Francis's morality instead speaks vaguely to issues of resource allocation. Like Obama who radically altered health care in the United States, Pope Francis promises change. His is to be a papacy of joy (e.g., *Evangelii Gaudium*), change (no more harping on abortion), and social justice.

Those who are not committed to right worship and right belief, those who are not committed to being faithful to an unbroken church reaching to the

Apostles (i.e., those who are not traditionalists or fundamentalists), have been long tired of, and indeed have never been committed to, the culture wars. Such persons also came to regard the loss of congregants and vocations after Vatican II as not stemming from the liturgical and theological disorientation that followed Vatican II, but from a failure to realize the liberalizing promises of a new Pentecost through Vatican II. This judgment has added a further urgency to ending the culture wars while again affirming an *aggiornamento*. Pope Francis's strategy is to weaken the affirmation of divisive dogmas, such as condemnations of reproduction outside of marriage, abortion, and homosexual acts, but without directly changing these dogmas. A change in the tone of discourse can work foundational changes. "[T]his new pope may have found a way out of the 20th century culture wars, which have left the church moribund in much of Western Europe and on the defensive from Dublin to Los Angeles" (Chua-Eoan & Dias 2013, p. 53). Pope Francis is attempting to be a peacemaker for the culture wars. Of course, a crucial demographic question is whether cultural accommodation instead of fundamentalist commitments attract and keep communicants. If Pope Francis succeeds in imposing a new and comprehensive theological paradigm on Roman Catholicism, is it likely to attract believers and produce vocations? Whatever implications the changes may have for stemming or accelerating the loss of congregants, Pope Francis appears to have a principled commitment to his doctrinal course.

Pope Francis's views appear to have an important root in The Pact of the Catacombs, which may have been styled The Pact of the Servant and Poor Church. This pact was signed on November 16, 1965, by forty bishops, the majority of whom were from Latin America. The full text remains only in the writings of the Franciscan bishop Bonaventure Kloppenburg. Subsequently, Cardinal Roger Etchagaray, president of the Pontifical Council for Justice and Peace, also signed it. The pact reflected Pope John XXIII's admonition at the opening of Vatican II that the Council should make Roman Catholicism a "church of the poor." Although Pope Francis has never cited the Pact of the Catacombs, the language he has engaged and the principles he has underscored reflect a common wish that the church become a "poor church, for the poor." Cardinal Walter Kasper, who is a retired German theologian close to Pope Francis, has stated that the pope is bringing the Pact of the Catacombs back after it was long forgotten.

Although the pact was largely forgotten in most of the world, its influence continued to have life in Latin America.

In many of his remarks, Pope Francis manifests the envy born of countries marked by chronic economic and political dysfunction for those countries that are prosperous and stable.[30] That is, Pope Francis fails to attribute the economic problems of much of the dysfunction of such countries to uncertain property rights, over-regulation of markets, and corruption, which hamper growth and produce high unemployment, including high youth unemployment. Instead, he lays the problems of the poor at the feet of the market and capitalism, rather than to blame populist socialist polities that create malfunctioning economies such as that of Argentina. With this approach, he places a major emphasis on economic problems without addressing the actual problems of uncertain property rights and constraints on the market that lead to chronic high youth unemployment. All the while he also avoids addressing the spiritual roots of the weakening of Christian commitments (i.e., the de-Christianization of which John Paul II spoke). For example, on October 1, 2013, in an interview published in *La Repubblica*,[31] Pope Francis laments:

> The most serious of the evils that afflict the world these days are youth unemployment and the loneliness of the old. The old need care and companionship; the young need work and hope but have neither one nor the other, and the problem is they don't even look for them any more. They have been crushed by the present. You tell me: can you live crushed under the weight of the present? Without a memory of the past and without the desire to look ahead to the future by building something, a future, a family? Can you go on like this? This, to me, is the most urgent problem that the Church is facing (Scalfari 2013a).

One is struck by the religious poverty of the pope's remarks: there is no indication of the traditional Christian exhortation that all worldly problems in order to be rightly addressed must be placed within the pursuit of the Kingdom of Heaven (Mt 6:33). There is in fact nothing particularly Christian about the pope's concerns. His interviewer, Eugenio Scalfari, the founder of *La Repubblica*, responds in evident amazement: "Your Holiness, I say, it is largely a political and economic problem for states, governments, political parties, trade unions" (Scalfari 2013a).

Pope Francis surely knows that out of love of God and neighbor one ought to give to the poor. However, as Scalfari implies, what basis is there for anyone's holding that Pope Francis, or Roman Catholic theologians in general, have any useful insights into the problems of youth unemployment?[32] After all, the problems of youth unemployment tend to be greater in Roman Catholic countries in Western Europe than in countries with a substantial proportion of Protestants.[33] The countries of southern Europe, the inheritors of a Graeco-Roman culture, appear much less able to remedy the problem of youth unemployment than the relatively more capitalist, less-regulated nations of northern Europe, such as Germany and Austria.[34] In addressing economic issues in *Evangelii Gaudium*, one is then left with the question of how to understand Pope Francis's statements on economic issues. The difficulty lies in part with Pope Francis's penchant for attacking straw men, such as the "absolute autonomy of the marketplace" (Francis 2013, p. 47, #56), when an unregulated market exists nowhere on the face of the earth. With Scalfari, one can only wonder why a pope from an economically and politically marginally functional country such as Argentina, who makes cliché-like populist remarks, would have something useful to say regarding how one ought politically and economically to address the problems of youth unemployment, indeed economic problems generally. Probably to Scalfari's amazement, Pope Francis does not call on Christians individually, like the individual good Samaritan, to turn to those who they know are in need.

Pope Francis in many of his public statements, ratified and developed further in *Evangelii Gaudium* (Francis 2013), adopts a rhetoric with family resemblances to a political campaign speech. His statements, if placed within a populist context, are attractively misleading and rhetorically powerful generalizations marked by unjustified hyperbole ("today everything comes under the laws of competition and the survival of the fittest" [Francis 2013, p. 45, #53]), which are combined with vague but anxiety-provoking warnings of possible civil violence ("inequality provokes [a] violent reaction" [Francis 2013, p. 50, #59]). While avoiding as far as possible issues such as homosexual marriage that would place him among the politically incorrect, fundamentalist religious, he emphasizes joy. At the same time, he plays on class divisions through references to economic inequalities and to economic forces not necessarily being tied to justice. Pope Francis speaks of being joyful while supporting a hermeneutic of distrust regarding the market and those who have succeeded in the market. Without providing grounds for informed judgments about those economies that are more market friendly, Pope Francis advances vague grounds for distrust and envy. In particular, he criticizes "trickle-down" economics as having "a crude and naïve trust in the goodness of those wielding economic power and in the sacralized workings of the prevailing economic system" (Francis 2013, p. 46, # 54).

"Trickle-down" economics is grounded on the view that if high earners earn more, they will be more likely to expand their businesses and to hire more workers independently of any views these high earners might have regarding social justice, solidarity, and/or concerns for others. After all, the rhetorically negative term "trickle-down economics" is used to refer to a theory about how to generate greater wealth, including greater wealth for the poor, not about any view of justice for the poor, whatever this might mean. The pope does not acknowledge the possibility that programs to redistribute wealth will discourage the creation of new jobs through increasingly costly bureaucracies and regulations, as is the case in Argentina and much of Latin America. Reality is different from what Pope Francis indicates. As Terry Miller points out,

> Countries achieving higher levels of economic freedom consistently and measurably outperform others in economic growth, long-term prosperity and social progress. Botswana, for example, has made gains through low tax rates and political stability.
>
> Those losing freedom, on the other hand, risk economic stagnation, high unemployment and deteriorating social conditions. For instance, heavy-handed government intervention in Brazil's economy continues to limit mobility and fuel a sense of injustice (Miller 2014, A13).

Pope Francis's position appears to be grounded in a political and economic vision that is largely independent of the facts. For example, the pope, rather than advancing concrete evidence against economic claims on behalf of capitalism and the market, mounts the economically irrelevant but politically powerful charge that "trickle-down" economics will not bring about "greater justice and inclusiveness in the world" (Francis 2013, Sec. 54). His Apostolic Exhortation is not a well-reasoned opinion piece.

Because Pope Francis is an intelligent and able person, his statements might at first blush seem puzzling, not only because of what he says, but because of what he does not say. Although it is clear that Pope Francis wishes to reach out to the poor, it is striking that he does not address how one might support an ethos of charity or philanthropy. Such an ethos, one must note, is more prominent in the capitalist United States than in predominantly Roman Catholic countries. In the United States, personal charity involves 1.6% of the GDP, the highest in the world, followed by the United Kingdom (0.73%), Canada (0.72%), and Australia (0.69%), with only 0.14% given in France (Clegg & Pharaoh 2006). Roman Catholic countries do not distinguish themselves as countries with a prominent ethos of personal charity. Pope Francis gives considerable space to concerns for the poor, but he does not ask the rich to tithe to the poor, personally to reach out through charity to the poor. He is not that interested in the individual charity of individual persons.

How, then, is one to understand Pope Francis's remarks? What is he trying to do? Why has he chosen the rhetoric he employs? Some are of the opinion that Pope Francis's remarks are simply ill-considered and sophomoric. For example, R. R. Reno writes:

> Unfortunately Francis' sweeping generalizations about economics are inaccurate, and even irresponsible. He ignores the ways in which state-dominated economies encourage corruption and often deepen rather than alleviate poverty while singling out trickle-down theories for harsh criticism. He effectively demonizes economic conservatives as moral cretins "in thrall to an individualistic, indifferent, and self-centered mentality." This rhetoric contributes to our already degraded political culture (Reno 2014b, 4).

This explanation requires one to hold that a person with a lifetime of public speaking and giving interviews has suddenly lost his grip on what messages he intends to send. Unlike Reno, Michael Novak has attempted to defend Pope Francis (although the text suggests that Novak's sub-text is to neutralize the danger that Pope Francis would be correctly interpreted by Roman Catholics as requiring a greater intervention by the state in the market [Novak 2013]). Novak does this by pointing out that the exact equivalent of "trickle-down" economics occurs nowhere in the Spanish version of the Apostolic Exhortation.[35] "Trickle-down" economics, Novak contends, is an incorrect translation of the Spanish *derrame*, which should be rendered as "spillover" or "overflow." This would allow one to attribute part of the character of Pope Francis's Apostolic Exhortation to the ideological bias of his translators, rather than to him. Second, Novak tries to account for Pope Francis's views of capitalism, economics, and the market in terms of Pope Francis's having spent his life for the most part in Argentina, so that it "might be understandable" that he evinces a lack of sympathy for the capacities of the market. As Novak observes, because Argentina has economically performed so poorly because of state interventions and the insecurity of property rights, Pope Francis may be biased against the market and capitalism.[36] The market, as Novak adds, when not hampered as it is in Argentina, does a splendid job of raising the poor to the middle class, as for example has occurred in Hong Kong, Singapore, South Korea, and Taiwan (Novak 2013), places largely innocent of the Roman Catholic vision of social justice.

There are good reasons to hold both of these assessments of Pope Francis to be wrong. There are instead good grounds to consider Pope Francis's populist and post-modern rhetoric not to be an error of expression or the result of a dismal ignorance of economic situations outside of Argentina (or for that matter, outside of Latin America), but as deliberately chosen. Again, Pope Francis is best read as actually knowing what he is doing and what he is saying. Although Pope Francis is an Argentine, he surely understands how different the market, property rights, and society are structured in Anglo-American countries and in much of northern Europe. It is not plausibly the case, *pace* Novak, that being an Argentine blinded Pope Francis or left him woefully ignorant of this state of affairs. Rather, it is much more plausible that Pope Francis has a widely left-of-center ideological view of capitalism, economics, and the market, which is integrated within a political-theological agenda that supports goals he holds should be pursued and should shape society whatever the economic costs. This political-theological agenda ranks equality before liberty, and both before economic security. It is this agenda that he is advancing through his *La Repubblica* remarks and in *Evangelii Gaudium*.

Pope Francis is opening up a new political-theological space. In part, the change of discourse is meant to attract left-of-center Roman Catholics and those moved by populist appeals so as to fill increasingly empty pews. To them he projects an image of humility and gentleness. This rhetorical turn has earned him "Person of the Year" by *Time* magazine (December 23, 2013). He appeals to mainstream journalists. More importantly, Pope Francis's rhetorical style and recent statements can be appreciated as aimed at reshaping the context and character of Roman Catholic morality and bioethics, a change pursued for its own sake, and only secondarily, albeit importantly, because he and others hold that his rhetoric will resonate with alienated Roman Catholics. No longer talking absolutely about what had been affirmed and believed absolutely changes the whole discourse of morality, thus changing the substance of that about which one speaks (Francis 2013). Through an indulgent pastoral approach, Pope Francis *de facto* alters moral constraints without having to do so *de jure*. Pope Francis rather than repeatedly condemning sin has engaged a powerful non-judgmental discourse: "Who am I to judge?" (Donadio 2013), which suggests more than it says. Pope Francis does this as well by indicating the possibility of significant changes in doctrine by alluding to God as a God of surprises.

In contrast with Pope Francis, the traditional Christian response is unconditional forgiveness to the repentant sinner. Christ's loving and compassionate forgiveness presupposes that the sinner recognizes his sin. Traditionally, there is also certainty about what one must preach. For example the Great Commission includes the injunction to teach "them to obey everything I have commanded you" (Mt 28:20). Francis steps back from Apostolic clarity with his non-judgmental rhetoric regarding sin, not just the sinner, that opens up an intellectual space for a Roman Catholicism sustained by weak theological presuppositions, including by a new way of locating morals, dogma, and social concerns. Pope Francis hints at this when he describes his God as a God of surprises. Francis is rebranding Roman Catholicism as a "big-tent" church. Pope Francis is not just a media pope like John Paul II and Benedict XVI; he is a pope at home in the non-judgmental sexual and reproductive moral discourse of the contemporary West. He can take a further step to a new bioethics. Again, the changes he seeks to effect are primarily pursued indirectly, through a change in tone and focus in order subtly but surely to redirect the energies of Roman Catholicism.

The post-traditional character of Pope Francis's position becomes clearer in his response to Scalfari's question as to whether the pope wants to convert him. Pope Francis sidesteps the issue of conversion by changing the subject through substituting the now politically incorrect term "proselytism" so that he can say "no." This shift of attention allows Pope Francis to advance a post-modern position that seems at the last moment to be withdrawn by his reference to "the Good."

> Proselytism is solemn nonsense, it makes no sense. We need to get to know each other, listen to each other and improve our knowledge of the world around us. Sometimes after a meeting I want to arrange another one because new ideas are born and I discover new needs. This is important: to get to know people, listen, expand the circle of ideas. The world is crisscrossed by roads that come closer together and move apart, but the important thing is that they lead towards the Good (Scalfari 2013).

Pope Francis carefully avoids recognizing the obligation given by the Great Commission to convert the world (Mt 28:19–20). He instead embraces a post-modern or "weak theological" position (i.e., he never explicitly references an objective good): "Each of us has a vision of good and of evil. We have to encourage people to move towards what they think is Good." It is important to observe that Pope Francis takes the same position in *Evangelii Gaudium* when he states: "Non-Christians, by God's gracious initiative, when they are faithful to their own consciences, can live 'justified by the grace of God'" (Francis 2013, Sec. 254). One way very plausibly to read these statements is that the criterion at stake is meant to be subjective: one is left with doing whatever feels right to one's conscience. One is in a post-modern world of moral pluralism. Of course, for those with a traditional morality, the difficulty is that the "consciences" of people often support them in doing what Pope Francis should recognize as wrong (e.g., physician-assisted suicide) and in doing what Pope Francis should condemn as evil (e.g., suicide bombing). However, no reference is made to an objective standard by which to judge the propriety of the different moral and dogmatic commitments that sit well with different consciences. There is no clear corrective to a subjective understanding. Pope Francis should not be seen as witless in these matters. This omission must be intended.

Pope Francis in the Scalfari interview repeatedly supports this weak theological reading. He says, for example, "And I repeat it here. Everyone has his own idea of good and evil and must choose to follow the good and fight evil as he conceives them. That would be enough to make the world a better place" (Scalfari 2013). Here and in *Evangelii Gaudium* Pope Francis avoids any clear acknowledgement that the good that many pursue in accord with their "own consciences" is often in reality very evil.[37] Very likely, Pol Pot held that he was killing millions of fellow Cambodians in the pursuit of his vision of the good.[38] So, too, many following their "own consciences" formed by their religious convictions, *pace Evangelii Gaudium*, engage in abortion, infanticide, euthanasia, and the beheading of captives. One should recall the words of Satan in *Paradise Lost*: "Evil be thou my Good" (Milton, Book IV, line 110). Pope Francis's statements, to say the least, are astonishing after the Holocaust. Doing what one thinks is proper can be very destructive. As with regard to his statements bearing on economics, one may be tempted to attribute them to a monumental lack of care. However, Pope Francis says what one would expect him to say, given a "weak" theology.

For Pope Francis, the *La Repubblica* interview was integral to his commitment to restructure the character of Roman Catholic theological and bioethical discourse. The interview sent an important message, even after it was withdrawn from the Vatican website. His remarks in the *La Repubblica* interview allowed an indirect affirmation of the post-Vatican II hermeneutic of rupture that acknowledges what is now obvious: Vatican II created, or at least led to, a new Roman Catholicism. As a consequence, a new theology, a new morality, and a new bioethics are needed for a new Roman Catholicism. This new Roman Catholicism will have first and foremost a new, softer approach to dogmatic commitments. The old dogmas will in some sense remain, but one will not be dogmatic about these dogmas. Again, there is a crucial change in tone with foundational implications. The old pre-Vatican II Roman Catholicism is dead (and in the case of the traditionalist Society of St. Pius X to be interred alive), so that, among other things, secular bioethics now not only replaces the medical ethics of the previous manualist tradition, but also demoralizes and redirects that bioethics. The major focus will be on social issues that will run against the sentiments of those who are right-of-center, but they will not be politically incorrect, as with the condemnation of abortion and homosexual marriage. An important step appears underway towards a substantial accommodation with the now-dominant secular culture. In Italy, this means that Roman Catholicism can step back from divisive issues such as *in vitro* fertilization and the condemnation of embryo wastage so as instead to join with mainstream, left-of-center politicians in criticizing capitalism. As Scalfari states, "You are and will be a revolutionary Pope" (Scalfari 2013a).

A useful interpretive framework within which to locate the remarks of Pope Francis, including both his *La Repubblica* interview and *Evangelii Gaudium*, can be found in the recent proposals for a "weak thought," especially for a "weak theology" (Engel 2001; Robbins 2004a and 2004b; Vattimo 1982 and 2002; Vattimo & Rovatti 1983). Core to "weak theology" is a radical toning down, even demoralization and deflation, of bioethical, moral, and theological claims. Bioethical, moral, and theological claims may still be made, but they are to be stated without a dogmatic or epistemic stridency, without an insistence on objectivity, but instead with an openness to the claims and positions of others that conflict with one's own. Different bioethical, moral, and theological claims become compatible in that they are reduced to different epistemic or theological life-style choices. Morality is not something to fight about. As Richard Rorty in summary of Vattimo's "weak" thought states:

> In a "weak" conception, morality is not a matter of unconditional obligations imposed by a divine or quasi-divine authority but rather is something cobbled together by a group of people trying to adjust to their circumstances and achieve their goals by cooperative efforts (Rorty 2005, p. xviii).

Within such a "weak" theology, Vattimo can both call himself a Christian (purportedly now a Waldensian) and say that "thanks to God I am an atheist" (Vattimo 2004, p. 63). Of course, Pope Francis is surely not likely to say, "I am a Roman Catholic, albeit an atheist." But he can say, "I am a Roman Catholic and a loyal son of the church and believe whatever Roman Catholicism teaches," while at the same time no longer underscoring the importance of Christianity's politically incorrect moral and bioethical dogmas about sexuality, reproduction, and end-of-life decision-making.

Pope Francis appears to embrace a new paradigm of bioethics and theology that allows him to accept enough of "weak" thought to say with Vattimo, of course with some important qualifications, "What project can I have in the world if I am a Christian? To defend the authority of the church and its dogmas, or to strive for a different situation, an ecumenical situation, a situation in which we really come together and feel mutual affection" (Vattimo & Girard 2010, pp. 41–42). Within such a "weak" theology, one substitutes "the term 'solidarity' for the term 'truth,' and I come right out and propose to make 'charity' the substitute because all the rest is just opinion" (Vattimo & Girard 2010, p. 51). Of course, charity will be translated into taxing the rich and providing welfare rather than asking all who have resources personally to give to the poor. The focus is on political action and intervention, not on individual almsgiving. Against this background, it makes sense to shift the accent from bioethical, moral, and theological truth, and to focus instead on youth unemployment and economic inequalities, with a view towards governmental regulation of the market. A whole new framework, a new comprehensive paradigm, for theology and bioethics appears to be re-shaping Roman Catholicism through a subtle but momentous change in tone and focus. A soft revolution is being softly or subtly introduced, a revolution that is nevertheless profound. The most plausible interpretation of Pope Francis's interviews and of *Evangelii Gaudium* is that Pope Francis has taken an important step towards a "weak" or "ambiguous" theology and bioethics.

Pope Francis is willing to accept the fact that his statements are a scandal or stumbling block for conservative Roman Catholics, for Roman Catholics who have not wanted to face how different post-Vatican II Roman Catholicism is.[39] He is also speaking to a new audience. Among the dwindling proportion of baptized Roman Catholics still regularly attending Mass, a substantial percentage holds approving views about the ordination of priestesses, abortion, homosexual acts, and homosexual marriage, which views are at odds with traditional and official Roman Catholic teaching. The bioethics of these Roman Catholics is not just at odds with traditional manualist Roman Catholic medical ethics, but even with the bioethics engendered in the 1970s, because this bioethics is beyond founda-tions and demoralized.[40] These congregants tend to embrace a post-modern view (i.e., incompatible and demoralized views of the good can be affirmed, indeed celebrated as reflecting the rich moral diversity of the human condition, no longer understood as fallen), such as those advanced by Pope Francis in the *La Repubblica* interview and in *Evangelii Gaudium* (Scalfari 2013). Lack of unity in morality and belief is no longer to be lamented but accepted. These Roman Catholics implicitly, if not explicitly, embrace the hermeneutic of rupture engendered by Vatican II; this rupture sets Roman Catholicism's past within a new interpretive structure which acknowledges post-Vatican II Roman Catholicism as substantively different from pre-Vatican II Roman Catholicism. These post-rupture Roman Catholics have also felt themselves estranged by Benedict XVI's support of "Tridentine" Roman Catholics, as well as alienated from Roman Catholicism due to conservative Roman Catholics constantly underscoring the wrongness of choices approved by the dominant culture, such as abortion and sexual acts outside of the marriage of a man and a woman. Pope Francis wishes to welcome home these alienated, post-rupture Roman Catholics. He wants to embrace a political-theological perspective through which their estrangement can be set aside.

It would be too much if Pope Francis explicitly changed such politically incorrect and "offensive" doctrinal commitments such as the condemnation of abortion and homosexual acts. It is safer, indeed it is enough, to avoid as far as possible addressing or emphasizing controversial issues, and instead quietly allowing their demoralization to occur. Politically incorrect theological and moral views will tend to be eroded and forgotten if the ecclesial community does not invest energies in supporting traditional doctrines, including parsing Christianity's counter-cultural sexual ethics, as well as acting as a doctrinal policeman (Chua-Eoan & Dias 2013, p. 53). Contemporary Roman Catholics have forgotten their once central focus on usury. As doctrinal concerns fell into desuetude, they were lost in the past. If one ignores a doctrine, it tends generally to pass from view. Hence, the importance for traditional Christianity of remaining in the mind of the Apostles and the Fathers. A change of focus and style that supports a weak theology provides the opportunity for those who wish to deflate politically incorrect dogmas and then remove them from view. Towards that end, it is best to proceed "Gently, but firmly and tenaciously" (ITV 2013, p. 21). Pope Francis supports a politically freighted hermeneutic of suspicion against conservative Christianity, capitalism, and the market. This hermeneutic of suspicion is not only politically correct, but in harmony with a major political power base.

In pursuing his goal of a new theological framework for Roman Catholicism, Pope Francis projects an image of gentleness and humility. However, reality is quite contrary to this image. When speaking regarding conservative Roman Catholics, liturgical traditionalists, and those concerned to maintain the integrity of traditional dogma, Pope Francis is acerbic and even vitriolic. He engages *ad hominem* rather than substantive arguments. For example, Pope Francis characterizes traditionalists as having an insidious worldliness.

> In some people we see an ostentatious preoccupation for the liturgy, for doctrine and for the Church's prestige, but without any concern that the Gospel have a real impact on God's faithful people and the concrete needs of the present time. In this way, the life of the Church turns into a museum piece or something which is the property of a select few (Francis 2013, Sec. 95).

To the post-Christian world, Pope Francis offers a warm embrace. He is willing to be kind in his rhetoric regarding their deviations. However, to Roman Catholic traditionalists, he responds with a strident rhetoric of cutting remarks unconnected to any careful analysis of what he is criticizing and why.

In *Evangelii Gaudiium* Pope Francis uses a strong but nevertheless incoherent rhetoric. He accuses those who wish to submit their wills to Christ so as to direct their lives in obedience to the mind of of the Apostles and Fathers of being narcissistic. Remarkably, he characterizes traditional Christians as "promethean neo-pelagians"

> who ultimately trust only in their own powers and feel superior to others because they observe certain rules or remain intransigently faithful to a particular Catholic style from the past. A supposed soundness of doctrine or discipline leads instead to a narcissistic and authoritarian elitism, whereby instead of evangelizing, one analyzes and classifies others, and instead of opening the door to grace, one exhausts his or her energies in inspecting and verifying (Francis 2013, Sec. 94).

Pope Francis not only radically misdescribes traditional Christians who wish to conform their lives to the unbroken mind of the Church, characterizing them as self-seeking rather than Christ-seeking, but he also fails to recognize that those who take the living God seriously are in fact those who tend to make converts. His rhetoric is well crafted to the goal of giving shape to a new understanding of Roman Catholicism in accord with politically acceptable populist goals.

> British Catholic Laurence England writes that, "in sifting through media reports, I was shocked by how often the Pope criticized Christians and by the severity of his insults" (CNN.com, Feb. 19, 2014). England lists some of Francis's more noteworthy nuggets of negativity, names the Pope has actually called people: "pickled pepper-faced Christians," "closed, sad, trapped Christians," "defeated Christians," "liquid Christians," "creed-reciting, parrot Christians," and "watered-down faith, weak-hoped Christians." He has even gone so far as to call Catholics who focus on Church traditions "museum mummies." Oh, how he despises those ill-starred traddies! ... Francis has built up such an arsenal of put-downs that [Laurence] England says he's been commissioned to write *The Pope Francis Little Book of Insults.* (He jests, of course, but if some publisher takes up the notion, the volume might soon become encyclopedic in length.) (Anonymous 2014, pp. 18–19).

To traditionalists, Pope Francis shows a face quite different from what he presents to post-traditional Christians, non-Christians, and atheists.

Pope Francis opposes those who would restore the old *lex orandi* (rule of prayer), because restoring the old Mass and the old pieties would act to restore the old *lex credendi* (rule of faith), along with its traditional mores and its quite different paradigm and understanding of the nature of morality. On the other hand, Francis supports a politically freighted hermeneutic of suspicion against capitalism and the market, which is not only not politically incorrect, but in harmony with a major political power base.

To ensure that his agenda succeeds, all must be placed securely within the new *lex orandi*. Towards this end, supporters of the old Mass must be marginalized, because they are also supporters of a theological paradigm that Pope

Francis wants fully past. The traditionalists' *lex orandi* undergirds a *lex credendi* that is to be rendered into a history that is before a profound rupture so as no longer to be integral to post-Vatican II Roman Catholicism. This is the case because Paul VI's Mass sustains a totally new liturgical life-world and pieties, which is to open up new ways of approaching dogmas. Nevertheless, because many bishops will find it useful to appeal to as many constituencies as possible, and because doctrinal conservatives still command congregants and money, no doctrinal deviations or changes will be clearly or explicitly stated. To accomplish this goal, Pope Francis makes sufficient statements seemingly contrary to his *La Repubblica* remarks so that they can be taken by devout conservatives as indicating that he is not really setting traditional dogmas aside.

This possibility for a re-interpretation of the pope's remarks is essential for conservative Roman Catholics who embrace a very strong view regarding their obligation to submit to the opinions of the pope (a view that did not develop until after Trent, but especially in the 19th century). Their view of papal authority highly discourages openly and directly protesting papal actions and/or statements, even when such actions and/or statements are potentially very harmful to Roman Catholicism. In order to calm such conservative Roman Catholics so that they remain relatively quiet, the circumstances of the *La Repubblica* interview allow plausible deniability. Because the text was produced by Scalfari from memory, even though it was then submitted to the Vatican, approved, placed on the Vatican's website, and published in *L'Osservatore Romano*, there are grounds for disavowal. This is the case despite similar, but not as forthright, views appearing in *Evangelii Gaudium*. This strategy gives room for conservative Roman Catholics to resituate his statements in *La Repubblica* without Pope Francis's having in detail explicitly to repudiate them. The bottom line is that there are reasons for Pope Francis to make statements such as those in his *La Repubblica* interview so as to affirm his new vision of Roman Catholicism in a way that conservative Roman Catholics if they wish can discount their significance. This sets the stage for a largely unnoticed but in the end substantial recasting of morality and bioethics as they are placed in a new, weak theological framing context.

Pope Francis's interview with *La Repubblica* in this light makes perfect sense as an expression of his commitment to a return to the revolutionary promises of Vatican II, while also pursuing reconciliation with an important constituent group, who have been alienated because of what they hold to be the unacceptable conservative character of the papacies of John Paul II and Benedict XVI. As the Roman Catholic philosopher John Caputo puts it, "I feel a common outrage at the pontifical authoritarianism and 'fundamentalism' of John Paul II" (Caputo & Vattimo 2007, p. 71). Caputo and others regard John Paul II and Benedict XVI as having betrayed the promise of Vatican II.

> John Paul II virtually extinguished every trace of the notion of the "people of God" that was the hallmark of the Second Vatican Council and thoroughly betrayed the spirit of that great council. He set back the legitimate aspirations of women in the Church a generation, intimidated Catholic scholars and free speech with inquisitorial violence, and left behind a Church in which it is impossible to imagine that its dangerous and reactionary teachings on birth control and homosexuality will be corrected in the foreseeable future. He suppressed open discussion in the Church of the legitimate civil rights of men and women in secular society to decide these and other matters, like abortion rights, without ecclesiastical intimidation (Caputo & Vattimo 2007, pp. 71–72).

Many in this group of Roman Catholic intellectuals yearn for a demoralization of morality and bioethics within Roman Catholicism. In order to reconcile those who sympathize with Caputo's position, Pope Francis gestures towards a post-modern "weak theology" or "ambiguous theology," combined with a political turn to the left (Engel 2001; Robbins 2004a, 2004b). Pope Francis also adroitly engages a "pastoral approach" that does not explicitly set traditional doctrine aside, but instead finds ways not to apply it in particular circumstances.[41]

For those with whom he seeks a rapprochement, the change of theological and bioethical paradigms begun with Vatican II must be completed, even though official doctrine may at times be affirmed, so that conservative Roman Catholics do not become so concerned as to consider going into schism, as did Archbishop Marcel Lefebvre. The result is that the general tenor and spirit of the Roman Catholic approach to theology and bioethics have for quite understandable reasons been rendered dogmatically soft or weak, subtly changing everything, even that which is still affirmed. The previous morality and bioethics, which had a firm faith in reason and a common morality, have been brought into question because the character of the framing approach has changed, with the result that Roman Catholic bioethics is not simply on its way to accommodating secular bioethics, but also to aiding its demoralization and to accepting a bioethics that is after God and after modernity.

For bishops who want to have broad influence on economic and social policy while avoiding the culture wars occasioned by traditional Christians and a traditional Christian bioethics (e.g., by the public condemnation of abortion), Pope Francis's statements can only be welcome.[42] The cardinals who elected Pope Francis and the bishops who supported them had grounds to hold him to favor the doctrinal liberalization that Pope Francis's friend, Carlo Cardinal Martini, had hoped to accomplish, had he become pope (Martini & Sporschill 2012). Pope Francis's remarks support this project. But bishops needed to be reassured on this point. Attempts by Benedict XVI to reconcile with traditionalists further alienated left-of-center Roman Catholics such as those sympathetic with Caputo, who hoped for a new vision of morality and bioethics following Vatican II. Consider the remarks that Archbishop Alois Kothgasser of Salzburg made in response to Benedict XVI's support for the wider celebration of the Tridentine mass, the mass of Pius V (Benedict XVI 2007). In reaction to Benedict XVI, Kothgasser asked: "Should the Catholic Church reduce herself to a cult, which only a few, but law-abiding, members practice, or should the Catholic Church of Jesus Christ leave room for diversity, be open and influence society from the inside?" (Archdiocese Salzburg 2009; Hull 2010, p. 341). The opposition to Benedict XVI's conservatism was so open and strident that "during the formal reception in Berlin for Pope Benedict, September 22, 2011, eleven of his fellow cardinals and bishops publicly rebuked the Holy Father by refusing to shake his extended hand—while television cameras from around the world recorded the spectacle" (Connolly 2014, p. 43). The celebration of the old Latin Mass had failed fully to extinguish or at least radically to marginalize that mass so as to sever all liturgical connection with the pre-Vatican II Roman Catholicism, which constitutes a threat in the eyes of such bishops to a softer, weaker moral theology. The rupture from pre-Vatican II Roman Catholicism is to be complete and final. The old *lex orandi* must not be allowed to bring the new *lex credendi* with its new approach to dogma, morality, and bioethics into question.

Those seeking to increase the influence of Roman Catholicism on left-of-center politics therefore affirm Archbishop Kothgasser's position and find support in Pope Francis's *La Repubblica* interview, even if it has been withdrawn from the Vatican website. The message of the interview allows them to look forward to being more effectively a part of the contemporary secular socio-political, as well as moral-bioethical movements they endorse. Pope Francis's change of discourse means that they will not be forced into a social ghetto with other religions that affirm politically incorrect dogmas. Pope Francis's *La Repubblica* statement, despite the discomfiture it may cause for conservatives, is from this point of view strategic, and indeed expertly crafted. So, too, in the case of *Evangelii Gaudium*. Conservative Roman Catholics are left attempting to blunt the difficulties posed by the text, using excuses such as Michael Novak's for Pope Francis's intemperate economic populism (Novak 2013). The change in discourse supported by Pope Francis allows Roman Catholic hierarchs and congregants to gain a place within those intellectual circles integral to the dominant and effective cultural elite of the age, what Hegel characterizes as 'Absolute Spirit.'

Hegel, a devout Christian atheist, could easily live with Pope Francis's Christianity and the bioethics it supports, save for Pope Francis's lack of sympathy for the market. Hegel presented himself, in all good conscience *pace* Pope Francis, as true to Lutheran doctrine, the meaning of which he understood to be enduring but the higher truth of which he had appreciated: all men are free. Hegel had produced a 'weak theology.' Pope Francis has taken his first, but nevertheless important, step towards establishing a Roman Catholic weak theological position. His view of theology has consanguinities with mainline Christianity's accommodation with the secular culture, a position in harmony with Hegel's claims. Conflicts with the secular dominant culture over abortion and homosexual marriage are to be overcome through eschewing strident dogmatism: "Who am I to judge?" It is not just that, and properly, the sinner will not be judged, but also the sin itself will not be firmly condemned but rather transformed into a life-style choice. The presence of traditional moral commitments will be recognized as in principle still existing, but only softly. When their subject is raised, one will change the subject and in a populist mode address matters of social

justice. As with many of the mainline Christianities, there remains an intimation of the transcendent, which intimation has been transformed into social
concerns and an 'ambiguous theology.'

Once again, where does all of this leave morality and bioethics and their
place in the culture wars? First, one must again note that the culture wars in
the Americas and in Europe have been driven by the opposition of fundamentalist Protestantism, traditionalist Roman Catholicism, Orthodox Christianity,
Mormonism, and Orthodox Judaism to the demoralization and deflation of
traditional morality and bioethics. The culture wars are in the main a function
of the rejection by traditional religious believers of the secular culture's embrace
and affirmation of a "weak" moral and theological understanding of sexuality,
reproduction, and end-of-life decision-making. The revolutionary character
of Pope Francis's papacy lies in his commitment to move gently and "weakly"
to a "weak" theology and bioethics of sexuality, reproduction, and end-of-life
decision-making, a circumstance quite clear to Scalfari in the *La Repubblica*
interview (Scalfari 2013). However, Pope Francis has hopes for a strong theology of social justice. Because of Roman Catholicism's social and economic
resources, this "weak" theological, moral, and bioethical turn, as well as his
remaining strong morality of socio-economic concerns (Pope Francis perhaps
does not acknowledge that this morality, too, is without rational foundations),
will have a major impact on the character of public policy and health care policy
debates in the Americas and in Western Europe. If this theological turn proves
as unsuccessful in maintaining and attracting congregants as did a similar turn
in the mid-20th century by the mainline Christianities in America (Dorrien
2013), then the decline in congregants and the low level of vocations in Roman
Catholicism will continue as clergy and congregants age, and as South America
becomes ever more fundamentalist Protestant[43] and Europe ever more agnostic.
The religious geography of the world will change. Secular morality and bioethics
will become demoralized regarding issues bearing on sexuality, reproduction,
and dying. Roman Catholicism will abet this development.

Yet, it is still possible that the concerns that created traditionalist movements
such as the Society of St. Pius X, founded by Archbishop Marcel Lefebvre (1905–
1991) to preserve the old Tridentine Mass as welll as pre-Vatican II theology, may
eventually lead Roman Catholics to reverse some of the profound changes in

Roman Catholicism since Vatican II so as to re-establish a Roman Catholicism not as distant as it now is from the Church of the first millennium.[44] The challenge to Pope Francis from Tridentine traditionalists, who would restore the philosophical-theological paradigm within which the medical ethics literature of the manualist tradition flourished, is that these traditionalists prevent the pre-Vatican II liturgy and pieties from becoming fully past. They maintain the life of pre-Vatican II Roman Catholicism, and this threatens post-Vatican II Roman Catholics with a return to the past. The old *lex orandi* supports the old *lex credendi* with its view of morality and medical ethics. As a consequence, as long as the pre-Vatican II Mass and its attendant pieties exist among an appreciable number of Roman Catholics, those Roman Catholics exist as a movement at odds with Vatican II and its consequences, so that there is always the possibility of a counter-revolution, a return to what had once been the prevailing norm. Given the still significant demographic size, financial resources, and influence of Roman Catholicism, such a return to traditional Christianity would have a major cultural impact. As unlikely as such an event now seems, it is traditional Christians who generally remain the most faithful churchgoers. It is conservative, traditional Christians who generally have large families (Hayford & Morgan 2008). Only through an appreciation of the great otherness of God and the seriousness of worshipping Him can one be moved to live a committed traditional Christian life with a large family, despite the self-centered social goals set by the current reigning secular culture (Longman 2004a, 2004b, 2006). Deep in their hearts, people generally know that if God exists, worshipping Him will be a serious matter. Perhaps this insight will finally drive a true renewal within Roman Catholicism, and perhaps even a return to the Orthodox Church, along with its bioethics different in spirit and content from post-Trent manualist medical ethics. As we will soon see, Orthodox Christianity represents the roots of traditional Christianity, a Church embedded in quite a different life-world. After all, Christianity is not a Western religion.

An authentic renewal of Roman Catholicism would require a pervasive reconstitution of its lost ascetic and liturgical character. Given the bond between the *lex credendi* and the *lex orandi*, this would demand monumental changes in ascetic and liturgical practices, not just in dogmas, so as to restore ecclesial, liturgical, and spiritual life to what had existed prior to Vatican II, indeed prior to Pope Gregory VII (Hildebrand). To go all the way back to the Church of the first thousand years, to Orthodox Christianity, would require a radical restoration of the ancient forms of piety and spirituality (e.g., fasting), so that through right worship Roman Catholicism could re-enter the mind of the Fathers. This would necessarily involve more than an intellectual acceptance of dogmas. After Vatican II's *aggiornamento* and the robust secularization of the life-world of most Roman Catholics, Roman Catholicism has become so distant from the Church of the Fathers that the gulf will be difficult to bridge. The barriers are deep, subtle, and multi-faceted. One need only consider the liturgical revolution in the rubrics of its Novus Ordo Mass to appreciate how distant Roman Catholicism has already become from the Church of the Apostles and the Fathers. The priest no longer prays *ad orientem, ad deum*, but gazes *ad occidentem, ad populum*, to the congregation. In Christian liturgies from the beginning, the priest led the congregation in looking toward Paradise, to the East.[45] The Roman Catholic priest now looks instead to his fellow mortals, who form a prayer circle in which the congregation directs its gaze to the priest looking back at them. In looking towards the congregation, the priest fashions and affirms a circle of immanent fellowship and meaning. Humans look to humans. Rituals disclose much more than words can ever say (Engelhardt 2012). A substantive change, a rupture from traditional Christianity, has taken place. A fundamental ritual immanentization of the community's life-world has occurred, shaped by a turn from the transcendent to the immanent. Any turn back to the infinite is now hindered, in that the rubrics of the Paul VI mass direct the gaze of the participants immanently, humans to humans, so that all remains within the horizon of the finite.

Within this circle, one can speak of social justice and human rights, as well as of a "weak morality and bioethics" set within a political and economic vision born of Argentine economics and politics. But this circle is not a place for all-night vigils, fasting, and personal almsgiving in one mind with the Fathers. In the liturgical prayer circle formed by post-Vatican II Roman Catholicism, one is not laboring to enter into the mind of the Fathers, but into a mind, a consciousness informed by Roman Catholicism's recent synthesis that followed its *aggiornamento*. The priest looking toward the congregation avoids encountering the politically incorrect truth that the Christian priest is the icon of the Second Adam, which icon of the Second Adam excludes *inter alia* the possibility of

Christian priestesses. The liturgy is not recognized as structured around Adam (i.e., the second Adam, Christ) finally on behalf of Eve offering everything back to God. Closed within this finite circle of the *versus ad populum*, the turn to the people, one can try to weave a narrative to sustain an immanent fellowship without the gender essentialism involved in the relation of Adam and Eve, the redemption of Adam and Eve's proper roles in the unfolding of salvation. Ritual shapes belief. Rite forms that which is recognized as right (Solomon et al. 2012).

This immanent gaze also ratifies the abandonment of the old paradigm of manualist medical ethics in favor of the bioethics that emerged in the 1970s, which is now being placed within the soft uncertainty of a post-modern vision. The liturgy of Paul VI, given its immanentization of focus, invites and supports the weak theological and bioethical paradigm that Pope Francis embraces. Before Pope Francis, Roman Catholicism was already a world away from pre-Vatican II Roman Catholicism and a universe away from the Church of the first millennium. Charles the Great, Pope Gregory VII (Hildebrand), the Fourth Lateran Council, Thomas Aquinas, and the Council of Trent had fashioned a radically new paradigm and life-world even before the impact of modernism and then Vatican II. *Aggiornamento* played a further and powerful transforming role through which post-Enlightenment early-modern commitments entered into Roman Catholicism. These post-traditional Christians born of Vatican II will not experience what it is like to turn to the East led by the priest, looking to a window behind the altar as the sun rises, just as the priest intones a cardinal battle cry in the culture wars that separates traditional Christianity from the dominant secular culture, including its post-traditional Christianities: "Blessed is the Kingdom of the Father, and of the Son, and of the Holy Spirit, now and ever, and unto ages of ages. Amen" (*Liturgikon* 1994, p. 258).

VIII. Encountering God: The Turn Towards Ultimate Meaning

What then can one make of Christianity at the beginning of the 21st century? What can one make of its current appreciation of morality and bioethics? Will Pope Francis lead Western Christianity to a widespread demoralization of its morality and its bioethics? What place can traditional Christianity have in

contemporary society, given traditional Christianity's politically incorrect gender essentialism and its prohibition of sexual acts outside of the marriage of a man
and a woman, not to mention abortion, the artificial insemination of unmarried
women, experimentation on human embryos, physician-assisted suicide, and
euthanasia? How should one acknowledge God in a culture that is attempting to
banish all reference to the transcendent? How will traditional Christianity and
traditional Christian bioethics be understood as much of Christianity embraces
weak theology or ambiguous theology? All such questions and more are nested
within a range of scandals that render Christianity implausible.

Turned in on itself, Protestantism is fragmented into a plurality of human
accounts of the meaning of Christianity, into thousands of sects, each of which
believes different things over space and time, across locations and over history.
Their views of bioethics are plural; their doctrines are legion. The Roman Catholics for their part have changed their dogmas over time, developing substantively
new understandings of theology and of church, along with new dogmas such as
papal universal jurisdiction, papal infallibility, and the immaculate conception.
Now after the liturgical and theological rupture created by Vatican II, Roman
Catholicism appears to be on the brink of further changes, this time a post-modern, weak theological transformation embedded in a political and economic
vision born of the South's failures of governance and economics. Beyond all
of this, the never-ending cacophony of new revelations of sexual abuse, many
involving pederasty, generally make serious reflection and discernment difficult
(Engel 2006). The scandals reported by the recent volume, *Sex and the Vatican*,
may have even motivated the resignation of Benedict XVI (Abbate 2011; Badash
2011; Benedict XVI 2013; Nadeau 2013).

Through its very size, Roman Catholicism dominates news about Christianity. The difficulties, indeed chaos, troubling Roman Catholicism influence how
many regard Christianity. The problems stem in part from Roman Catholicism's
doctrinal disorientation, much of which places Roman Catholicism at odds with
traditional Christianity. It is no longer clear how Roman Catholicism regards the
truth of Roman Catholicism, indeed of Christianity. Consider one conservative
Roman Catholic's indictment of Pope John Paul II's behavior that proved a major
scandal to traditional Christians.

In the remaining years of his pontificate Wojtyla did nothing to convince alarmed Catholics that he was any closer to recognizing the obvious relationship between the programme of heteropraxis over which he willingly presided and its disastrous effects on the life of the Church, a catastrophe which he paradoxically acknowledged and deplored. On the contrary, there is abundant evidence that the force which blinded his intellect was the actor's ego that propelled him into so much undignified and compromising public behavior, a problem aggravated by a somewhat worldly predilection for frequent travel and tours. . . . What was by far the most scandalous of John Paul II's "philanthropic" gestures occurred on 1 June 1999. At the end of an audience at the Vatican with an Iraqi delegation, he bowed to a copy of the Koran presented to him by an imam, and kissed it. This "sign of respect" would have been regarded by orthodox Christians of any other age as an act of apostasy, since Islam's holy book explicitly denies the divinity of Christ. . . . The thousands of early Christian martyrs who preferred gruesome deaths to offering a few grains of incense before images of deified Roman emperors evidently had a vastly different "faith vision" (Hull 2010, p. 325).

Similar behavior, repeated on many occasions, as for example with the incorporation of pagan rituals into Masses over which John Paul II presided (Hull 2010, p. 324), underscored the rupture of post-Vatican II Roman Catholicism from what had existed beforehand. John Paul II was taking implicit but nevertheless forceful steps towards a "weak" or "ambiguous" theology. It would be Pope Francis who would begin, *expressis verbis*, to articulate a weak theology along with its bioethics, thus beginning a further and widely significant recasting of the world's largest Christian denomination.

Does the collapse of much of traditional Christianity in the West, as well as its seeming intractable plurality, serve as a *modus tolens* for Christianity? Does the moral and theological chaos in Christianity bring Christianity radically into question? The chaos of Western Christianity stands in stark contrast with Orthodoxy. As Cardinal Ratzinger, later Pope Benedict XVI and now Pope Emeritus, remarked,

> If today the entire liturgy has become the playground of private "creativity,"
> which can romp at will just as long as the words of consecration are kept in

place, at work is the same reduction of vision whose origin lies in an erroneous development typical of the West but quite unthinkable in the Eastern
Church. . . . Both in doctrine and in liturgy, what really matters is lost when
one feels obliged to distill a juristical minimum, beyond which everything
is left subject to arbitrariness. Here too we would do well to learn to look
once more beyond the fence of Western thinking and to make the attempt
to understand anew the original vision which has remained largely intact in
the East (Ratzinger 1995, p. 112).

In contrast with Western Christianity, the Orthodox Church shows the remarkable, if indeed not miraculous, character of being one over space and time—all
without a pope of Rome or a Roman curia. It is a historical wonder. But is this
state of affairs *sensu stricto* a miracle? Can Orthodox Christianity in fact promise a God's-eye perspective able to avoid the demoralization and deflation of its
morality and bioethics? Could God in fact have broken into history in Palestine?
Could the Messiah to Whom so many have turned in hope have been born
two thousand years ago in a village in the Levant? Could He have established
a Church that remains in its fullness, unbroken und unbranched, even today?
Could all of existence in the end *not* be meaningless, but instead grounded in
an infinite, transcendent, personal God? If this is the case, what sort of theology
would that Church need to possess in order not to fracture into the intractable
pluralism of Protestantism, or be beset by the development of new doctrines, as
with Roman Catholicism? It would need to have a theology that could unite the
Church over time and space in an unbroken experience of God. In anticipation
of what will now follow, its theology in the strict sense could not be grounded
in a philosophical theology.

Orthodox Christian theology is in its strict sense not a philosophical undertaking. It is not grounded in philosophical reflection on experience, on revelation, on the Bible, and/or on the notion of God. Instead, theology in the strict
sense is grounded in an empirical, albeit not sensible empirical, experience of
God. Of course, it also involves a sensible empirical encounter with God when,
for example, icons weep. Orthodox Christianity claims that its theologians in
the strict sense know God, that they do not simply know about Him (Engelhardt
2008). Quite against the expectations of the contemporary culture, theology

requires as a necessary condition praying well,[46] not necessarily an academic preparation. As a consequence, the majority of the great Orthodox Christian theologians of the 20th century never completed college.[47] Instead, they turned from self-love to an all-consuming love of God and, in the light of that love, to a love of one's neighbor as oneself. They by violence conquered their passions so that they might enter into the Kingdom of Heaven (Mt 11:12). If one wishes to test the truth of what they say they know, one must conduct this same experiment and live as they lived. One must oneself become a theologian as they have become theologians.

Of course, that asks for a lot, and usually more than what most self-loving persons (including myself) are willing to give. Indeed, it asks for everything. Still, even if one has not paid that price, even if one has not given up one's terrible self-love, one can be granted, if God wills, the gift of seeing and encountering the power of true theology. In the spring of 2002, after just returning from lecturing in Australia, and after the birth of my second granddaughter (my fourth grandchild), I found a message from a priest I knew: he had been called by the owner of an icon shop in Houston, Texas, when an icon in his inventory had begun to weep oil. The priest had gone to the shop and chanted the *paraklesis*, and the icon wept oil. With the blessing of the bishop, the priest asked to buy the icon at once and to bring it to the safety of an Orthodox church. The icon shop's owner agreed, but only if he could keep it in his shop for at least two weeks. With a reckless and even presumptuous boldness (that I hope, God forgive me, was not too sinful), I went to my four research assistants and asked them, "Do you want to watch a miracle occur like throwing a light switch? Do you want to kick David Hume and Immanuel Kant where it hurts?" Three of the four begged off with various excuses. At some level, these three sensed that if they came, their lives would forever be changed. Only one said she would come. It was as I thought—there was a purity about her. I then called a priest I knew visiting from out of state, a convert from Judaism and also a Cohen, an ascetic but married priest who prayed earnestly. He said he would come.

The priest, my wife, the graduate student, and I entered the icon shop. The priest walked up to the icon and proceeded to chant the paraklesis. Oil came out of the icon. When he had finished, he took the oil with his finger and anointed the graduate student, saying, "You have now seen the power of God." (She later converted to the Orthodox Church.) The shop owner was shaken (as were my wife, the graduate student, and I). The shop owner gave the priest an old and expensive icon of the priest's patron saint. Then we walked out. We had seen the fruit of true theology. After numerous such miracles, it no longer makes sense for me to say that I believe in God. I *know* that God exists. I have seen His power. I have experienced His presence. He is a Given, before any concept. Orthodox Christianity "has no concept of God. It views God not as an essence to be grasped intellectually, but as a personal reality known through His acts, and above all by oneself sharing in those acts" (Bradshaw 2004, p. 275). However, it does make sense to say that I have faith in Him, in the sense that I trust Him. As is sung after Communion, "We have beheld the true light; we have received the heavenly Spirit; we have found the true faith" (Hapgood 1996, p. 120). After such events, one's relationship to God, indeed to the Church is no longer simply intellectual or even volitional. Something has happened, Someone has broken through all usual expectations. The transcendent personal God has entered into time and space. One is beyond morality in the sense that for Orthodox Christianity "morality is not primarily a matter of conformance to law, nor (in a more Aristotelian vein) of achieving human excellence by acquiring the virtues. It is a matter of coming to know God by sharing in His acts and manifesting His image" (Bradshaw 2004, pp. 175–176).

All of this establishes a context that frames a bioethics not only different from the demoralized and deflated bioethics that has emerged in the West, but different as well from the medical ethics of the manualist tradition of Roman Catholicism. Orthodox Christian morality and bioethics understand the right, the good, and the virtuous in terms of the holy. Morality and bioethics are about approaching God, not about natural law apart from God or about canons of morality and bioethics disclosable and justifiable through a secular moral-philosophical rationality (as if such had ever been possible). Instead, the Orthodox Christian bioethical focus remains within an unbroken theological experience of proper action, which recognizes that sexual activity and reproduction are permitted only within the marriage of a man and a woman, that the use of donor gametes is prohibited in having a child, that the killing of zygotes, embryos, or fetuses is forbidden, and that a family- and salvation-oriented understanding of consent to treatment is endorsed (i.e., strict truth-telling is not always obligatory). There is as well an openness to germline genetic engineering, as long as this does not set aside the differences between men and women, or the marks of being human (Delkeskamp-Hayes 2012). There is also a robust understanding of the obligations of charity, which include providing health care to those in need. There is in addition a clear recognition of the prohibition of the use of medical treatment when it distracts from the pursuit of salvation, along with a prohibition of the killing of patients (e.g., infanticide, passive euthanasia, active euthanasia, and physician-assisted suicide). Orthodox Christian bioethics thus has some family resemblances to the traditional Christian bioethics of Western Christianity. However, the bioethics of the Christianity of the first millennium is set within a non-sensible empirical or noetic theology that remarkably spans diverse cultures. There are a number of important particular differences with Roman Catholicism (e.g., indirect abortion still counts as killing an innocent unborn child), but the most important difference is global. The framing theological context or paradigm is different.

This volume does not explore Orthodox Christian bioethics in any detail, in that this has already been done elsewhere (Engelhardt 2000). Here it is enough to indicate that Orthodox Christian bioethics is not grounded in a particular view of moral rationality. For example, the prohibition of zygote and embryo destruction will not depend on a doctrine of ensoulment, truth-telling to patients will not be required out of an absolute prohibition against lying or from an absolute respect required by forbearance rights, and there will not be the affirmation of a social-democratic redistribution of resources towards the realization of social justice in health care allocation. Instead, the focus is on what is a barrier to approaching God. Most significantly, because the holy locates the right, the good, and the virtuous, the bioethics affirmed will be spiritual and therapeutic rather than moralistic and legalistic. What is important for this volume is whether the context for this bioethics involves a God's-eye perspective that can in principle avoid the intractable pluralism, demoralization, and deflation that has transformed secular bioethics and the moral theology of Western Christianity.

IX. *Theology Reconsidered:*
Orthodox Christianity as the Enduring Faith

The theology and bioethics of the Orthodox Church are radically different from those of the West, which were shaped by the cathedral schools, especially those of Chartres and Notre Dame in the 12th century, as well as the University of Paris, founded in 1208, all of which led to a radical recasting of Christian thought under the influence of Aristotle. This dramatic change was associated *inter alia* with the introduction by Dominicus Gundissalinus (1110–1190) of a view of metaphysics shaped by Avicenna (Fidora 2013). As already indicated, the translation of Aristotle's works into Latin (A.D. 1210) marked a watershed in Western Christian theology and in Western culture generally. The result is that for the West the office of the theologian in the strict sense became that of a philosophically trained scholar in the academy, reflecting on and analyzing texts and ideas. For the West, theology in the strict sense became an academic undertaking. For Orthodox Christianity, theology in the strict sense remains located in the unbroken noetic experience of God, which unites all true theologians over time and over space. It is the unity of the Church in one mind with the Fathers and the Apostles, one in Christ in the Holy Spirit. Orthodox Christianity also has theologians in the secondary sense of theologian, who function something like theological science writers reporting on what real theological scientists experience and know (i.e., on what those who have noetic experience know). Theologians in the secondary sense are usually academics such as myself. But the truth of even this secondary theology is at its core not a set of propositions, but the Persons of the Trinity. For Orthodox Christianity, theology and the bioethics it supports are not philosophical. In the Church as the Body of Christ in the Holy Spirit, theology is and lives—it does not develop new doctrines. The veridical theological experience unites all right-believing and right-worshipping Christians over space and time.

The non-Orthodox are not here invited to concede the truth of Orthodoxy's claims, but only to examine whether, if the claims were true, they would show a way beyond our intractable moral and bioethical pluralism, as well as beyond the demoralization and deflation of morality and bioethics. The claim is not just that one can envisage a God's-eye perspective as Kant did for morality, but that one can experience the existence of that God's-eye perspective with a compelling force of truth distantly like what occurs in first-person reports such as "I see blue." The claim is that humans have a *nous*, a capacity non-empirically to see reality, and that this is realized by theologians in the strict sense. This is not to deny that such knowledge does not require techniques for its successful development such as attention to whether the results remain the same over time, indeed through history, as well as whether one is being distracted by self-love and pride (which opens the way to diabolic deception, regarding which there will also be techniques to test its presence). There will also be techniques to engage so as to focus and refine one's noetic experience. What is at stake are three claims. The first claim is that there is a God's-eye view. The second claim is that this perspective can be experienced. The third claim is that if one knows experientially that there is a God's-eye perspective, as well as what this perspective requires, then one can avoid bioethical and moral pluralism as well as the demoralization of morality and bioethics. This approach to theology has led to an Orthodox Christian theology that contrasts on a number of key points with that of the Western Christianities. Roman Catholicism, given its greater doctrinal coherence, will be used as the exemplar Western Christianity to display the difference from traditional Christianity.

Orthodox Christianity is distinguished from Western Christianity in not having accepted the novel dogmas that developed in the West, most of which (save for the *filioque*) Protestants rejected in their protest against Roman Catholicism. These include (1) the Western teaching that the Father is not the origin of all. As indicated in chapter four, Orthodoxy rejects the *filioque*, the Western teaching affirmed at the Second Council of Lyon (A.D. 1274) that the Holy Spirit proceeds eternally from the Father *and* the Son, rather than *just* from the unique person of the Father alone, as taught in John 15:26 as well as at Constantinople I in A.D. 381. This difference changes how one orients in prayer to God and how one is open to experiencing the Father. As a logical point, the views of God in the two cases are conceptually in profound contrast. The West has a different concept of God. They indeed have a concept of God, just not an experience of Him.

The second major difference bears on ecclesiology, (2) the rejection of what became the Roman Catholic claims of papal universal original jurisdiction. One bishop indeed has been recognized as having primacy as the successor of Peter, although the office of primacy is like the Speaker of the House (i.e., speaker of the synod of all bishops), all along remaining the bishop of one diocese and having only one vote.[48] Moreover, the place of this bishop's see is not necessarily tied to any particular city (e.g., Rome), as is clear from Canon 28 of Chalcedon (A.D. 451).

> Following in all things the decisions of the holy Fathers, and acknowledging the canon, which has been just read, of the One Hundred and Fifty Bishops beloved-of-God (who assembled in the imperial city of Constantinople, which is New Rome, in the time of the Emperor Theodosius of happy memory [Constantinople I, A.D. 381]), we also do enact and decree the same things concerning the privileges of the most holy Church of Constantinople, which is New Rome. For the Fathers rightly granted privileges to the throne of old Rome, because it was the royal city. And the One Hundred and Fifty most religious Bishops, actuated by the same consideration, gave equal privileges to the most holy throne of New Rome, justly judging that the city which is honoured with the Sovereignty and the Senate, and enjoys equal privileges with the old imperial Rome, should in ecclesiastical matters also be magnified as she is, and rank next after her; so that, in the Pontic, the Asian, and the Thracian dioceses, the metropolitans only and such bishops also of the Dioceses aforesaid as are among the barbarians, should be ordained by the aforesaid most holy throne of the most holy Church of Constantinople; every metropolitan of the aforesaid dioceses, together with the bishops of his province, ordaining his own provincial bishops, as has been declared by the divine canons; but that, as has been above said, the metropolitans of the aforesaid Dioceses should be ordained by the archbishop of Constantinople, after the proper elections have been held according to custom and have been reported to him (Schaff & Wace 1994, vol. 14, p. 287).

The Church could in the future acknowledge the leading city of the world as the capital of Texas (perhaps Santa Fe, once the original boundaries of Texas are restored), as the fourth Rome after old Rome, Constantinople, and Moscow.[49] The Orthodox Church rejects the Roman Catholic ecclesiological and epistemological doctrine of (3) papal infallibility out of hand as having no root in the

Church of the Apostles and the Fathers. The legates from the pope of Rome, for example, were examined for their Orthodoxy at the Council of Chalcedon.

(4) Claims are also rejected regarding purgatory where, according to Roman Catholics, one is punished in order to make up for supposed temporal punishment due to sin. At stake is the Roman distinction between the forgiveness of guilt and a remaining penalty due to sin, which distinction led to the conclusion that absolution in confession relieves the guilt of sin but not the penalties due to sin, the temporal punishment due to sin.[50] However, the gift of the forgiveness of sins given by Christ to the Apostles is unqualified. When Christ forgives sin, there is no sense that the person forgiven may still owe punishment in purgatory due to the penalties owed for sin, even though the sins have been absolved. Quite to the contrary, the priest in giving absolution absolves absolutely:

> My spiritual child, who hast confessed to my humble self, I, humble and a sinner, have not power on earth to forgive sins, but God alone; yet through that divinely spoken word which came to the Apostles after the Resurrection of our Lord Jesus Christ, saying: Whosoever sins ye remit, they are remitted, and whosoever sins ye retain, they are retained, we too are emboldened to say: Whatsoever thou hast said to my most humble self, and whatsoever thou hast not succeeded in saying, either through ignorance, or through forgetfulness, whatever it may be: God forgive thee in this present world, and in that which is to come.
>
> God it was Who forgave David through Nathan the Prophet, when he confessed his sins, and Peter weeping bitterly for his denial, and the sinful woman in tears at His feet, and the Publican, and the Prodigal Son: May that same God forgive thee all things, through me a sinner, both in this present world, and in that which is to come, and set thee uncondemned before His dread Judgment Seat. And now, having no further care for the sins which thou hast declared, depart in peace (Pocket Prayer Book 1956, pp. 44–45).

The forgiveness of sin given is whole and complete.

(5) Because there is no recognition of purgatory (a place for the purging of the temporal punishment due to sin), there is no recognition of indulgences. Also, due to the absence of a treasury of excess merits of the saints,[51] only Christ merits our redemption, and even then not in terms of an understanding under

which His excess merits would be stored in a spiritual treasury to be given out by the pope. Even today, Roman Catholicism emphasizes the role of indulgences, as for example when during Pope Francis's visit to Brazil, July 23–29, 2013, he declared that those who could not physically attend World Youth Day would receive a plenary indulgence by participating in the week's devotions "via the new means of social communication," including the pope's Twitter feed (Kidd 2013, p. 64).[52] The differences lie also in the quite disparate views of the significance of suffering that took shape in Western Christianity. As a consequence, the Orthodox Christian appreciation of suffering and its understanding of the propriety of medical interventions in many ways contrast with those of Western Christianity. Before the Reformation, Western Christianity came to place suffering within an economy of sin, propitiatory punishment, and salvation, in which suffering plays a central role in paying off a penalty, namely, temporal punishment due to sin. One's personal suffering, the suffering offered up on one's behalf, or an indulgence can free one from purgatory as a temporal punishment due to sin. This view of suffering, when combined with the view that the penance a priest imposes in confession serves as a punishment merited by the temporal punishment due to sin, created a background spiritual currency in which the penalties due to sin can be set aside by current tribulation, pain, and suffering. None of this exists in Orthodox Christianity. Again, the Orthodox priest at the end of confession absolves the penitent of the sins confessed so as to make pain and suffering to avoid purgatory beside the point. Any penance imposed serves a therapeutic goal focused on the particular needs of the penitent. So, too, with suffering generally: it offers an opportunity for repentance and humble submission to the will of God.

(6) The Roman Catholic prohibition of remarriage before the death of the spouse and after divorce when the first marriage has been broken by adultery (more broadly *pornoi*, see Mt 19:9) is not recognized. The Orthodox know that sacramental marriage is not a contract, but is conveyed by the Church through the priest to the couple. Christian marriage restores the icon of the unique union of husband and wife. Abraham and other patriarchs, as well as kings, had not just multiple wives, which was allowed to all before Christ, but also lawful concubines (see, for example, Gen 25:6).[53] But now even a second and surely a third spouse after the death of the first spouse are generally discouraged (and

forbidden to a priest and his wife). What is so shocking for those around Jesus is not just His setting aside the usual easy grounds for divorce, but that His changing the rules for divorce announced that He is the Messiah. There had been a dispute regarding the grounds for divorce. Hillel had accepted as *pornoi* anything that displeased a husband (e.g., his wife's bringing the students of the rabbi to laugh at their teacher), while Shammai had accepted only the strong ground approved by Jesus. When the question was asked as to whom they should follow, the answer was generally to follow Hillel until the Messiah came, whom Jesus announced Himself as being.

(7) The immaculate conception is rejected, because if the Theotokos were born without the consequences of original sin, then no one could be saved, because Christ would not have taken on our sinful flesh and redeemed it. Moreover, it is because Christ did take on our sinful flesh that the Letter to the Hebrews states: "For we do not have a high priest who is unable to sympathize with our weaknesses, but we have one who has been tempted in every way, just as we are—yet was without sin" (Heb 4:15). Adam before the Fall was not tempted as we are. Both the Theotokos and the Body of Christ before the Resurrection were touched by the consequences of "original sin."[54] The great triumph of the Theotokos is that, despite her sharing with all men the fallen flesh of Adam, she submitted to the will of God. Within the second millennium, Western Christendom had embraced radically new dogmas, separating itself not just through schism, but through heresy from the Church of the Apostles and the Fathers.

This short list of *some* of the important doctrinal differences separating the Christian community that emerged in the West from the original Christianity[55] does not include a very important and indeed cardinal difference, one not maintained by Protestantism: Orthodox Christianity understands the Church as the Body of Christ in the Holy Spirit, so that the Church is united in history (i.e., apostolic succession) and belief with the Church of the Apostles and the Fathers. Those without apostolic succession, who are separated by heresy (e.g., the Roman Catholics) are not within the Church. St. Basil draws the following important distinction between heretics, schismatics, and unlawful congregations.

> By *heresies* they meant men who were altogether broken off and alienated in matters relating to the actual faith; by *schisms* men who had separated

for some ecclesiastical reasons and questions capable of mutual solution; by *unlawful congregations* gatherings held by disorderly presbyters or bishops or by uninstructed laymen. . . . So it seemed good to the ancient authorities to reject the baptism of heretics altogether (Basil 1994, Letter CLXXXVIII. I, vol. 8, pp. 223–224).

Protestantism could not maintain the sense of the church as an actual community of believers that is one and apostolic in its origins and over time, possessing theological continuity with the Church of the Apostles and the Fathers. In addition, because the Protestants were protesting against what appeared factually in the West to be the exemplar of church, namely, Roman Catholicism, the meaning of church had to be revised. The ecclesial body of Roman Catholicism they knew to have created doctrinal novelties such as purgatory, as well as disciplinary novelties such as compulsory clerical celibacy. Their reaction against Roman Catholicism encouraged a new *lex orandi*, which grounded a new *lex credendi*. In order plausibly to attempt to start Christianity anew in the 16th century, one was forced to abandon the recognition of the church as one and apostolic, as a real ecclesial body that was the Body of Christ in the Holy Spirit (Eph 1:23). As Protestantism fragmented into a plurality of denominations in bitter disagreement, Protestantism had to abandon the claim to being catholic.

The Orthodox Church lives across history in the same dogmas, that is, without any development of new dogmas (e.g., the immaculate conception). The Orthodox Church invites all into the mind of the Apostles and the Fathers so as to live at one with Christ. The preservation of the traditional fasts (e.g., the fast on Wednesdays and Fridays, known since the time of the Fathers[56]) aids the control over our self-love and also allows one to be united in common ascetical struggle over time with the Apostles. The result is that Orthodox Christians experience reality, morality, and bioethics in categories that have not been available for Western Christians for 1200 years. There is, for example, the appreciation of involuntary sins, that to be causally involved in the death of another human (e.g., as with a spontaneous abortion[57]), even without any intention or negligence, often harms the heart so as to require ascetical support by the Church (e.g., before communion one asks for the forgiveness of sins, both voluntary and involuntary[58]). Among the other differences, there is no recognition of the doctrine of double effect, as in Roman Catholicism, that would allow one to consider "indirect" therapeutic abortions to be without moral harm (Engelhardt 2000, pp. 277–280). Double effect, however, is implicitly invoked by Roman Catholics in other circumstances. The result is that sin is approached more medicinally and less juridically, with the focus on using fasting, almsgiving, and vigils not as a punishment, but as a treatment for the consequences of sin.

The view of sexuality is also other than what became salient in parts of Western Christianity. The Church is rich with holy monks, as well as with priests who are usually married. As mentioned in chapter four, it is a Church that affirms marital sexuality. It emphasizes the chastity of the marriage act. The Church of the Apostles and the Fathers affirms that the marriage bed is undefiled as in Canon LI of the 85 Apostolic Canons.

> If any Bishop, or Presbyter, or Deacon, or anyone at all on the sacerdotal list, abstains from marriage, or meat, or wine, not as a matter of mortification, but out of an abhorrence thereof, forgetting that all things are exceedingly good, and that God made man male and female, and blasphemously misrepresenting God's work of creation, either let him mend his ways or let him be deposed from office and expelled from the Church. Let a layman be treated similarly (Sts. Nicodemus and Agapius 1994, p. 91).

Indeed, in describing the marriage act, St. John Chrysostom affirms the goodness of the orgasm of the wife. As he states,

> And how become they one flesh? As if thou shouldest take away the purest part of gold, and mingle it with other gold; so in truth here also the woman as it were receiving the richest part fused by pleasure, nourisheth it and cherisheth it, and withal contributing her own share, restoreth it back a Man. And the child is a sort of bridge, so that the three become one flesh, the child connecting, on either side, each to other (Chrysostom 1994, vol. 13, p. 319).

Man is to be redeemed in flesh and spirit, body and soul. When married, the wife and the children under the husband and father constitute the family as a domestic church. All is to be transformed by the uncreated energies of God. All is to be rendered holy.

How, then, is one to locate Orthodox Christianity along with its morality and bioethics in terms of the history of Christianity? The Orthodox share with Western Christianity the first seven ecumenical councils. However, Orthodoxy recognizes a different eighth council, namely, the Council in the Temple of Holy Wisdom held in Constantinople 879–880, which was attended by legates of Pope John VIII. This Council during the reign of Emperor Basil I (reigned 867–886) affirmed the actions of St. Photios the Great (c. 820–891), who excommunicated Pope Nicholas I (c. 800–867) for having inter alia accepted the filioque, the Western dogma that the Holy Spirit proceeds in His existence not just from the Father but also from the Son. The West instead accepts a council held in Constantinople in 869–870, which Orthodoxy rejects as a Robber Council. The last ecumenical council assembled in Constantinople in 1341, 1344, and 1347 under Emperor John V Palaiologos (reigned 1341–1376). This Ninth Ecumenical Council articulated the position of Orthodoxy inter alia over against a Scholasticism that would render theology into a philosophical academic endeavor. The Council supported St. Gregory Palamas (1296–1356), who defended the Christian epistemology of the first millennium from a recasting in the image and likeness of a philosophically grounded theology. It reaffirmed the recognition that theologians are those with hesychia[59] who have through asceticism overcome their self-love so as to love God with their whole heart, soul, and mind, so as to be able to love their neighbor in the light of this love (Mt 22:37–40) and be allowed to experience God. Real theologians know God. They do not merely know about God.

The cardinal importance of this last ecumenical council is that it resisted the rational horn of Plato's Euthyphro. It rejected the view that the good, the right, and the virtuous can rightly be known without the holy, without an experience of God. It affirmed instead that that which is good, right, and/or virtuous is good, right, and/or virtuous because it leads to holiness, to God. Theology in the strict sense, in the primary sense, is not discursive reflection on God but an actual relationship with Him and an actual experience of Him. This theology is not about abstract principles, but about persons, about our relationship with the Persons of the Trinity. That is, this theology is not primarily reflection about God, but about knowing and being united to God. The theologies of Orthodoxy and the West thus involve fundamentally different understandings of the nature and of the sociology of theology (i.e., as to who is a theologian in the strict sense), which has very important implications for what one will recognize as the foundation of a Christian bioethics. In the West, one came to expect that theologians in the strict sense would be found in the Academy, so that theology became an academic profession, one of the four faculties of the university. Such theologians shaped the magisterium of Western Christianity. In stark contrast, in the Church of the first millennium one expects to find most real theologians among ascetics. This would not necessarily rule out academicians being theologians, for academicians can live ascetic lives and know God. However, all things being equal, one would expect that the majority of theologians in the strict sense would be found in holy monasteries among those who with violence against their passions turned to wholehearted love of God. Holding honorary doctorates is not necessarily an impediment to being a theologian in the strict sense, but it is not a support towards being a theologian in the strict sense and indeed might through inciting pride constitute a stumbling block. As John Romanides has put it: "The Fathers do not say anything about God on the basis of philosophical reflection. They do not sit at their desks like the Scholastics in order to do theology, because when the Church Fathers theologize, speculation or reflection is strictly forbidden" (Romanides 2008, p. 85).

Among other things, this means that the morality and bioethics of the Orthodox Church are not grounded in the moral-philosophical project that has shipwrecked with the collapse of philosophical foundations. It is grounded instead in an encounter and experience of God. Its discursive dimension will be an analysis of the content delivered and maintained by the experience of its theologians who are theologians in the strict sense (Engelhardt 2011). As a consequence, this morality and bioethics will increasingly contrast with the morality and bioethics of the dominant secular culture, as well as with the "rationalized" Christian morality and bioethics of the Western Christianities (Engelhardt 2000). Orthodox Christian bioethics is integral to a way of life.

Theology in the strict sense is always nested in prayer, most particularly in the prayer of the Church assembled in Liturgy. The Liturgy compasses all true theologians in the strict sense. Because of this, as Archimandrite Vasileios of Stavronikita Monastery on Mount Athos stated, "The Gospel cannot be understood outside the Church nor dogma outside worship" (Vasileios 1984, p. 18).

It is for this reason that biblical scholarship is of such marginal significance in the Orthodox Church, for "outside the Church the Gospel is a sealed and incomprehensible book" (Vasileios 1984, p. 18). Those outside the Church will approach the Bible in a fashion not at one with the mind of the Apostles and the Fathers, generating various and diverse interpretations as within Protestantism. The result will be a legion of Christian bioethics. The Liturgy provides the privileged epistemic standpoint that unites. Because the Liturgy unites all who are truly theologians, the Liturgy provides the place for appreciating the Bible. After all, the Bible is the record of revelation, and the Church, which is the Body of Christ, is revelation. Consider, for example, Archbishop Hilarion's [Alfeyev] remarks, who on October 22, 2008, at the University of Toronto stated:

> For an Orthodox theologian, liturgical texts are not simply the works of outstanding theologians and poets, but also the fruits of the prayerful experience of those who have attained sanctity and *theosis*. The theological authority of liturgical texts is, in my opinion, higher than that of the works of the Fathers of the Church, for not everything in the works of the latter is of equal theological value and not everything has been accepted by the fullness of the Church. Liturgical texts, on the contrary, have been accepted by the whole Church as a 'rule of faith' (*kanon pisteos*), for they have been read and sung everywhere in Orthodox churches over many centuries. . . .
>
> The *lex credendi* grows out of the *lex orandi*, and dogmas are considered divinely revealed because they are born in the life of prayer and revealed to the Church through its divine services. Thus, if there are divergences in the understanding of a dogma between a certain theological authority and liturgical texts, I would be inclined to give preference to the latter. And if a textbook of dogmatic theology contains views different from those found in liturgical texts, it is the textbook, not the liturgical texts, that need correction (Hilarion 2008).

A very similar point is also made by Archimandrite Vasileios:

> among the creedal and dogmatic monuments of the Orthodox Catholic Church [are] . . . the liturgies of St. John Chrysostom and St. Basil the Great, complete with their *typikon* or liturgical rubrics and the actual manner of

their celebration. For it is not only prayers with dogmatic content but the whole liturgical action and life of the Church that constitutes a unique theological witness and grace (Vasileios 1984, p. 19).

With the recognition of the importance of the Liturgy comes the appreciation of Tradition, including the accretion of traditions that serve as insights about how to live the faith in a hostile, post-Christian, secular world. The Liturgy involves an understanding not anchored in a faith in philosophical rationality, but in the presence of God. As a consequence, Orthodox Christianity, which did not embrace the Enlightenment, is rooted in the transcendent.

Western Christianity and its bioethics have largely disengaged from this traditional life-world and the theology of the Fathers. In particular, Roman Catholicism's life-world is a novum. The *lex orandi* has radically changed, leading to fundamental changes in its *lex credendi*. Fish-on-Friday-eating Christians of the West are no more (or at least very few). Western Christians live in a post-ascetic life-world, which contrasts with that of Orthodox Christians, and which is different from that of the Church of the first millennium. The theological substance, character, and "style" of the Church of the first millennium is incompatible with that which emerged in the early second millennium in the West. The latter first produced the medical ethics of the manualist tradition, then the bioethics that took shape in the West at the end of the second millennium, and it is now supporting the emergence of a weak bioethics.

Following the Reformation and the Enlightenment, worship and belief were transformed in the mainstream culture of the West, eventually producing a low-church Kantian moral domain and a high-church Hegelian cultural domain. The first, as with reformed Judaism and secularized low-church Protestantism, emphasizes the moral life, while generally minimizing ritual, even ritual without metaphysical force. The second, with the high-church Hegelians, supports ritual as integral to culture, but without metaphysical force.[60] All this led to a secular culture vastly different from the Church of the first millennium, as well as different even from the Western Christianities prior to the Enlightenment and prior to the subsequent death of God in Western culture. Although, at its inception, the bioethics of the 1970s still had an early medieval and Enlightenment faith in reason, this is now being lost. Such a faith is now being recognized as clearly unfounded, leading to the demoralization and deflation of bioethics. The Roman Catholicism that had generated a manualist medical ethics and the transformed, post-Vatican II Roman Catholicism that then replaced it with the bioethics of the 1970s is now on its way to a further transformation and a bioethics framed by a weak theology congenial in important ways with a bioethics after God. The result is a secular culture *cum* morality and bioethics at odds with that of traditional Christianity. The bioethics battles in the culture wars will be ever more complex.

X. A Conflict of Life-Worlds: Morality, Bioethics, and the Culture Wars

The moral as well as metaphysical geography just sketched brings one back to the character of morality and bioethics after God, as well as to a better appreciation of the likely future character of the bioethical battles in the culture wars. Traditional Christianity is alive and well not only in fundamental Protestantism, but in Orthodox Christianity. Traditional Christianity gives good grounds to hold that the culture wars over bioethical issues between the now-dominant secular culture of the West and traditional Christianity will not go away. This is the case even though the mainline Christianities have become deeply secularized, and even though Roman Catholicism, which still holds that the gulf between Christianity and the secular culture can be bridged by philosophy, is being further radically secularized by that surrounding culture. The more the secular culture attempts to force traditional Christians to violate their obligations to God (and not merely what in more secular terms is referred to as violating the integrity of their conscience), the more this cultural gulf between the dominant secular culture and traditional Christianity becomes a place of intense disagreement. This will especially be the case in health care, as chapter five showed. Health care and the ethics of health care professionalism will constitute the cultural equivalent of a fault line along which major cultural tectonic plates will collide, eliciting earthquakes of cultural reaction. The more that Western cultures recognize the foundationless character of their secular moralities and bioethics, the more fundamentalist and threatening the morality and bioethics of traditional Christians will appear.

The dominant secular culture will continue to respond vigorously to the presence of traditional Christianity. Given traditional Christianity, these conflicts will fuel the culture wars. Nevertheless, the secular culture will seek as far as possible to make the presence of traditional Christianity, and of traditional religion generally, seem invisible. One might note, for example, how infrequently the dominant secular media, in analyzing Vladimir Putin's role in the social changes of contemporary Russia, avoid calling attention to the role of religious and moral differences in defining Russia over against the European Union. Little attention is paid to the circumstance that Putin has made Orthodox Christianity the *de facto* established religion of Russia. An exception to the silence of the Western press is Patrick J. Buchanan (2014; also Reno 2014a). In analyses of Putin and contemporary Russia, recognition of the importance of Orthodox Christianity in Russia and of Russia's support of Bashar al-Assad of Syria (Syria has an ancient Orthodox Christian population that looks to Russia for protection) is minor at best.[61] The marginalization of the role of Christianity from public reflection and from health care policy is thus achieved at the price of a highly skewed and inaccurate account of the contemporary conflict between civilizations (Huntington 2011). This disturbed picture is demanded by an established secular culture that seeks to be after Christendom, Christianity, and a Christian bioethics. This attempted secular reinterpretation can only intensify the disagreements. If traditional Christianity responds, then the attempt to make traditional Christianity invisible will make it only more visible.

Where does all of this leave us? The answer is: with irreconcilable moral and bioethical controversies. We do not share common ground. Christianity has ancient roots that are immune from the consequences of the collapse of the Western moral-philosophical project. The culture wars about matters moral and bioethical are rooted deeply in contrary and incompatible views about the ultimate meaning of reality and the character of moral as well as bioethical knowledge. The contemporary normative geography within which the moral and bioethical culture wars are waged has taken its current shape due to wide-ranging changes in the dominant culture of the West. These include changes from the 1960s and onward, many due to the consequences of Vatican II, which have reached far beyond Roman Catholicism. As this chapter argues, popes John XXIII and Paul VI did not appreciate the destabilizing forces they helped unleash. Popes John Paul II and Benedict XVI then failed to appreciate the character and depth of the de-Christianization that is occurring. They regarded the current cultural crisis as one of philosophical rationality rather than of Christian faith. They did not fully appreciate that the bioethical battles in the culture wars are due to the widening gulf between the dominant culture and traditional Christianity. Faith in reason discounted the depth of the gulf and supported the presumption that reason can bridge it.

Matters are different with Pope Francis. He appears ready to embrace the cultural changes underway, thus further refashioning Roman Catholic morality and bioethics. Unlike his predecessors, he seems to be attempting to change Roman Catholicism's focus by internalizing the post-modern character of the contemporary moral and bioethical terrain so as to move towards a weak theology and bioethics. This agenda, which has wide-ranging consequences for bioethics, is in deep tension with traditional Christianity, as this chapter shows. This new focus will likely strengthen the grounds for disagreement between traditional and post-traditional Christians, not to mention the disagreements between the traditional Christian and the fully secularized post-Christian culture, along with its morality and bioethics. The moral and bioethical battles in the culture wars will not just involve a conflict of Christianity with a post-Christian culture, but traditional with post-traditional Christians. Our contemporary moral and bioethical disputes are set within a collision of life-worlds. Our views of morality and bioethics are inextricably defined by controversy and disagreement. Secular morality and bioethics are firmly after God. Because of regarding its medical ethics as rationally equivalent to secular medical ethics, Roman Catholicism will be at peace with a secular bioethics after God. In addition, in having made peace with its bioethical battles in the culture wars, Roman Catholic intellectuals will also aspire to being part of Hegel's Absolute Spirit. Such will not be the case for Orthodox Christians.

Notes

[1]This chapter is drawn from the following ancestral presentations: "Bioethics after Foundations: Feeling the Full Force of Secularization," conference on Secularization and Bioethics,

sponsored by the Centro Evangelico di Cultura "Arturo Pascal" and Consulta di Bioetica Onlus, Turin, Italy, January 31, 2012, and "Religion, Politics, and the State in Modern Secularized Societies," presented to the Comune di Napoli on 6 February 2012.

[2]For an account of the decline of mainline Protestantism in the United States, see Bottum 2008. See also Hutchison 1989. In part, this decline was driven by serious divisions within Western Christian denominations that arose around the ordination of priestesses, the acceptance of homosexual acts and homosexual marriage, along with other elements of post-traditional morality generally. The post-traditional Christianities declined in contrast with those Protestant churches that remained closer to Christian tradition (Cadge et al. 2008; Nemeth & Luidens 1989). An important factor in the decline of the mainline churches is that conservative Protestants reproduced more than the liberals (Hout et al. 2001). Recently, there has been a decline in attendance at those evangelical churches that appear not to have adequately catechized the next generation. See Hinch 2013.

[3]The complex set of circumstances that made it plausible for Jews to abandon traditional Judaism included the robust anti-Semitism of the day and the exclusion of Jews from a wide range of civil and other positions. At least from Canon 69 of Lateran IV (A.D. 1215), Jews had been excluded throughout Western Christianity from public offices and by Canon 68 been required to wear distinctive dress. As the Protestant Christianity of the late 18th and 19th centuries came to have ever less dogmatic substance, a conversion to Christianity became less off-putting. As Jacob Katz summarizes:

> Participation in salon life generally led Jews to join the non-Jewish society outright, to the point even of adopting its religion and its church. If the new converts required ideological backing for their decision, they could find it in the idea of a common positive core to all religions, a notion that denied any importance to the specifics of the historical religions. The theory of the positive nucleus common to all religions discredited completely the claims to uniqueness of each religion. A person who accepted this theory could believe that in changing his religion he was simply altering the external trappings, which were unimportant in any case. On the basis of this theory, one public figure, David Friedländer, thought it possible for the entire Jewish community to be absorbed into Christianity without having to renounce what really constituted its fundamental beliefs. For those individuals who were enticed by social inducements to accept the prevailing religion, his theory no doubt served to soothe their conscience and remove their psychological inhibitions (Katz 1993, p. 223).

Michael Meyer, by using the travails of Heinrich Heine (1797–1856), illustrates the pressure brought on Jews of the 19th century to convert to Christianity. "In an atmosphere increasingly unfriendly to Jews, marked by the Prussian law of 1822 that definitively excluded Jews from academic teaching positions and in Heine's own life by Christian acquaintances turning against him as a Jew, he began to think seriously of conversion" (Meyer 1997, p. 210).

[4]For further reflection on unitarian and congregational Christianity, as well as on liberal Judaism, see Engelhardt 1991, esp. pp. 181–182. One should also underscore the influence of

Moses Mendelsohn (1729–1786) and Hermann Cohen (1842–1918) on liberal Judaism, which rendered it a child of the Enlightenment.

[5]New England intellectual life already in the 18th century was influenced by British free-thought movements such as those associated with Anthony Collins (1676–1729) and his work *A Discourse of Free Thought* (1713) and Thomas Paine's (1737–1809) *The Age of Reason* (1794–96). Denying any link to atheism, Collins claims, "If there is any such rare Monster as an Atheist, David has given us his Character in these words, The Fool hath said in his heart, there is no God; that is, no one denies the Existence of a God but some idle, unthinking, shallow Fellow" (Collins 1713, p. 104). By the mid-19th century, many Free Thinkers were atheists, as shown by the association of the London Atheistical Society with the Freethought movement. Free thought was also associated with Holyoake's secularism and his Secular Guild, which anticipated the 20th-century phenomenon of atheistic secular humanism and the new atheist movement. By the end of the 19th century, the border between Unitarians and free thinkers had in many areas become unclear. The result was that the British free thought associations lacked crisp points of difference from many Congregationalist and Unitarian communities. This state of affairs was in part shaped by what had become a culture in reaction against traditional Christian culture. As Lionel Trilling (1905–1975) appreciated, "Between the end of the first quarter of this century and the present time there has grown up a populous group whose members take for granted the idea of the adversary culture" (Trilling 1966, p. xiii). The Renaissance, the Age of Reason, the Enlightenment, have all been adversary cultures, cultures opposed to the traditional Christian culture of the West, which for more than a millennium held cultural and political hegemony over Europe.

[6]Christian fundamentalism under this name emerged as part of a larger effort to stem a modernist re-interpretation of Christianity. It thus has consanguinities with Pope Pius IX's and Pius X's reactions against modernism. The term *fundamentalist* originated in American Protestantism with the American Bible League, which beginning in 1909 produced twelve pamphlets entitled "The Fundamentals" directed against that higher biblical criticism that sought to deconstruct the authority of the Bible. In contrast, fundamentalism stressed the authority of the Bible for Christian life. This defense of the fundamentals of Christianity was tied to a 19th-century millenarian movement, which emphasized the inerrancy of the Scriptures, the literal interpretation of the Bible, the Virgin Birth, the Atonement, the Resurrection, and the imminent Second Coming of Jesus Christ.

[7]Regarding the phenomenon of post-theistic and post-religious Jews, Edward Shapiro opines,

> a Jew who rejects Judaism, and many of the fiercest critics of Judaism have been Jews, remains a Jew in good standing in the eyes of fellow Jews. Elaine Marks, a professor of French at the University of Wisconsin, indicated just how far notions of Jewishness could be stretched. Central to her sense of Jewishness was her apostasy. "I am Jewish precisely because I am not a believer," she said paradoxically, "because I associate . . . the courage not to believe with being Jewish." The non-Jewish Jew, to use Isaac Deutscher's terminology, becomes in Marks' telling the most committed of Jews (Shapiro 2014, pp. 42–43).

Within the secular culture there has been a rejection of the transcendent God, which is so thoroughgoing that it affirms the Christian or Jew who rejects God. Being a non-theistic Christian or Jew fits securely within the dominant secular culture's horizon of the finite and the immanent.

[8]For a study of some of the struggles with modernism in Roman Catholicism, see Motz-kin 1992.

[9]Regarding the prohibition of vernacular translations of the Latin rite, that is, of printing what later became lay missals, Joseph Jungmann reports that

> even as late as 1857 the prohibition to translate the Ordinary of the Mass was renewed by Pius IX, although, to be sure, its enforcement was no longer seriously urged. However, it was not openly and definitely rescinded until near the end of the century. In the revision of the *Index of Forbidden Books*, issued under Leo XIII in 1897, the prohibition was no longer mentioned. After that the spread of the Roman Missal in the vernacular took on greater and greater proportions (Jungmann 1951, vol. 1, pp. 161–162).

As Jungmann notes, "The most popular missal in the German tongue was the *Messbuch der hl. Kirche* by Anselm Schott, O.S.B., which first appeared in 1884; in 1906, in its 10th edition it had reached 100,000 copies and by 1939, in its 45th edition some 1,650,000 copies" (Jungmann 1951, p. 162, fn 12). The reader should observe that the Schott *Messbuch* appeared after the pontificate of Pope Leo XIII began, but before such books were officially removed from the *Index*. They continued to be published at least up until Vatican II. See, for example, Schott 1961.

[10]In 1955 there were 137,310 adult conversions to Roman Catholicism, in 1960 146,212, in 1970 92,670, and in 1975 75,123 (Jones 2003, p. 67).

[11]The "renewal" produced by Vatican II was not so much predicated on the view that the state of Roman Catholicism needed address and specific reform, but represented a global collapse of philosophical-theological paradigms, resulting in an encompassing change in the view of liturgy, piety (e.g., the nearly total abolishment of the Lenten fasts), and medical ethics.

[12]Geoffrey Hull has given an extensive account of why few Roman Catholics other than Archbishop Lefebvre and his followers responded decisively and forcefully against the liturgical and theological revolution of Vatican II. As he has argued, this is due to a very strong view of papal authority, which arose after the Reformation.

> The cult of the Pope promoted by the Jesuits, and Ignatius' willingness to obey to the letter every papal command, attributed to the visible head of the Church a personal sanctity and wisdom never in fact guaranteed by the *Tu es Petrus* ('Thou art Peter': Christ's affirmation of Peter's potential charism of infallibility). Loyola went so far as to aver that 'if the Holy Father were to order me to abandon myself to the sea without a mast, without sails, oars or rudder . . . I would obey not only with alacrity but without anxiety or repugnance, and even with great internal satisfaction' (Hull 2010, p. 141; quoting Mitchell 1980, p. 65).

Such concepts of absolute and mindless obedience were to become a permanent feature of modern Latin Catholicism, as can be seen from the following testimony of Monica Baldwin, who once consulted the well-known English Dominican, Bede Jarrett, on the matter. Fr Jarrett related how he had once taken to his novice master this very problem of whether or not to comply with the unwise and unjust command of a superior:

> He asked me to re-read *The Charge of the Light Brigade*. The idea, you see, is that you do what you're told, no matter how certain you feel that someone has blundered. To ride fearlessly into the jaws of death without reasoning adds splendour to your obedience (Hull 2010, p. 142).

This cult of the papacy grew dramatically in the 19th century. "One of Pius IX's most dangerous extravagances was his equation of Catholic tradition itself with the authority of the successors of Peter, a claim that stripped the bases of belief and practice of all objective reality outside the will (or whim) of the reigning pontiff" (Hull 2010, pp. 146–147). The result was, as Hull argues, unavoidable.

> It will be clear by now that there was a direct cause-and-effect relationship between the spirit of ultramontanism and the general acquiescence of Latin Catholics in the Pauline liturgical revolution. . . . In the last analysis the instinct of blind obedience to ecclesiastical authority proved stronger than the moral dictate of fidelity to the truth or patrimonial loyalties. In any case the possibility of papal error was by now a fact ably suppressed in ordinary Catholic education. If the average man in the pew knew nothing of the occasions when past popes had erred dogmatically outside the *Tu es Petrus*, it is understandable how a mere prudential judgement on the part of the reigning Pontiff could have been claimed as an 'infallible' (and hence irreformable) act of the Papacy (Hull 2010, p. 150).

[13]Yves Congar rued his reference to the October Revolution. "The integrists have outrageously abused a phrase, admittedly ill-judged, which I used when writing about the voting on the College at the Council, 30 October 1963: 'The Church has undergone, peacefully, her October Revolution'" (Congar 1976, p. 94).

[14]The quotation is taken from Hull 2010, p. 251. For an Italian report on Pope Paul VI's address of June 29, 1979, see http://www.vatican.va/holy_father/paul_vi/homilies/1972/documents/hf_p-vi_hom_19720629_it.html. Despite Virgilio Cardinal Noè's gloss, the plain sense of Pope Paul VI's address indicates a chaos much broader than merely liturgical confusion (Noè 2008). As Robert Fastiggi remarks, "This statement in itself is most remarkable. The Roman Pontiff who confirmed each of the sixteen documents of Vatican II was stating—less than seven years later—that 'something preternatural' was in the world seeking to disturb and suffocate the intended fruits of the Council" (Fastiggi 2012, p. 63).

[15]As one can imagine, the abrupt removal of Archbishop Annibale Bugnini from his ability to influence further liturgical changes provoked numerous speculations. One such account by a conservative Roman Catholic is worth noting:

> I have made my own investigation into the affair and can vouch for the authenticity of the following facts. A Roman priest of the very highest reputation came into

possession of evidence which he considered proved Archbishop Bugnini to be a Freemason. He had this information placed into the hands of Pope Paul VI with the warning that if action were not taken at once, he would be bound in conscience to make the matter public. Archbishop Bugnini was then removed by means of the dissolution of his entire Congregation. I have verified these facts directly with the priest concerned, and the full facts can be found in Chapter XXIV of my book *Pope Paul's New Mass* (Davies 2003, p. 17).

[16]In English, this literature of medical-moral manuals included: Bonnar 1944; Bouscaren 1933; Capellmann 1882; Coppens 1897; Ficarra 1951; Finney 1922; Flood 1953–54; Hayes, Hayes & Kelly 1964; Healy 1956; Kenny 1952; La Rochelle & Fink 1944; McFadden 1946a, 1946b; O'Donnell 1956; Sanford 1905.

[17]For an overview of this remarkable medical ethics literature in North America, see Kelly 1979.

[18]For an account of the history of the developments of the "Code of Ethics–1948" see Griese 1987, pp. 1–19.

[19]There seems to be some dispute regarding exactly what Bugnini stated (Bugnini 1965). It may have been the case that he only spoke against retaining the seventh prayer for Good Friday: "Oremus et pro haereticis et schismaticis" (Schott 1961, p. 391). See, for example, Roberts 2011, p. 21.

[20]One must as well note the role played by the Institute of Society, Ethics, and the Life Sciences that would become the Hastings Center, which was founded in 1969 by Daniel Callahan and Willard Gaylin. Callahan had once been a practicing Roman Catholic and was also looking for a guiding secular moral perspective.

[11]Some non-traditionalist Roman Catholics have attributed the continued demographic decline of their denomination to the failure adequately to reach out to liberal Roman Catholics by adapting Roman Catholicism's sexual morality and its bioethics of end-of-life decision-making to the requirements of the now-dominant culture. Such Roman Catholics are of the view that the conservative "constituency cannot sustain the church in the long term, and the church now needs a figure able to bridge the gap between its rightward movement and the reality that Westerners are leaving the church in droves" (D'Antonio 2013). This figure is seen to be Pope Francis. One should note the criticism of this position of liberal Roman Catholics and members of the Western mainline Christianities by traditional Christians, including Archbishop Kyrill (Gundiayev), now patriarch of Russia, when in 2000 he observed:

> Can you or anyone else tell me that as a result of modernization (*aggiornamento*) there has been a strengthening of Christianity in the Western world? Can you say that as a result of modernization there are more believers, that your churches are fuller, that the role of the Church has become more active, visible and necessary for people? Have more people been going to Catholic churches since Vatican II? Have more people started going to Anglican churches since they began ordaining women? Unless you can give me convincing statistics to reflect on, I shall continue to think that all these drastic reforms have done nothing to strengthen church life in Western society (Hull 2010, p. 352).

In short, there is the view on the part of many that the liberalization of Roman Catholicism, like the liberalization of mainline Christianity, will not fill the pews but further empty them.

[22]Within traditional Christianity, love of one's neighbor is to be placed within the context of an all-enveloping love of God. "'You shall love the Lord your God with all your heart, and with all your soul, and with all your mind.' This is the greatest and first commandment. And a second is like it: 'You shall love your neighbor as yourself.' On these two commandments hang all the law and the prophets" (Matthew 22:37–40).

[23]Moses Maimonides underscores the need to act out of obedience to God. He states, for example,

> Anyone who accepts upon himself the fulfillment of these seven mitzvoth [the seven laws given to Noah and his sons] and is precise in their observance is considered one of "the pious among the gentiles" and will merit a share in the world to come.
>
> This applies only when he accepts them and fulfills them because the Holy One, blessed be He, commanded them in the Torah and informed us through Moses, our teacher, that Noah's descendants had been commanded to fulfill them previously.
>
> However, if he fulfills them out of intellectual conviction, he is not a resident alien, nor of "the pious among the gentiles," nor of their wise men (Maimonides 2001, p. 582, *Hilchot Melachim U'Milchamoteihem*, ch 8.11).

[24]Traditionally, Christians recognize an essential difference between taxing in order to provide resources to feed the poor, and Christian charity, which requires that each freely give money and/or goods to persons in need. Charity encourages a personal relationship to those in need, which is blessed by responding in love to a command of God. In a secular culture, to support taxation in order to underwrite welfare is to support funding a welfare system that will always be post-Christian, if not anti-Christian in its character.

[25]For a recent reflection on Camosy's arguments regarding the harmonies between Peter Singer and Christian ethics, see Wicks 2013a and 2013b, as well as Perry 2013.

[26]Of course, it is possible that Roman Catholicism will abandon all concerns with foundations and re-constitute itself as a religious group making room for both atheists and theists (Zabala 2005). The choice will likely be either the path taken by the liberal Anglican community or that of the more traditional believers, including the Priestly Fraternity of St. Peter, which was founded in 1988 in order to draw priests and laity from the Society of Saint Pius X founded in 1970 by Archbishop Marcel Lefebvre (1905–1991), which had not submitted fully to papal authority.

[27]Christ reminds us that salvation is from the Jews, not from the Greeks or others (John 4:22).

[28]As has become clear, the Western faith in reason is unfounded. The project of a rationally grounded morality, a project first shaped by Plato as well as Aristotle and then further developed by the West especially after the 12th century, has failed. Contemporary, content-full, secular moral views have become recognized as freestanding moral positions framed out of various collages of moral intuitions sustained by diverse moral narratives all floating

within the horizon of the finite and the immanent. This state of affairs comes as no surprise to Orthodox Christianity, which embraces the theocentric horn of Euthyphro's dilemma. In contrast, Roman Catholicism has tended to consider the integrity of morality and moral philosophy to be independent of a rightly-ordered relationship with God. Orthodox Christianity lacks a morality in the sense that, for Orthodox Christianity, morality is not a third thing between God and man, an independent set of norms open to philosophical refinement and development.

For Western Christianity, and for Roman Catholicism in particular, morality is a set of intellectually justifiable norms constituting a third thing between God and man, a third thing rationally disclosable and justifiable. It is for this reason that Roman Catholicism supports an intellectual account of the aggressive secularization of the dominant culture in holding that secularization stems from intellectual mistakes that have led to a false view of morality, bioethics, and reality. It does not recognize that the contemporary secularization of culture derives primarily from a failure of Christians to live a traditional Christian life, to turn in right worship to God, and thus to transform themselves and their culture. Given Roman Catholicism's background commitments, it will appear plausible to them to attempt through moral foundational arguments to reconnect morality with being-as-it-is-in-itself, and thus philosophically to re-orient the dominant secular culture with its morality and bioethics. The contemporary Roman Catholic position, if it remains true to its rationalist commitments held since the beginning of the second millennium, and given its break from Christian asceticism with Vatican II, will not be to call all to fasting and repentance, as did the king of the repentant city of Nineveh. Crucially, the king of Nineveh does not rely on philosophy, but on asceticism in order to respond to the corruption of his people.

"By the decree of the king and his nobles:
    Do not let any man or beast, herd or flock, taste anything; do not let them eat or drink. But let man and beast be covered with sackcloth. Let everyone call urgently on God. Let them give up their evil ways and their violence. Who knows? God may yet relent and with compassion turn from his fierce anger so that we will not perish."
    When God saw what they did and how they turned from their evil ways, he had compassion and did not bring upon them the destruction he had threatened (Jonah 3:7–10).

[29]Roman Catholicism, given its traditional faith in reason, has been of the conviction that one can by reason alone ground nearly all of its bioethical claims. The result is that medical-moral commitments that many recognize to be uniquely Roman Catholic (e.g., the natural-law prohibition of artificial contraception) have been held to be defensible by reason alone. The "reason" invoked by Roman Catholics is obviously already endowed with a very particular content. Here the criticism directed against Thomas Aquinas and other "natural lawyers" is similar to that which Hegel directed against Kant, namely, that crucial premises have been given more content from a particular community than the arguments as general rational arguments can justify (see the section "Moralität" in *The Philosophy of Right*).

[30]In addition to Pope Francis's unsympathetic remarks regarding capitalism and the market, such as in his speech at Cagliari, the capital of Sardinia, on September 22, 2013, one might also consider the remarks of his chief adviser, Cardinal Maradiaga, in Dallas, Texas, on October 25, 2013. Rather than criticizing how socialist government policies have retarded economic growth, as well as encouraged corruption, thus imposing constraints on productivity in countries such as Argentina, Brazil, Italy, Mexico, Portugal, and Spain, thus leading to high unemployment, in particular high youth unemployment in contrast to sovereignties such as Hong Kong and Singapore, he lays the blame at the feet of free-market capitalism. See: http://www.opposingviews.com/i/religion/christianity/catholicism/pope-francis-criticizes-global-economy-worshipping-god-called# and http://whispersintheloggia.blogspot.com/2013/10/the-councils-unfinished-business.html. One can but be struck by a discourse that suggests a South American, if not particularly Argentinian, left-of-center populist rhetoric.

[31]As already observed in the text, the circumstances of the *La Repubblica* article (i.e., although the text of Pope Francis's interview was not transcribed by Eugenio Scalfari from notes or from a recording but taken from memory, the text that appeared in print was approved by the Vatican and published in *L'Osservatore Romano*) created the best of all possible worlds: a text that could send a message and then be qualified as would prove expedient. In the wake of persistent criticism, the interview was removed from the Vatican website, although in the meantime it appeared elsewhere in the Roman Catholic press. See, for example, ITV Staff 2013. Regarding the grounds to rely on the general accuracy of Pope Francis's statements in his *La Repubblica* interview, one might consider the remarks of Michael S. Rose, the associate editor of *New Oxford Review*.

> Now, some might want to respond by saying that the Vatican eventually took this interview off its official website, where it was posted with pride of place alongside other official papal writings, due to alleged errors in Scalfari's transcription of the interview. However, it was not removed until it became obvious that much of what Francis reportedly said during the interview was recognized as egregiously flawed from the point of view of basic eighth-grade-level theology. Before the interview was scrubbed from the Vatican website, it was published in the Italian daily *Corriere della Sera*, defended by Vatican spokesman Federico Lombardi, S.J., and quoted in mass media outlets the world over (Rose 2014, p. 14).

[32]As Michael Novak observes with regard to the impact of Pope Francis's remarks, "Ever since Max Weber, Catholic social thought has been blamed for much of the poverty in many [Roman] Catholic nations. Pope Francis inadvertently adds evidence for Weber's thesis" (Novak 2013).

[33]In December 2015 the lowest rates of youth unemployment in Western Europe were in Germany (7.0%), Austria (11.2%), the Netherlands (11.2%), and Denmark (10.3%), all countries with a substantial Protestant population or a historical and cultural connection to such a country (e.g., Austria with its special ties to Germany). In southern Europe, youth unemployment was much higher: Spain (46.0 %), Italy (37.9%), and Portugal (31%). There is no evidence that approaches to social justice inspired by Roman Catholicism have had a positive impact

on youth unemployment in Western Europe. Available at: http://www.statista.com/statis-tics/266228/youth-unemployment-rate-in-eu-countries/ [accessed February 8, 2016]. The youth unemployment in Texas is 13.5%. Available at: http://www.governing.com/gov-data/youth-employment-unemployment-rate-data-by-state.html [accessed February 8, 2016].

[34]The Roman Catholic thinker Michael Novak in a recent article titled "Agreeing with Pope Francis" offers a highly qualified defense of Pope Francis's *Evangelii Gaudium*. He admits that the Exhortation has a skewed character, given its radical political-theological character.

About six of [Pope Francis's] swipes are so highly partisan and biased that they seem outside this pope's normal tranquility and generosity of spirit. Exactly these partisan phrases were naturally leapt upon by media outlets such as Reuters and the *Guardian*. Among these are "trickle-down theories," "invisible hand," "idolatry of money," "inequality," and trust in the state "charged with vigilance for the common good" (Novak 2013).

[35]Novak attempts to excuse Pope Francis's account of capitalist economics by in part appealing to problems of translation.

Note first that "trickle-down" nowhere appears in the original Spanish, as it would have done if the pope had meant to invoke the battle-cry of the American Democrats against the American Republicans. Professional translators of Spanish say the correct translation of *derrame* is "spillover" or "overflow." Instead, the English translation introduces both a sharply different meaning and a harsh new tone into this passage. Only those hostile to capitalism and Reagan's successful reforms, and to the policies of Republicans in general after the downward mobility of the Carter years, use the derisive expression "trickle-down," intended to caricature what actually happened under Reagan, namely, dramatic upward mobility (Novak 2013).

[36]As an excuse for Pope Francis's distorted economic assertions, Novak also argues that the realities of Argentina gave the pope a false understanding of economic and social realities.

As the 20th century began, Argentina was ranked among the top 15 industrial nations, and more and more of its wealth was springing from modern inventions rather than farmland. Then a destructive form of political economy, just then spreading like a disease from Europe—a populist fascism with tight government control over the economy—dramatically slowed Argentina's economic and political progress. Instability in the rule of law undermined economic creativity. Inflation blew to impossible heights. . . . Human energies are drained by dependency on state benefits, the visible result has been a largely static society, with little opportunity for the poor to rise out of poverty. A great inner humiliation comes over the poor as they see their lack of personal achievement and their dependency. If this is what Pope Francis was painfully visualizing as he wrote this exhortation, it is exactly what the eyes of many other observers have seen (Novak 2013).

Surely, if the pope has such a wrongheaded view of economics, many would argue that he is responsible for not having better informed himself. They would hold Pope Francis's ignorance to be vincible.

[37]Christ Himself addresses the issue of people thinking they are pursuing the good when they are actually doing evil. Christ warns that those who will martyr Christians will think they are acting rightly without in any way implying that this is good. "[I]n fact, a time is coming when anyone who kills you will think he is offering a service to God" (John 16:2).

[38]Anent Pope Francis's endorsement of the goodness of everyone pursuing his own view of the good, Merleau-Ponty points out that Stalin in killing millions of people surely was pursuing the good as he understood it.

For it is certain that neither Bukharin nor Trotsky nor Stalin regarded Terror as intrinsically valuable. Each one imagined he was using it to realize a genuinely human history which had not yet started but which provides the justification for revolutionary violence. In other words, as Marxists, all three confess that there is a meaning to such violence—that it is possible to understand it, to read into it a rational development and to draw from it a humane future (Merleau-Ponty 1969, p. 97).

[39]One should recall Christ's warning regarding those who are stumbling blocks for the faith of the weak. "Things that cause people to sin are bound to come, but woe to that person through whom they come. It would be better for him to be thrown into the sea with a millstone tied around his neck than for him to cause one of these little ones to sin" (Luke 17:1–2).

[40]There appears to be a view that if one appeals to the liberal disaffected Roman Catholics, they will return to fill the pews, the experience of mainline Protestantism to the contrary notwithstanding. See D'Antonio 2013. There remains the question as to whether left-of-center populist rhetoric can fill Roman Catholic churches, as it fills the streets of South America.

[41]A pastoral approach can allow Pope Francis de facto to change doctrine without changing it de jure. For example, homosexual couples can quietly be allowed to receive communion by appealing to pastoral considerations. The result is to go against the need for the sinner to repent before the sinner is forgiven.

[42]Because of his affirmation of left-of-center populist issues, Pope Francis has received praise from the media establishment. See, for instance, Dionne 2013; Anonymous 2013a, 2013b, and 2013c. Pope Francis's positions will make him more acceptable in many intellectual and political circles. A major question is whether media acceptance and popularity will translate into more congregants and more congregations.

[43]An indication of the rapid spread of conservative Protestantism in South America is given by the circumstance that it is estimated that one out of every four Brazilians is evangelical, and that by 2020 perhaps half the population will be evangelical (Madambashi 2010).

[44]The Society of St. Pius X has been successful worldwide in acquiring vocations, supporting the traditional morality of its members, and building churches. Despite a number of very reckless statements by some of its clerics, the bond to tradition has maintained congregants. Traditional belief generally produces children and converts. See http://www.sspx.org.

[45]St. Basil states with regard to praying *ad orientem*, to the east: "Thus we all look to the East at our prayers, but few of us know that we are seeking our own old country, Paradise, which God planted in Eden in the East . . ." (St. Basil 1994, Letter XXVII, vol. 8, p. 42).

Although the so-called reforms of the Roman Catholic Mass with its orientation *ad populum* were justified by some on the basis that it represented an ancient practice, this is clearly not the case. As László Dobszay in his study of the Roman rite remarks, "the prevailing (in fact almost universal) situation was that both the priest and the congregation prayed regularly turning towards the east" (Dobszay 2010, p. 90).

Since in the great basilicas of Rome celebration facing the people was the general practice (because the basilicas themselves faced west, not east, so that in order to face east the pope turned in to the body of the building), many supposed that this had been the original and authentic tradition, and the Liturgical Movement had to return to that. Pius XII in his encyclical *Mediator Dei* criticized the one-sidedness of this argument, and called it a manifestation of extreme archaism (Dobszay 2010, p. 91).

[46]As already noted, the Church of the first millennium understood that "If you are a theologian, you will pray truly. And if you pray truly, you are a theologian" (Evagrios 1983, vol. 1, p. 62).

[47]Recent examples of Orthodox Christian theologians in the strict sense include St. John of San Francisco (1894–1966), Elder Joseph the Hesychast, the Cave-Dweller of the Holy Mountain (1897–1959), Elder Paisios of Romania (†1993), St. Paisios of Mt. Athos (1924–1994), St. Porphyrios (1906–1991), St. Silouan the Athonite (1866–1938), and Archimandrite Sophrony (1896–1993).

[48]Regarding the nature of proper papal authority, one might consider the famous letter (A.D. 1386) of Nikitas, Archbishop of Nicomedia, to the German bishop Anselm of Havelberg.

My dearest brother, we do not deny to the Roman Church the primacy amongst the five sister Patriarchates; and we recognize her right to the most honourable seat at an Ecumenical Council. But she has separated herself from us by her own deeds, when through pride she assumed a monarchy which does not belong to her office . . . How shall we accept from her decrees that have been issued without consulting us and even without our knowledge? If the Roman Pontiff, seated on the lofty throne of his glory, wishes to thunder at us and, so to speak, hurl his mandates at us from on high, and if he wishes to judge us and even to rule us and our Churches, not by taking counsel from us but at his own arbitrary pleasure, what kind of brotherhood, or even what kind of parenthood can this be? We should be the slaves, not the sons, of such a Church, and the Roman See would not be the pious mother but a hard and imperious mistress of slaves (Runciman 1955, p. 116).

[49]For a discussion of where the fourth Rome should be established, see Engelhardt 2000, pp. 393–396.

[50]On November 25, 1551, during the 14th session, the Council of Trent published the following canons concerning the doctrine of the temporal punishment due to sin:

12. If anyone says that the entire punishment is always remitted by God along with the sin, and that the satisfaction made by penitents is nothing else but the faith by which they grasp that Christ has made satisfaction on their behalf: let him be anathema.

13. If anyone says that, for temporal punishment for sins, no satisfaction at all is made to God, through the merits of Christ, by the sufferings imposed by God and patiently borne; or by the penances enjoined by a priest; or, further, by those voluntarily undertaken such as fasts, prayers, almsgiving or other additional works of devotion; and consequently that the best penance is only a new life: let him be anathema. . . .

15. If anyone says that the keys have been given to the church only for loosing and not also for binding; and that, consequently, when priests impose penalties on those who confess, they are acting contrary to the purpose of the keys and to the institution of Christ; . . . : let him be anathema (Tanner 1990, vol. 2, p. 713).

See also Brzana 1953.

[51]The Roman Catholic doctrine of indulgences developed out of a practice of commuting or ameliorating severe penances, such as years of strict fasting, if the penitent engaged in some good act such as building a monastery.

[52]A more complete statement concerning the July 2013 indulgences granted by Pope Francis is provided by the news service Zenit, sponsored by the Legionaries of Christ.

A plenary indulgence will also be granted for those who cannot attend World Youth Day. "The faithful who on account of a legitimate impediment cannot attend the aforementioned celebrations may obtain Plenary Indulgence under the usual spiritual, sacramental and prayer conditions, in a spirit of filial submission to the Roman Pontiff, by participation in the sacred functions on the days indicated, following the same rites and spiritual exercises as they occur via television or radio or, with due devotion, via the new means of social communication," the decree states.

See: http://www.zenit.org/en/articles/pope-francis-decrees-plenary-indulgence-for-world-youth-day [accessed October 17, 2015]

[53]In commenting on the prerogative of kings to have concubines, Maimonides remarks: "The Oral Tradition states that he may take no more than eighteen wives. The figure eighteen includes both wives and concubines" (Maimonides 2001, p. 518).

[54]For a study of the difference between the Roman Catholic doctrine of original sin and the Orthodox view of ancestral sin, see Romanides 2002. The Vulgate inaccurately translates the Greek of Romans 5:12 as: "Propterea sicut per unum hominem peccatum in hunc mundum intravit, et per peccatum mors; et ita in omnes homines mors pertransiit, in quo omnes peccaverunt" (Romans 5:12, *Biblia Sacra* 1956). The correct translation of the Greek original into English is: "Therefore, even as through one man sin entered into the world, and death through sin, thus death passed to all men, on account of which all have sinned" (Holy Apostles 2000, p. 98). The key issue in the Latin translation is the *quo* (by which), which does not adequately translate the Greek that refers to death, which is indeed passed on, along with the inclination to sin to which all except Christ have succumbed. John Romanides makes clear that the Patristic tradition was of one mind about the fact that the original Greek is "because of

which," where "which" refers to death. Thus, the fact that "all have sinned" is the case through their exposure to death and the resulting omnipresent inclination to sin: "death was viewed as the root from which sin springs up" (Romanides 2002, p. 166f). See also Sopko 1998.

[55]There are numerous other differences in dogma separating Orthodox Christians from Roman Catholics, such as whether grace is created.

[56]*The Didache,* a text from the early second century, but perhaps from as early as A.D. 60, enjoins that one "fast on Wednesdays and Fridays" (*Didache* viii.1, vol. 1, p. 321).

[57]Consider, for example, the absolution for the involuntary miscarriage of an unborn child, which absolution recognizes the need for God's grace when our bodies fall short of the mark.

O Master, Lord our God, Who was born of the Holy Theotokos and Ever-virgin Mary, and Who, as an infant, lay in the manger: According to Your great mercy, be merciful to Your servant, N., who is in sin, having been involved in the loss of a life, whether voluntary or involuntary, for she has miscarried that which was conceived in her. Forgive her transgressions, both voluntary and involuntary, and protect her from every snare of the Devil. Cleanse her stain and heal her infirmities. And grant to her, Lover of Mankind, health and strength of soul and body. Guard her with a shining Angel from all assaults of the unseen demons; Yea, O Lord, from sickness and infirmity. Purify her from bodily uncleanness and the various troubles within her womb. By Your many mercies lead her up in her humbled body from the bed on which she lies. For we all have been born in sins and transgressions, and all of us are defiled in Your sight, O Lord. Therefore, with fear we cry out and say: Look down from heaven and behold the feebleness of us who are condemned. Forgive this, Your servant, N., who is in sin, having been involved in the loss of a life, whether voluntary or involuntary, for she has miscarried that which was conceived in her. And, according to Your great mercy as the Good God Who loves mankind, be merciful and forgive all those who are here present and who have touched her. For You along have the power to remit sins and transgressions, through the prayers of Your Most-pure Mother and of all the Saints (Monk 1987, pp. 6–7).

[58]The prayer before communion includes a petition that one be absolved of one's involuntary sins. "Wherefore I pray thee, have mercy upon me and forgive my transgressions both voluntary and involuntary, of word and of deed, of knowledge and of ignorance; and make me worthy to partake without condemnation of thine immaculate Mysteries, unto remission of my sins and unto life everlasting" (*Pocket Prayer Book* 1956, p. 98). See also Petrà 2011.

[59]Hesychasm (from *hēsychia,* "stillness, rest, quiet, silence") is the ascetical practice that follows Christ's injunction that "when thou prayest, enter into thy closet, and when thou hast shut thy door, pray" (Matthew 6:6), so that in prayer (especially through the Jesus Prayer: *Lord Jesus Christ, Son of God, have mercy on me, a sinner*) one turns away from the world and the senses to experience God (i.e., *theōria*). Hesychasm is the process of retiring within oneself in order that through prayer one may cease to be misdirected by the senses, so that one may be granted an experiential knowledge of God.

[60]For a Roman Catholic approach to ritual as valuable in itself apart from God, see Perniola 2001. As a fully cultural matter, one can state, "I am an atheist, I am not a Christian, but I am surely Roman Catholic," thus affirming the culture and/or ritual form but not the metaphysical or dogmatic dimension of Roman Catholicism. The atheist Marcello Pera, a friend of Benedict XVI, in his portion of their jointly authored *Without Roots* endorses a Christian morality, but without recognizing God, much less Christ as the Redeemer (Ratzinger & Pera 2006). Indeed, Pera has become well known for endorsing a Christianity without God, arguing for an essential tie between Christianity and liberal democracy. He endorses the importance of the Christian heritage or tradition (Pera 2011). In short, there are a number of ways in which atheists, agnostics, and deists can be cultural Christians. This persistence of a "religious" culture as a moral commitment after the traditional religious core is gone exists in forms of Judaism as well. One might think, for example, of Ethical Culture, which was founded by Felix Adler (1851–1933), a former Reform Jewish rabbi, who convoked the initial members of the movement on May 15, 1876. He had already espoused many of its foundational ideas in a sermon at Temple Emanu-El on October 11, 1873, in New York under the title "The Judaism of the Future" (see Kraut 1979). It was not until February 21, 1877, that the New York Society for Ethical Culture was incorporated. Adler's influence was also significant in Europe. With his inspiration, the Deutsche Gesellschaft für ethische Kultur was established in 1892. In 1894 Die ethische Gemeinde was founded in Vienna and in 1896 the International Ethical Union (IEU) was formed. See Friess 1981. There is as well a high church or ritual form of the persistence of a "religious" community after it has passed beyond belief. For example, in addition to Perniola's reflections, one might consider high-church Anglicans who might not recognize that Jesus Christ physically rose from the dead or even that God exists, but who can be committed to a substantive ritualism. One encounters agnosticism celebrated in good Christian cultural style, all without having to belabor traditional belief. One must distinguish such post-Christian, ritual-friendly Christianity from the late-19th-century Anglican ritualism movement, which under Queen Victoria led to Anglican ministers being arrested, convicted, and imprisoned for excessive high-church ritualism, and which appeared to many as flagrantly "Romish." For an account of this 19th-century phenomenon, see Reed 1970.

[61]As an example of the discounting by the secular media of the role that religion plays in public affairs, see Simon Shuster's recent article concerning Vladimir Putin, which makes only two brief mentions of Orthodox Christianity (Shuster 2013).

References

Abbate, Carmelo. 2011. *Sex and the Vatican*. Milan: Piemme.

Abel, Francesc. 1999. Bioethical dialogue in the perspective of the third millennium. Unpublished paper delivered in Barcelona, May 9.

Altizer, Thomas J. J. 1966. *The Gospel of Christian Atheism*. Philadelphia: Westminster Press.

Altizer, Thomas J. J. & William Hamilton. 1966. *Radical Theology and the Death of God*. Indianapolis: Bobbs-Merrill.

Anonymous. 2014. Pope Francis: put-down artist? *New Oxford Review* LXXXI.3 (April): 17–20.

Anonymous. 2013a. Pope Francis, *Foreign Policy* (December): 86.

Anonymous. 2013b. Pope Francis and the primacy of conscience, *New Oxford Review* 80 (December): 18–21.

Anonymous. 2013c. Pope Francis: Delight of the world, *New Oxford Review* 80 (December): 21–23.

Aquinas, Thomas. 1947. *Summa Theologiae*, 2nd Part of the 2nd Part, Question 154, Article 12, trans. Fathers of the English Dominican Province. New York: Benziger Brothers.

Archdiocese Salzburg. 2009. Bei Gott und den Menschen bleiben! Ein Interview mit Erzbischof Alois Kothgasser zur Lage der Kirche (February 10). Available: http://www.kirchen.net/portal/page.asp?id=13622 [accessed October 7, 2015]

Badash, David. 2011. "Sex and the Vatican" claims thousands of priests in illicit relationships. http://thenewcivilrightsmovement.com/sex-and-the-vatican-claims-thousands-of-priests-in-illicit-relationships/news/2011/04/20/19057 [accessed February 3, 2016]

Basil, St. 1994. *Basil: Letters and Select Works*, in *Nicene and Post-Nicene Fathers*, Second Series, eds. Philip Schaff and Henry Wace, vol. 8. Peabody, MA: Hendrickson Publishers.

Benedict XVI. 2013. Benedict XVI leaves the papacy, *L'Osservatore Romano* 46.7 (February 13): 1.

Benedict XVI. 2007. *Summorum pontificium*, 7 July.

Biblia Sacra. 1956. Rome: Typis societatis S. Joannis Evang.

Bottum, Joseph. 2008. The death of Protestant America: A political theory of the Protestant mainline, *First Things* 186 (Aug/Sept): 23–33.

Bouyer, Louis. 1970. *Der Verfall des Katholizismus*. Munich: Kösel.

Bradshaw, David. 2004. *Aristotle East and West*. New York: Cambridge University Press.

Brzana, Stanislao J. 1953. *Remains of Sin and Extreme Unction According to Theologians after Trent*. Rome: Catholic Book Agency.

Buchanan, Patrick J. 2014. Vladimir Putin, Christian crusader? *The American Conservative* (April 4). www.theamericanconservative.com/vladimir-putin-christian-crusader/ [accessed October 25, 2015]

Buckley, Michael. 1987. *At the Origins of Modern Atheism*. New Haven: Yale University Press.

Bugnini, Annibale. 1990. *The Reform of the Liturgy 1948–1975*, trans. Matthew J. O'Connell. Collegeville, MN: Liturgical Press.

Bugnini, Annibale. 1965. Le "variationes" al alcuni testi della Settimana Santa, *L'Osservatore Romano* 65 (March 19): 6.

Burtchaell, James T. 1998. *The Dying of the Light: The Disengagement of Colleges & Universities from their Christian Churches*. Grand Rapids, MI: Wm. B. Eerdmans.

Cadge, Wendy, Laura R. Olson, & Christopher Wildeman. 2008. How denominational resources influence debate about homosexuality in mainline Protestant congregations, *Sociology of Religion* 69.2: 187–207.

Cahill, Lisa Sowle. 2005. *Theological Bioethics: Participation, Justice, and Change*. Washington, DC: Georgetown University Press.

Camosy, Charles. 2012. *Peter Singer and Christian Ethics*. New York: Cambridge University Press.

Caputo, John D. & Gianni Vattimo. 2007. *After the Death of God*, ed. Jeffrey W. Robbins. New York: Columbia University Press.

Chrysostom, St. John. 1994. Homily XII on Colossians iv.12,13, in Philip Schaff (ed.), *Nicene and Post-Nicene Fathers*, First Series, vol. 13. Peabody, MA: Hendrickson Publishers.

Chua-Eoan, Howard & Elizabeth Dias. 2013. The people's pope, *Time* 182.26: 46–75.

Clegg, Sally & Cathy Pharaoh. 2006. International comparisons of charitable giving: November 2006. https://www.cafonline.org/PDF/International%20Compariso ns%20of%20Charitable%20Giving.pdf Comparisons of Charitable Giving.pdf [accessed December 20, 2015]

Collins, Anthony. 1713. *A Discourse of Free-thinking*. London.

Congar, Yves. 1976. *Challenge to the Church: The Case of Archbishop Lefebvre*, trans. Paul Inwood. Huntington, IN: Our Sunday Visitor.

Connolly, Ronald G. 2014. The beautiful bride of Christ, our church, 2014: One perspective, *Latin Mass* 23.2 (Summer): 42–46.

Curran, Charles E. 1976. *Catholic Moral Theology in Dialogue*. Notre Dame, IN: University of Notre Dame Press.

D'Antonio, Michael. 2013. More catholic than the pope? *Foreign Policy* (July 30). http://www.foreignpolicy.com/articles/2013/07/30/more_catholic_than_the_ pope-Francis_homosexuality_reform [accessed October 2, 2015]

Davies, Michael. 2003. *Liturgical Time Bombs in Vatican II*. Rockford, IL: TAN Books.

Delkeskamp-Hayes, Corinna. 2012. Rethinking the Christian bioethics of human germ line genetic engineering: A postscript against the grain of contemporary distortions, *Christian Bioethics* 18.2 (August): 219–230.

Denzinger, Henricus. 1965. *Enchiridion Symbolorum*, 33rd ed. Freiburg im Breisgau: Herder.

Didache, The. 1965. Trans. Kirsopp Lake, in *Apostolic Fathers*, 2 vols. (vol. 1, pp. 303–333). Cambridge, MA: Harvard University Press.

Dionne, E. J., Jr. 2013. Resurrection, *Foreign Policy* (December): 88–89.

Dobszay, László. 2010. *The Restoration and Organic Development of the Roman Rite*, ed. Laurence Paul Hemming. New York: T&T Clark.

Donadio, R. 2013. On gay priests, Pope Francis asks, 'Who am I to judge?' New York Times (July 30): A1.

Dorrien, Gary. 2013. America's mainline, *First Things* 237 (November): 27–34.

Durkheim, Émile. 1947. *The Elementary Forms of the Religious Life*, trans. Joseph Swain. Glencoe, IL: Free Press; 1st ed., 1915.

Ellard, Gerald. 1948. *The Mass of the Future*. Milwaukee: Bruce Publishing.

Engel, Randy. 2006. *The Rite of Sodomy*. Export, PA: New Engel Publishing.

Engel, Ulrich. 2001. Religion and violence: Plea for a weak theology *in tempore belli*, *New Blackfriars* 82: 558–560.

Engelhardt, H. T., Jr. 2012. Ritual, virtue, and human flourishing: Rites as bearers of meaning, in *Ritual and the Moral Life: Reclaiming the Tradition* (pp. 29–51), eds. David Solomon, Ping-Cheung Lo, Ruiping Fan. Dordrecht: Springer.

Engelhardt, H. T., Jr. 2011. Orthodox Christian bioethics: Some foundational differences from Western Christian bioethics, *Studies in Christian Ethics* 24.4 (November): 487–499.

Engelhardt, H. T., Jr. 2010a. Political authority in the face of moral pluralism: Further reflections on the non-fundamentalist state, *Notizie di Politeia* 26.97: 91–99.

Engelhardt, H. T., Jr. 2010b. Religion, bioethics, and the secular state: Beyond religious and secular fundamentalism, *Notizie di Politeia* 26.97: 59–79.

Engelhardt, H. T., Jr. 2000. *The Foundations of Christian Bioethics*. Salem, MA: Scrivener Publishing.

Eppstein, John. 1971. *Has the Catholic Church Gone Mad?* New Rochelle, NY: Arlington House.

Erlandson, Greg, Msgr. Owen F. Campion, Beth McNamara, & Gretchen R. Crowe. 2015. A year of mercy, *Our Sunday Visitor* 103.48: 19.

Evagrios the Solitary. 1983. On prayer, in St. Nikodimos and St. Makarios, *The Philokalia*, trans. and eds. G. E. H. Palmer, Philip Sherrard, & Kallistos Ware (pp. 55–71). Boston: Faber and Faber.

Fackenheim, Emil. 1967. *The Religious Dimension in Hegel's Thought*. Bloomington: Indiana University Press.

Fastiggi, Robert. 2012. Paul VI and the smoke of Satan forty years later, *Latin Mass* 21.2 (Summer): 62–63.

Fidora, Alexander. 2013. Dominicus Gundissalinus and the introduction of metaphysics into the Latin west, *Review of Metaphysics* 67.4 (June): 691–712.

Francis, Pope. 2013. *Evangelii Gaudium*. Vatican City: Vatican Press.

Friess, Horace L. 1981. *Felix Adler and Ethical Culture*. New York: Columbia University Press.

Fuchs, Josef. 1980. Is there a specifically Christian morality? In *Readings in Moral Theology No. 2: The Distinctiveness of Christian Ethics* (pp. 3–17), eds. Charles Curran and Richard McCormick. New York: Paulist Press.

Gilbert, Alan D. 1980. *The Making of Post-Christian Britain*. London: Longman.

Gleason, Philip. 1995. *Contending with Modernity: Catholic Higher Education in the Twentieth Century*. New York: Oxford University Press.

Greeley, Andrew M. 1990. *The Catholic Myth*. New York: Scribner's Sons.

Griese, Orville N. 1987. *Catholic Identity in Health Care: Principles and Practice*. Braintree, MA: Pope John Center.

Halivni, David W. 1997. *Revelation Restored*. Boulder, CO: Westview Press.

Hamilton, William. 1966. American theology, radicalism, and the death of God, in Thomas J. J. Altizer & William Hamilton, *Radical Theology and the Death of God* (3–7). Indianapolis: Bobbs-Merrill.

Hapgood, Isabel (ed. and trans.). 1996. *Service Book of the Holy Orthodox-Catholic Apostolic Church*, 7th ed. Englewood, NJ: Antiochian Orthodox Christian Archdiocese.

Harvey, John Collins. 2013. André Hellegers, the Kennedy Institute, and the development of bioethics: The American-European Connection, in *The Development of Bioethics in the United States*, eds. Jeremy Garrett, Fabrice Jotterand, & D. Christopher Ralston (pp. 37–54). Dordrecht: Springer.

Hauerwas, Stanley. 1995. How Christian ethics became medical ethics: The case of Paul Ramsey, *Christian Bioethics* 1(1): 11–28.

Hauerwas, Stanley. 1979. Theological reflections on *in vitro* fertilization, in *HEW Support of Research Involving Human* In Vitro *Fertilization and Embryo Transfer* (pp. 1–20). Washington, DC: U. S. Government Printing Office.

Hauerwas, Stanley & John H. Westerhoff (eds.). 1992. *Schooling Christians: "Holy Experiments" in American Education*. Grand Rapids, MI: Wm. B. Eerdmans.

Hayek, Friedrich. 1976. *The Mirage of Social Justice*. Chicago: University of Chicago Press.

Hayford, Sarah R. and S. Philip Morgan. 2008. Religiosity and fertility in the United States: The role of fertility intentions, *Social Forces* 86.3: 1163–1188.

Hellegers, André. 1969. A scientist's analysis, in *Contraception: Authority and Dissent*, ed. C. E. Curran (pp. 216–239). New York: Herder and Herder.

Hengel, Martin. 1989. *The Johannine Question*, trans. John Bowden. London: SCM Press.

Hess, Jonathan M. 2002. *Germans, Jews and the Claims of Modernity*. New Haven, CN: Yale University Press.

Hilarion [Alfeyev]. 2008. Theological education in the 21st century, lecture given at Wycliffe College, University of Toronto, October 22. Available at: http://www.interfax-religion.com/?act=documents&div=134 [accessed September 30, 2015]

Hildebrand, Dietrich von. 1969. *Trojan Horse in the City of God*. Chicago: Franciscan Herald Press.

Hinch, Jim. 2013. Where are the people? *The American Scholar* (Winter). http://theamericanscholar.org/where-are-the-people/#.UrMOLSfw2ko [accessed December 20, 2015]

Holy Apostles Convent. 2000. *Acts, Epistles, and Revelation*. Buena Vista, CO: Holy Apostles Convent.

Hout, Michael, Andrew Greeley, & Melissa J. Wilde. 2001. The demographic imperative in religious change in the United States, *American Journal of Sociology* 107.2: 468–500.

Hull, Geoffrey. 2010. *The Banished Heart: Origins of Heteropraxis in the Catholic Church*. London: T&T Clark.

Hunter, James Davison. 1991. *Culture Wars*. New York: Basic Books.

Huntington, Samuel P. 2011 [1966]. *The Clash of Civilizations and the Remaking of World Order.* New York: Simon & Schuster.

Hutchison, William R. 1989. *Between the Times: The Travail of the Protestant Establishment in America, 1900–1960.* New York: Cambridge University Press.

Index to International Public Opinion, 1978–1978. 1980. Westport, CN: Greenwood Press.

ITV Staff. 2013. The interview that shook the world, *Inside the Vatican* 21.9 (November): 17–21.

John Paul II. 1998. *Fides et ratio.* Vatican City: Libreria editrice vaticana.

John Paul II. 1993. *Veritatis splendor.* Vatican City: Libreria editrice vaticana.

Jones, Kenneth C. 2003. *Index of Leading Catholic Indicators: The Church since Vatican II.* Fort Collins, CO: Roman Catholic Books.

Jungmann, Joseph A. 1951. *The Mass of the Roman Rite: Its Origins and Development,* trans. Francis A. Brunner. New York: Benziger Brothers.

Kant, Immanuel. 1960. *Religion within the Limits of Reason Alone,* trans. Theodore Greene & Hoyt Hudson. New York: Harper Torchbooks.

Katz, Jacob. 1993. *Tradition and Crisis: Jewish Society at the End of the Middle Ages,* trans. Bernard Cooperman. New York: Schocken Books.

Kelly, David F. 1979. *The Emergence of Roman Catholic Medical Ethics in North America.* New York: Edwin Mellen Press.

Kelly, Gerald. 1949. *Medico-moral problems,* Part I. St. Louis, MO: Catholic Hospital Association.

Kelly, Gerald. 1950. *Medico-moral problems,* Part II. St. Louis, MO: Catholic Hospital Association.

Kelly, Gerald. 1951. *Medico-moral problems,* Part III. St. Louis, MO: Catholic Hospital Association.

Kelly, Gerald. 1953. *Medico-moral problems,* Part IV. St. Louis, MO: Catholic Hospital Association.

Kelly, Gerald. 1954. *Medico-moral problems,* Part V. St. Louis, MO: Catholic Hospital Association.

Kelly, Gerald. 1958. *Medico-Moral Problems.* St. Louis, MO: Catholic Hospital Association.

Kenny, John P. 1962. *Principles of Medical Ethics,* 2nd ed. Westminster, MD: Newman Press.

Kidd, Thomas. 2013. Papal homecoming, *World* 28.17 (August 24): 64.

Kraut, Benny. 1979. *From Reform Judaism to Ethical Culture: The Religious Evolution of Felix Adler*. Cincinnati: Hebrew Union College Press.

Leigh, Edward. 2009. Grave symptoms, in *The Nation that Forgot God*, eds. Edward Leigh & Alex Haydon (pp. 11–21). London: Social Affairs Unit.

Liguori, Alphonsus de. 1862. *Theologia moralis*, ed. Michael Heilig. 6 vols. Paris: Adrianus le Clere.

Liturgikon, The. 1994. Englewood, NJ: Antakya Press.

Longman, Phillip. 2006. The return of patriarchy, *Foreign Policy* 153 (March/April): 56–65.

Longman, Phillip. 2004a. *The Empty Cradle*. New York: Basic Books.

Longman, Phillip. 2004b. The global baby bust, *Foreign Affairs* 83.3 (May/June): 64–79.

Luckmann, Thomas. 1990. Shrinking transcendence, expanding religion? *Sociological Analysis* 51.2: 127–138.

Ludwig, Robert A. 1996. *Reconstructing Catholicism: For a New Generation*. Spring Valley, NY: Crossroad Publishing.

Madambashi, Andrea. 2011. Half of Brazil's population to be evangelical by 2020, *Christian Post U.S.* [On-line] http://www.christianpost.com/news/half-of-bra-zils-population-to-be-evangelical-christian-by-2020–49071/ [accessed February 3, 2016]

Maimonides, Moses. 2001. *Mishneh Torah*. New York: Moznaim Publishing.

Marsden, George M. 1994. *The Soul of the American University*. New York: Oxford University Press.

Marsden, George M. & Bradley J. Longfield (eds.). 1992. *The Secularization of the Academy*. New York: Oxford University Press.

Martini, Cardinal Carlo & Georg Sporschill. 2012. *Night Conversations with Cardinal Martini*, trans. Lorna Henry. New York: Paulist Press.

Mascall, E. L. 1966. *The Secularization of Christianity*. New York: Holt, Rinehart and Winston.

McClory, Robert. 1995. *Turning Point: The Inside Story of the Papal Birth Control Commission*. New York: Crossroads.

McCormick, Richard. 1981. *Notes on moral theology, 1965 through 1980*. Washington, DC: University Press of America.

Merleau-Ponty, M. 1969. *Humanism and Terror*, trans. John O'Neill. Boston: Beacon Press.

Meyer, Michael (ed.). 1997. *German-Jewish History in Modern Times*, vol. 2, *Emancipation and Acculturation 1780–1871*. New York: Columbia University Press.

Miller, Terry. 2014. America's dwindling economic freedom, *Wall Street Journal* 263.11 (January 14): A13.

Mitchell, Peter. 1980. *The Jesuits: A History*. London: Macdonald.

Monk of St. Tikhon's Monastery. 1987. *Book of Needs*. South Canaan, PA: St. Tikhon's Seminary Press.

Motzkin, Gabriel. 1992. *Time and Transcendence: Secular History, the Catholic Reaction, and the Rediscovery of the Future*. Dordrecht: Kluwer.

Moynihan, Daniel Patrick. 1965. *The Negro Family: A Case for National Action*. Washington, DC: U.S. Department of Labor.

Nadeau, Barbie. 2013. Did a cross-dressing priest sex ring bring down Benedict XVI? *The Daily Beast* (February 22). http://news.yahoo.com/did-cross-dressing-priest-sex-ring-bring-down-174300640—politics.html [accessed February 22, 2016]

Nemeth, Roger J. & Donald A. Luidens. 1989. The new Christian right and mainline Protestantism: The case of the Reformed Church in America, *Sociological Analysis* 49.4: 343–352.

Nicodemus and Agapius, Sts. (eds.). 1983. *The Rudder of the Orthodox Catholic Church*, trans. D. Cummings. Chicago: Orthodox Christian Educational Society.

Nietzsche, Friedrich. 1974. *The Gay Science*, trans. Walter Kaufmann. New York: Random House.

Noè, Cardinal Virgilio. 2008. CWNEws.com, 16 May 2008; www.catholicculture.org/news/features/index.cfm?recnum=58473 [accessed September 23, 2015]

Novak, Michael. 2013. Agreeing with Pope Francis, *National Review Online*; http://www.nationalreview.com/node/365720/ [accessed January 25, 2016]

Ottaviani, Alfredo & Antonio Bacci. N.d. *Breve esame critica del "Novus Ordo Missae."* Rome: Fondazione "Lumen gentium".

Overbeck, Franz. 1919. *Christentum und Kultur*. Basel: Schwabe.

Paz, Octavio. 1974. *Children of the Mire*, trans. Rachel Phillips. Cambridge, MA: Harvard University Press.

Pera, Marcello. 2011. *Why We Should Call Ourselves Christians: The Religious Roots of Free Societies*. Jackson, TN: Encounter.

Perniola, Mario. 2001. *Ritual Thinking*, trans. Massimo Verdicchio. Amherst, NY: Humanity Books.

Perry, John. 2013. Utility of utility, *First Things* 231: 17.

Petrà, Basilio. 2011. *I limiti dell'innocenza*. Bologna: Edizioni Dehoniane Bologna.

Pocket Prayer Book for Orthodox Christians. 1956. Englewood, NJ: Antiochian Orthodox Christian Archdiocese.

Ramsey, Paul. 1970. *The Patient as Person*. New Haven, CT: Yale University Press.

Ratzinger, Joseph. 1998. *Milestones*. San Francisco: Ignatius Press.

Ratzinger, Joseph. 1995. *The Nature and Mission of Theology*, trans. Adrian Walker. San Francisco: Ignatius Press.

Ratzinger, Joseph & Marcello Pera. 2006. *Without Roots*, trans. Michael F. Moore. New York: Basic Books.

Reed, John Chelton. 1970. *The Glorious Battle: The Cultural Politics of Victorian Anglo-Catholicism*. Nashville: Vanderbilt University Press.

Reich, Warren. 2003. Shaping and mirroring the field: the *Encyclopedia of Bioethics*, in *The Story of Bioethics*, eds. J. Walter & E. Klein (pp. 165–196). Washington, DC: Georgetown University Press.

Reno, R. R. 2014a. Global culture wars, *First Things* 242 (April): 3–4.

Reno, R. R. 2014b. Francis and the market, *First Things* 240 (February): 3–5.

Roberts, Jason A. 2011. *Reasons for Resistance: The Hierarchy of the Catholic Church Speaks on the Post-Vatican II Crisis*. Raleigh, NC: Queen of Martyrs Press.

Robbins, Jeffrey W. 2004. Weak theology, *Journal of Cultural and Religious Theory* 5.2: 1–4.

Romanides, John S. 2008. *Patristic Theology*, trans. Hieromonk Alexios (Trader). Dalles, OR: Uncut Mountain Press.

Romanides, John S. 2002. *The Ancestral Sin*, trans. George S. Gabriel. Ridgewood, NJ: Zephyr Publishing.

Rorty, Richard. 2004. Foreword, in Gianni Vattimo, *Nihilism & Emancipation*, ed. Santiago Zabala, trans. William McCuaig (pp. ix–xxiii). New York: Columbia University Press.

Rorty, Richard. 1999. Religion as conversation-stopper, in *Philosophy and Social Hope*. London: Penguin.

Rorty, Richard. 1991. *Objectivity, Relativism, and Truth*. New York: Cambridge University Press.

Rose, Michael S. 2014. The associate editor replies, *New Oxford Review* 81.1 (Jan.–Feb.): 13–14.

Rose, Michael S. 2002. *Goodbye, Good Men: How Liberals Brought Corruption into the Catholic Church*. Washington, DC: Regnery.

Rubenstein, Richard L. 1966. *After Auschwitz: Radical Theology and Contemporary Judaism*. Indianapolis: Bobbs-Merrill.

Runciman, Stephen. 1955. *The Eastern Schism*. Oxford: Oxford University Press.

Scalfari, Eugenio. 2013a. The pope: how the church will change, *La Repubblica* (October 1) http://www.repubblica.it/cultura/2013/10/01/news/pope_s_conversation_with_scalfari_english-67643118/ [accessed October 3, 2014]

Scalfari, Eugenio. 2013b. http://www.vatican.va/holy_father/francesco/speeches/2013/october/documents/papa-francesco_20131002_intervista-scalfari_en.html [accessed April 12, 2015 - no longer available]

Schaff, Philip & Henry Wace. 1994. *Seven Ecumenical Councils*, vol. 14 of *Nicene and Post-Nicene Fathers*. Peabody, MA: Hendrickson Publishers.

Schotsmans, Paul. 2005. Integration of bio-ethical principles and requirements into European Union statutes, regulations and policies, *Acta Bioethica* 11: 37–46.

Schott, Anselm. 1961. *Das vollständige Römische Messbuch*. Freiburg im Breisgau: Herder.

Sgreccia, Elio Cardinal. 2012. *Personalist Bioethics: Foundations and Applications*, trans. John di Camillo & Michael Miller. Philadelphia: National Catholic Bioethics Center.

Shapiro, Edward S. 2014. The decline and rise of secular Judaism, *First Things* 241 (March): 41–46.

Sheehan, Thomas. 1984. Revolution in the church. *The New York Review of Books* 13.10 (June 14): 35–45.

Shuster, Simon. 2013. The world according to Putin, *Time* 182.12 (September 16): 30–35.

Singer, Peter. 2011. *Practical Ethics*, 3rd ed. New York: Cambridge University Press.

Sloan, Douglas. 1994. *Faith and Knowledge: Mainline Protestantism and American Higher Education*. Louisville: Westminster John Knox.

Sloan, Douglas. 1973. *The Great Awakening and American Education*. New York: Teachers College Press.

Solomon, David, Ping-Cheung Lo, Ruiping Fan, & H. Tristram Engelhardt, Jr. 2012. Ritual as a cardinal category of moral reality: An introduction, in *Ritual and the Moral Life*, eds. David Solomon, Ping-Cheung Lo, & Ruiping Fan (pp. 1–13). Dordrecht: Springer.

Sopko, Andrew J. 1998. *The Theology of John Romanides*. Dewdney, B.C., Canada: Synaxis Press.

Tanner, Norman P. (ed.). 1990. *Decrees of the Ecumenical Councils*, 2 vols. Washington, DC: Georgetown University Press.

Taylor, Charles. 1975. *Hegel.* Cambridge: Cambridge University Press.

Taylor, Mark C. 1984. *Erring: A Postmodern A/theology.* Chicago: University of Chicago Press.

Trilling, Lionel. 1966. *Beyond Culture.* London: Secker & Warburg.

Vasileios [Gontikakis]. 1984. *Hymn of Entry*, trans. Elizabeth Briere. Crestwood, NY: St. Vladimir's Seminary Press.

Vattimo, Gianni. 2005. What is religion's future after metaphysics? in Richard Rorty and Gianni Vattimo, *The Future of Religion*, ed. Santiago Zabala (pp. 55–81). New York: Columbia University Press.

Vattimo, Gianni. 2002. *After Christianity*, trans. Luca D'Isanto. New York: Columbia University Press.

Vattimo, Gianni. 1982. Ornamento monumento, *Rivista di estetica* 12: 36–43.

Vattimo, Gianni & René Girard. 2010. *Christianity, Truth, and Weakening Faith*, ed. Pierpaolo Antonello, trans. William McCuaig. New York: Columbia University Press.

Vattimo, Gianni & Pier Rovatti (eds.). 1983. *Il pensiero dobele.* Milan: Feltrinelli.

von Hartmann, Eduard. 1874. *Die Selbstzersetzung des Christenthums.* Berlin: Duncker's.

Walters, Leroy. 2003. The birth and youth of the Kennedy Institute of Ethics, in *The Story of Bioethics*, eds. J. Walter & E. Klein (pp. 215–231). Washington, DC: Georgetown University Press.

Weidemann, Siggi. 1989. Altäre unter dem Hammer, *Süddeutsche Zeitung*, April 18.

Wicks, Peter. 2013a. Utility's deceptions, *First Things* 229 (January): 59–61.

Wicks, Peter. 2013b. Peter Wicks replies, *First Things* 231 (March): 17.

Wiltgen, Ralph. 1967. *The Rhine Flows into the Tiber.* New York: Hawthorn Books.

Woodward, Kenneth L. 2013. Reflections on the revolution in Rome, *First Things* 230 (February): 25–31.

Zabala, Santiago. 2005. A religion without theists or atheists, in Richard Rorty and Gianni Vattimo, *The Future of Religion*, ed. Santiago Zabala (pp. 1–27). New York: Columbia University Press.

CHAPTER EIGHT

Living Without God[1]

I. Hegel and Post-Modernity

We turn again to Hegel. Hegel is so important because he diagnosed and widened the intellectual point of rupture from which the now-dominant secular culture has emerged. Without a further examination and assessment of Hegel, we cannot adequately appreciate the significance of the severance of the dominant culture from any anchor in the transcendent. In the first decade of the 19th century, Hegel more clearly than any other recognized and then abetted a revolution in the significance of morality, religion, and the authority of the state. As noted in chapter two, Hegel is best interpreted as having resolutely fashioned a post-metaphysical view of reality (Hartmann 1972). This chapter draws on latter-day Hegelians such as Alexander Kojève (1902–1968, the nephew of Wassily Kandinsky), Francis Fukuyama, and Gianni Vattimo in order to gauge better the significance of the loss after God of moorings for morality and political authority. This chapter and this book close with reflections on the instability of a society severed from ultimate meaning. En passant, the challenge of the growing Muslim populations in Europe and whether they constitute a threat to European secular dreams of peace and laicism are considered. The book closes by addressing an issue confronted in the previous chapter: our knowledge of God. To the dismay of non-believers, and despite the best efforts of the dominant secular culture, God can unexpectedly break in on our lives.

As chapter two showed, we face the culture after God that Hegel foresaw. This book has explored this state of affairs and its implications for morality, bioethics, law, and public policy. It has examined how very different reality and morality cum bioethics and health care policy appear without God.[2] As we have seen, before the Enlightenment, the regnant culture recognized God and immortality. With dramatic implications, God and immortality are now widely forgotten: morality is both demoralized and deflated. Kant attempted, without really acknowledging God's existence, to hide from these implications by affirming as practical moral postulates God and immortality.[3] In fact, Kant hoped to secure all of the content of traditional Western Christian morality without acknowledging Christ as God, indeed without even recognizing an actually existing God.[4] The intellectual descendants of these Kantians took for granted that they could have a well-developed culture along with a morality and bioethics grounded in human dignity and human rights. As Rorty put it, Kantians "are the people who think there are such things as intrinsic human dignity, intrinsic human rights, and an ahistorical distinction between the demands of morality and those of prudence" (Rorty 1991, p. 197). Such intellectual descendants of Kant presume a rational substitute for a God's-eye perspective. The difficulty is, as we have seen, that such supporting foundations do not exist. Without God, there is only a quicksand of foundationless moral speculations into which one sinks.

Hegel embraced the implications of the post-theistic Christian culture that broke upon Europe after the Enlightenment and the French Revolution. As chapters two and three demonstrated, Hegel approached this state of affairs by philosophically resituating the significance of Christianity, God, and morality (and thus implicitly bioethics), through renouncing any claims about a canonical, content-full morality transcending time and place. As Rorty summarized matters, Hegelians recognize "that there is no human dignity that is not derivative from the dignity of some specific community, and no appeal beyond the relative merits of various actual or proposed communities to impartial criteria which will help us weigh those merits" (Rorty 1991, p. 197). Where Kant moralized religion, Hegel rendered religion after God in even the deistic sense of God. Hegel both diagnosed the roots of post-modernity and contributed to the loss of the remnants of modernity's faith that reason is one and canonical. Hegel marked a crucial turning point in world history.

> If the Hegelians are right, then there are no ahistorical criteria for deciding when it is or is not a responsible act to desert a community, any more than for deciding when to change lovers or professions. The Hegelians see nothing to be responsible to except persons and actual or possible historical

communities; so they view the Kantians' use of 'social responsibility' as misleading (Rorty 1991, p. 198).

It is now apparent that all secular moral categories are socio-historically conditioned, with the consequence that not only is secular moral pluralism intractable and bioethics a plural noun, but the meaning of morality and political authority have been transformed. Hegel is at the roots of post-modernity,[5] the recognition of the unavoidable condition of secular moral and bioethical pluralism, as well as the loss of any ultimate, transcendent point of orientation. Hegel allows one to appreciate the unavoidability of secularism's solipsism of a world floating within the horizon of the finite and the immanent, without an anchor in God, in being, or indeed in canonical rationality.

In 1802 in "Glauben und Wissen," Hegel confronted the significance of the growing cultural salience of "the feeling that 'God Himself is dead,' upon which the religion of more recent times rests" (Hegel 1977, p. 190; Hegel 1968, pp. 413–4).[6] The fabric of Western civilization was changing radically. All being, all culture, all reality would need to be rethought as now within a context after God. This cultural watershed loss of transcendence constituted "the Golgotha of Absolute Spirit" of which Hegel in 1807 speaks on the last page of *The Phenomenology of Mind* (Hegel 1910, p. 808). Hegel proclaimed that all that had been anchored in the transcendent must die to the beyond and be relocated within the ambit of immanence.[7] Hegel, wishing to establish a culture cut free from transcendence, affirmed that this radical shift in perspective "must re-establish for philosophy the Idea of absolute freedom and along with it the absolute Passion, the speculative Good Friday in place of the historic Good Friday. Good Friday must be speculatively re-established in the whole truth and harshness of its God-forsakenness" (Hegel 1977, p. 190; Hegel 1968, p. 414). Using Christian language, he aimed to turn Christianity on its head. God and the Resurrection were to be relocated within a philosophical vision, in which God has been rendered fully immanent. This is the kenosis of which Vattimo speaks and to which we will shortly turn: the kenosis of a "god" now incarnate within immanence who is dead to any hint of the transcendent (Rorty & Vattimo 2005). Hegel accepted that, once God's transcendent standpoint is no longer recognized within a culture, reality along with morality (and by implication bioethics) is cut loose from moorings in anything beyond our immanence. When a culture is deaf and blind to God's existence, when God is dead in a culture, all is by default embedded in being-as-it-is-for-us, cut off from being-as-it-is-in-itself apart from us. All is without ultimate meaning. Not being able to settle "the most profound human disagreements" (Owen 2001, p. 2), a culture after God must try to make do with attempting to deflate those questions into terms compassable by a dominant immanent narrative.

An implication of this state of affairs for Hegel is that philosophers and, more broadly, intellectuals, including bioethicists, who are in accord with and articulate the dominant culture of the age, become an immanent surrogate for God. In self-conscious reflection, they constitute the final standpoint, the final criterion for reality and morality. They are as close as it gets within the horizon of the finite and the immanent to a God's-eye perspective. In the absence of a God's-eye perspective for the secular culture, they serve the function of God by being the final criterion for reality and morality. The view of reality affirmed by these intellectuals becomes reality. This is the force of Hegel's acknowledgement of philosophers as Absolute Spirit or God conscious of himself: "God is God only so far as he knows himself: his self-knowledge is, further, a self-consciousness in man and man's knowledge *of* God, which proceeds to man's self-knowledge *in* God" (Hegel 1971, p. 298, §564). Once locked within the horizon of the finite and the immanent, there is no perspective beyond the perspective of these intellectuals. It is these intellectuals within a secular culture who self-reflectively articulate the final (albeit always provisional and historically conditioned) answers to the questions of the age, including all the questions raised in secular bioethics. These intellectuals complete the circle of being and thought. They reflect on how thought thinks about thought thinking about being, which in the end is what thought thinks it is. The truly philosophical of the philosophers who explicitly engage in categorial philosophical reflection constitute the final reflective standpoint within the horizon of the finite and the immanent. One must recall that the first two major categories of Hegel's Absolute Spirit are art and religion. It is philosophy, the third category, which is the higher truth or full explicit realization of Absolute Spirit. Its standpoint is that of the community that can appreciate and judge its own one-sidedness and incompleteness and thus transcend that one-sidedness. For Hegel, this transcendence is as good as it gets.

Peter Berger in a Hegelian fashion recognizes the cardinal role of those intellectuals who define the reality of the age (and are thus Absolute Spirit). These secular pundits who take the standpoint of Absolute Spirit both shape and define our now-dominant secular culture. He observes:

There exists an international subculture composed of people with Western-type higher education, especially in the humanities and social sciences, that is indeed secularized. This subculture is the principal "carrier" of progressive, Enlightened beliefs and values. While its members are relatively thin on the ground, they are very influential, as they control the institutions that provide the "official" definitions of reality, notably the educational system, the media of mass communication, and the higher reaches of the legal system. They are remarkably similar all over the world today, as they have been for a long time (though, as we have seen, there are also defectors from this subculture, especially in the Muslim countries). Again, regrettably, I cannot speculate here as to why people with this type of education should be so prone to secularization. I can only point out that what we have here is a globalized *elite* culture (Berger 1999, p. 10).

This Absolute Spirit of the early 21st century includes not just philosophers and bioethicists, but also members of the media, as well as artists and theologians, especially liberal theologians.[8] This standpoint of Absolute Spirit does not include traditional Christian theologians who have been placed by the post-Christian culture in an intellectual exclave because they hold a set of moral and intellectual viewpoints considered superceded, politically incorrect, and beyond the pale. Such are excluded because they recognize the sinfulness of homosexual acts, as well as for having a politically "insensitive" bioethics that condemns such actions as abortion and the insemination of lesbians. Traditional Christianity is thus placed as beyond the pale by the dominant secular culture. However, this dominant and leading intellectual class includes post-Pope-Francis Roman Catholic bioethicists and their bioethics, insofar as they have embraced a weak theology and thus softly distanced themselves from the intellectual ghetto into which traditional Christians are placed. Their position is enhanced insofar as they endorse populist socio-economic concerns.

This global secular intellectual class incarnates the final, secular, intellectual perspective on contemporary reality, morality, and bioethics. As the explicitly self-reflective class, as those who in self-reflection reason about reason in fully immanent terms, philosophers are the higher truth of all there is within the horizon of the finite and the immanent. They are Absolute Spirit's full and final meaning. All discursive rational questions within the dominant culture are in the end settled by and within this intellectual class, insofar as these questions within any age, and within the horizon of the finite and the immanent, can be rationally raised and settled. For Hegel, Absolute Spirit is the final and highest instance of the "true infinite," philosophical reflection that appreciates the one-sidedness and incompleteness of all finite or particular perspectives, insofar as this can be done. Without a transcendent God's-eye perspective to relativize the perspective of philosophy, there is no reality to be recognized beyond the sphere of human reflective thought.[9] There are only relative perspectives, post-modern Absolute Spirits, particular historically embedded accounts that recognize their own embeddedness in history. All immanent perspectives, including all moral-ity and bioethics, are always socio-historically conditioned.

The perspectives are always in principle plural. One confronts "[t]he disap-pearance of a unitary sense of history, conceived as objective rationality, [which] is a consequence, an aspect, or rather the true and proper meaning, of the death of God" (Vattimo 2004, p. 52). Any secular view of reality is always one among a plurality of possible socio-historically-embedded understandings. Philosophy can at best provide an overview of this pluralism. Philosophy cannot through rational analyses and sound rational argument set this pluralism aside. The dom-inant intellectual class, especially philosophers, can recognize and intellectually place post-modernity. They can recognize that moral pluralism in bioethics is intractable, and that post-modernity is entrenched in the fallen human condi-tion, because after God there is no canonical secular perspective. Nevertheless, secular philosophers thinking about thought thinking about reality are Absolute Spirit, because they rationally, self-consciously apprehend reality as best as pos-sible after God. They perform this function specially when they undercut the rationality undergirding foundationalisms such as Kant's. Within the horizon of the finite and the immanent, they are "the self-thinking Idea, the truth aware of itself" (Hegel 1971, p. 313, §574).

In the spirit of Hegel, one can even have a Christianity that is after God, after any ultimate answers, after any "truths" that point beyond the horizon of the finite and the immanent and towards the transcendent. Consequently, the now-dominant secular culture is after God, even when it talks about God. Hegel stands out in that he recognized the emergence of a post-Christian world-view. He endorsed this state of affairs and supported its development, including a Christianity after God, although he preserved a superficially Christian discourse. Such Christianities after God step beyond Kant's "as-if" God and beyond his postulated God. One can in this context after God appreciate the place of post-theistic Christian theologians such as Paul Tillich (1886–1965), regarding whom Rorty mused:

> when people asked why he [Tillich] didn't stop pretending to be a Christian theologian and instead bill himself as a Heideggerian philosopher . . . [h]e would say, in effect, that it was precisely the job of a Christian theologian these days to find a way of making it possible for Christians to continue using the term "Christ" even after they had given up supernaturalism (as he hoped they eventually would) (Rorty 1991, p. 70).

As Santiago Zabala observed, such a "Christianity without God represents a faith free from the objectivistic metaphysics that believed in its own ability to demonstrate, on the basis of 'sound natural reason,' the existence of a Supreme Being" (Zabala 2005, p. 14). The very notion of a Supreme Being is recast within the compass of human culture. Religion, following Ronald Dworkin, becomes without God (Dworkin 2013). The truth of the dominant culture of the contemporary age is rendered fully immanent.

The force of Hegel's claim that "thought and being are one" is vertiginous (Hegel, 1977, p. 190; Hegel 1968, p. 413). Everything is seen in terms of what we make of it. There is no reality that is not being-for-us. There is no secular morality or bioethics that is not the morality or bioethics of a particular community. After God, the notion of the reality we face and within which we live is recast in immanent terms. One can reflect on the post-modern context within which we find ourselves, but secular philosophy cannot transcend it. Philosophy cannot disclose any unconditioned ultimate meaning. It is not simply that philosophy cannot show us a way free from our socio-historically conditioned context, but as Hegel appreciated, philosophy has been recast so as to cut off any reference to the truly transcendent. The result is not simply that for post-modernity God is immanentized and obscured within the perspective of the dominant philosophical, intellectual class, but that all reality and morality (including bioethics) are to be regarded as existing fully within the dominant culture's grand narrative. Because one is to eschew reference to, or even thought about, a thing-in-itself, much less thought about a truly transcendent God, morality is recognized as fully socio-historically conditioned and therefore falling fully within the horizon of the finite and the immanent. It is for this reason that the dominant secular cultural narrative, including any particular secular bioethics, is always one freestanding account among others that floats unanchored in sociohistorically conditioned being within the horizon of the finite and the immanent, supported by Hegel's very immanent Absolute Spirit. In this way, Hegel sought to undermine what he took to be the half-measures of Kant. As James Kreines correctly puts it,

> Hegel seeks to advance yet farther Kant's revolution *against* pre-critical metaphysics. . . . Hegel denies all need to even conceive of Kant's things in themselves, leaving no contrast relative to which our own knowledge could be said to be merely limited or restricted. That is, Hegel aims not to *surpass* Kant's restriction so much as to *eliminate* that restriction from the inside (Kreines 2007, p. 307).

There are no constraints beyond the constraints or grammar of thought, and even these are socio-historically conditioned. Not only is God dead in the secular culture, but so, too, is the possibility of a canonical secular grammar. Once God is no longer recognized, all in the end floats freely without any anchor in being or in a canonical rationality.

The result is that, after God, within the horizon of the finite and the immanent all changes when the categories of the dominant culture change. There is no socio-historically independent standard of reality and morality. Absolute Spirit as the final available self-reflective perspective not only registers but affirms the depth and breadth of these changes in reality. The question is then how deep the changes go. The answer is not just that the changes go to the roots, but that the roots do not transcend being as it is for us, or reach beyond the horizon of the finite and the immanent. Hegel argues, for example:

All cultural change reduces itself to a difference of categories. All revolutions, whether in the sciences or world history, occur merely because spirit has changed its categories in order to understand and examine what belongs to it, in order to possess and grasp itself in a truer, deeper, more intimate and unified manner (Hegel 1970, p. 202).

One might be tempted to construe Hegel's position in conformity with a weak reading of Thomas Kuhn (1962), taking the full force of changes of categories as involving only changes in the categories of knowing. However, Hegel's claim is far more radical than a claim only about the categories of the knower. Within a particular culture, the dominant ideology, its "paradigm," *is* reality. At stake are the categories not just of appearance, but of being, because all being is regarded as being for us. After God, a change of paradigms involves a change in the ontology of the known, a change in being insofar as one can refer to being, because insofar as being is, being is for us. Kuhn did not dare explicitly to go quite that far.

As thought changes, reality changes, because within the horizon of the immanent, thought and being are one. As the major ways in which thought apprehends being (i.e., the categories of thought) change, so, too, does being (i.e., the categories of being), for after God all being is being as it is for us; being can only be insofar as it is for thought. All is embedded in, exists in, an all-encompassing solipsism. The ways in which being is for thought are congruent with the ways in which thought apprehends being, for again thought and being are one. This recognition lies as well behind the linguistic turn of analytic philosophy, as Arthur Danto appreciates in his reflections on Nietzsche.

The pages of *Mind* would have been one of the forums in which what we think of today as analytical philosophy took shape, with its central teaching that the problems of philosophy are *au fond* problems of language, however heavily disguised. But just this, I came to believe, was Nietzsche's own view, that the structures of language determine what are the structures of reality for those whose language it is, and that the deep order of the world, so sought by philosophers of the past, is but the cast shadow of the deep order of their grammar (Danto 1980, p. 8).

Because after God there is no reality beyond the reality that is for us, then there is no structure of reality beyond the grammar of our language and our thought. On this point, Dupré embraces a similar viewpoint that captures the force of Hegel's position.

> Cultural changes, such as the one that gave birth to the modern age, have a definitive and irreversible impact that transforms the very essence of reality. Not merely our thinking about the real changes: reality itself changes as we think about it differently. History carries an ontic significance that excludes any reversal of the present. Nor is it possible to capture that changing reality in an ahistorical system (Dupré 1993, p. 6).

As we saw in chapter two, it is for this reason that, being deaf and blind to God's existence and cut off from any anchor in being-as-it-is-in-itself apart from how being-as-it-is-for-us, morality is demoralized and deflated. Each particular secular bioethics with its account of abortion, third-party-assisted reproduction, health care resource allocation, informed consent, physician-assisted suicide, euthanasia, etc., constitutes a fabric of life-style choices framed by the macro life-style choices regarding morality and bioethics themselves, which are always framed by a particular morality and bioethics.

Within this account, at least in broad categorial terms, reality, morality, and bioethics are as the dominant culture construes them. It is a moral and intellectual landscape in which there is no ultimate meaning. Again, the narrative of the dominant culture, along with the morality and reality it sustains, floats free of any ultimate anchor beyond the horizon of the finite and the immanent. For this reason, secular moral philosophers, bioethicists, and intellectuals generally can invoke their own moral intuitions as normatively decisive for the dominant secular morality and bioethics. Their intuitions are normative for their immanent culture, because their intuitions disclose reality for us. Again, as Absolute Spirit, secular intellectuals are those who articulate the cardinal intuitions of the dominant narrative. For their culture, indeed for the dominant global culture, these people are the final judges of immanent reality, along with the dominant morality and bioethics. They reveal what is the case. They disclose the meaning of what is law and public policy, or at least of what within that dominant culture they hold law and public policy to be. Within the dominant culture, these intellectuals as Absolute Spirit consider themselves able on their own to exposit the character of their morality, politics, and reality after God. Their reality, though socially constructed, appears to them as a fact of the matter. As a consequence, Hegel can be characterized as defending a naturalism with family resemblances to Aristotle (Pinkard 2012).

Given the demoralization and deflation of morality (and therefore of bioethics), as well as the delegitimization of political authority (and therefore of health care policy), along with any canonical grounds for liberal constitutionalism, the members of this intellectual class are by default also the defenders of the dominant secular and liberal-democratic faith against those who challenge it. They articulate the political agenda, including the health care policy agenda, of the secular fundamentalist state (Engelhardt 2010a and 2010b), as a taken-for-granted reality, even though they are unable by conclusive sound rational argument to justify their morality or their political agenda, including their vision of the politically reasonable and of the proper constitutional framework. In lieu of anything better, they articulate a political rhetoric that poses as moral truth, because they are the class that articulates and sustains the established culture, its morality, its view of bioethics, and its account of the state. One finds a secular culture in which bioethical, moral, and political claims regarding human rights, human dignity, and equality are advanced as if they were definitive and canonical, all without sufficient justification and despite a growing acknowledgement of the ethnocentrism of these claims (Rorty 1991, p. 2). Because there is no immanent view from nowhere, all immanent views are a view from somewhere and therefore socio-historically embedded, ethnocentric, and particular. In the absence of a God's-eye perspective, the boundaries are thereby erased that once separated morality and political ideology. With no final point of reference, in the absence of a God's-eye perspective, the expositors of the regnant morality, the community of intellectual reflection, become the god of the age. This community of intellectuals is the ground of the reality that this culture embraces. Those who disagree are not just "wrong" but crazy. As a consequence, those who fundamentally disagree with the dominant secular view of morality and reality are regarded, as Rorty puts it, as crazy because "the limits of sanity are set by what *we* [like-minded secular liberals] can take seriously" (Rorty 1991, pp. 187–188). They are "crazy" because they do not recognize the established reality.[10]

Hegel's thought marks the emergence of our contemporary secular culture without roots and without foundations. Much of what had only become apparent to a few at the beginning of the 19th century, but which Hegel recognized and affirmed, by the beginning of the 21st century had become widely manifest. Hegel by his mid-thirties had lived through the end of the Western Christian empire when the last emperor, Francis II, abdicated on August 6, 1806, the Feast of the Transfiguration. Hegel saw the death of what had been the political symbol of the unity of Western Christendom: the Western Christian empire. Hegel surveyed a Western Christendom left in shards. The surviving traditional Christians had been left to live in the ruins. What remains now is a radically transformed cultural context that is after Christianity and after God. Even now as then, over against the dominant secular culture, there remain various counter-cultures, such as traditional Christianity and Orthodox Judaism. These counter-cultures at times still unexpectedly invade the public forum. The dominant culture is also marked by a range of agnosticisms and atheisms of different levels of explicitness and passion. On the one hand, there are the militant new atheists such as Richard Dawkins, Daniel Dennett, Sam Harris, and Christopher Hitchens. On the other hand, there are those who have a "spirituality" to various degrees separated from traditional religious roots. They include post-traditional, indeed post-theistic Christians, who in the spirit of Hegel are committed to being "believers" but without the affirmation of any transcendent truth. In any event, for them canonical objectivity and traditional Christianity are gone.

The result is a post-theistic Christianity born of Hegel's turn to immanence. For example, Vattimo articulates his Christianity through a substantial recasting of the kenosis of Christ.[11] Vattimo construes Christ's Incarnation as a rejection of transcendence, as Christ's becoming only human, thus allowing a "nihilistic rediscovery of Christianity" (Vattimo 1999, p. 34). Christ's kenosis becomes for Vattimo "God's renunciation of his own sovereign transcendence" (Rorty & Vattimo 2005, p. 51). Vattimo uses this radical and distorted reading of Philippians (Phil 2:7) as a way of forwarding his claim that "postmodern nihilism (the end of meta-narratives) is the truth of Christianity" (Rorty & Vattimo 2005, p. 51). Vattimo's post-theistic Christianity, which grows out of Hegel, eschews the metaphysics of the new atheists (Rorty & Vattimo 2005, p. 63), while rendering explicit what is implicit in Hegel. A shadow of Christianity is allowed to remain, explicitly emptied of any claims to objective truth, such that the force of its images is set within a particular, post-metaphysical narrative. The goal is to render Christianity into a belief without metaphysical substance, guided by a "theology of secularization" (Vattimo 1999, p. 63). As with Habermas's "non-destruction secularization" of religion (Habermas & Ratzinger 2006, p. 29), religion will be allowed to be seen in public, but only as long as it appears without any substance, as merely cultural. Religion, and in particular Christianity, is to be detheologized, while being allowed to persist in secularly transformed "religious" images and rituals. This was all affirmed by Hegel. Is it obliquely suggested by Pope Francis?

Thomas J. Altizer (1927–) in the mid-20th century rode the crest of the "death of God" reflections of the 1960s (Altizer 1966; Vahanian 1961). He became a major figure in the emergence of radical theology, a happening publicly recognized on the April 8, 1966, cover of *Time*: "Is God dead?" *Time* appreciated that the everyday lifeworld within the dominant secular culture of the West had been radically cut loose from its roots in reality-in-itself. There was no longer a recognizable point of orientation in terms of a canonical God's-eye perspective. Altizer addressed this foundational severance of reality along with culture from God's presence. This severance possesses similarities to what Hegel reported in the first decade of the nineteenth century when he reflected on the death of God in Western European thought. Altizer further developed ideas already voiced by William Hamilton:

> The experiences of many men in our time have suggested that the traditional sovereign and omnipotent God is a difficult God to perceive or to meet. In place of this God, the impotent God, suffering with men, seems to be emerging. . . . I am not referring to a belief in the non-existence of God. I am talking about a growing sense, in both non-Christians and Christians, that God has withdrawn, that he is absent, even that he is somehow dead. . . . This feeling ranges from a sturdy unbelieving confidence in God's demise to

the troubled believer's cry that he is no longer in a place where we can call upon him (Hamilton 1961, pp. 54–56).

This radical change in the dominant culture, which Hamilton and others acknowledged, rests on a foundational change in the character of theological discourse, which was occurring as alterations in the worship and beliefs of Western Christianity were taking place. Much of Christianity was being severed from its historical and dogmatic roots, leaving most of traditional Western Christianity in decline, if not also in chaos (Cox 1965; Küng 1966; Macquarrie 1961; Mascall 1966; Ogden 1961; Robinson 1963; van Buren 1963). The changes were so radical as to support a substantively new genre of religious lifeworlds. Various Christianities are now affirming what Christianity had from its beginnings condemned (e.g., living in concubinage, homosexual liaisons, and the ordination of priestesses). Altizer, who epitomized much of this turning of tradition on its head, was even recognized as having "converted to Satan" (Taylor 2006, p. xii). Many no longer knew where they stood. Everything seemed in transition, unsure, adrift.

In the early 1960s, one encountered a foundational transformation of the meaning of Western Christian theology that was the outcome of the loss of a recognition of God that became widespread in the 19th and early 20th centuries, as well as the changes in the sexual and reproductive mores, which have been explored in chapter 3. One confronts the emergence of an explicitly post-Christian Christianity, as is suggested by some of the remarks of Pope Francis noted in chapter 7. Consider, for example, van Buren's support for a secularized Christianity.

The path which we have described for the secular Christian in the secular world is clear and wide enough to carry the whole Gospel along it. Although we have admitted that our interpretation represents a reduction of Christian faith to its historical and ethical dimensions, we would also claim that we have left nothing essential behind. This claim stands or falls with our interpretation of the language connected with Easter (van Buren 1963, pp. 199–200).

When Jesus is no longer recognized as having physically risen from the dead, Christianity has been radically transformed. What followed was a period of great uncertainty and turbulence, indeed of revolutionary rage, ranging from the Weathermen in the United States (Burrough 2015) to the Baader-Meinhof Gang (also known as the Red Army Faction) in Germany.

Radical theology as an academic discipline was, as Altizer appreciated, deeply indebted to the contemporary mainline theology of the time, especially to Paul Tillich and his quasi-death-of-God idiom, which grew out of previous foundational changes in mainline Christianity. An essentially new way of living and experiencing Christianity was evolving within which even Christ and God were to be recast in Their significance.

> Paul Tillich is, as Thomas Altizer has suggested, the father of contemporary radical theology. Every one of today's radical theologians was either Tillich's student or was profoundly influenced by his writing. In the context of much of today's theological writing, Tillich seems almost conservative. Nevertheless, all radical theologians have elaborated on themes which are at least implicit in Tillich. After all, it was Tillich who asserted in *The Courage To Be* that the God whom Nietzsche said was dead was transcended in a "God above the God of theism" (Rubenstein 1966, p. 243).

In a discourse that was still characterized as theological, the very foundation of theology, *theos*, God, had been brought into question. Popular Christian theology was radically transformed. To use Martin Buber's (1878–1965) metaphor, God was eclipsed. There was an "[e]clipse of the light of heaven, eclipse of God— such indeed is the character of the historic hour through which the world is passing" (Buber 1952, p. 23).[12] This state of affairs was also anticipated by such as Rudolf Bultmann (1884–1976), who found much of the traditional vision of New Testament Christianity unacceptable to contemporary man (Bultmann 1984). These recastings of faith culminated in a culture after God, within which various theologies that treated God as in some sense dead took center stage. These theologies underscored the depth of the changes and the expanse of the gulf separating the contemporary dominant culture from traditional Christianity.

This was a time when persons who would later become prominent conservative Western Christian thinkers noted the vigor and breadth of the changes that followed Vatican II. For example, Michael Novak in 1967 remarked that "The evidence that profound ambiguity has stolen into contemporary Christian consciousness is so overwhelming that one hardly knows where to point" (Novak 1967, p. 237). There was a loss of a common point of orientation, if not the stark presence of disorientation. With conviction, members of the same denomination pointed in contrary directions, while many drew comfort from this chaos. Novak in this period of unclarity observed that "Certain Catholics are closer in spirit to some Presbyterians than either are to many members in their own religious communities" (Novak 1967, p. 259). In addition, Novak, caught in the ecumenical spirit of the 1960s, could even celebrate that "Christianity is ceasing to be sectarian; it is becoming more roundly human" (Novak 1967, p. 259). Vatican II had opened a novel vista of experience and practice that seemed to many to have set the commitments of traditional Christianity aside. As Harry Blamires put the matter,

> There is no longer a Christian mind. . . . [U]nfortunately the Christian mind has succumbed to the secular drift with a degree of weakness and nerveless-ness unmatched in Christian history. It is difficult to do justice in words to the complete loss of intellectual morale in the twentieth-century Church. One cannot characterize it without having recourse to language which will sound hysterical and melodramatic (Blamires 1963, p. 3).

After Vatican II, there was a shattering of past certitudes. A quite different age dawned in which Virginia Woolf's remark that human nature had changed in 1910 gained greater force (Blom 2008, p. 277). Perhaps human nature again changed during Vatican II. Persons in the 1960s came to live after God and increasingly reproduced outside of marriage (Murray 2012). Persons showed a different nature. A new world was present.

> The big change in the outlook of the intellectuals—as opposed to a change in human nature—that happened around 1910 was that they began to be confident that human beings had only bodies, and no souls. The resulting this-worldliness made them receptive to the idea that one's sexual behaviour did not have much to do with one's moral worth (Rorty 1999, pp. 168–169).

A truly post-Christian ethos is now center stage.

Altizer did not simply with Hegel acknowledge God's absence within, indeed exclusion from, the dominant, now secular culture; in addition, Altizer crucially celebrated the death of God as a kerygma to the effect that "everything we know as God is dead, and that this death is the gospel, is the 'good news'" (Altizer 2006, p. 16). The dramatic collapse of traditional Christian culture in the West with the resultant collapse of the mainline Western ecclesial communities led, as Altizer appreciated, to a culture in which "during the sixties . . . America discovered that it was not a Christian nation" (Altizer 2006, p. 17). A profound cultural transition was underway. The West had entered an age after God. The recognition of God in the dominant culture was radically transformed, indeed radically distorted, and then lost, so as to make plausible an aggressively post-Christian secular proclamation: "As my theological work approaches its culmination, I can see that the transfiguration of the Godhead has become its deepest center, and if its previous center was a *coincidentia oppositorum* of Christ and Satan, that, too, can be understood as a transfiguration of the Godhead" (Altizer 2006, p. 168). As Altizer frankly acknowledges, in the culture after God that has emerged, the force of what has occurred is that "the most actual name of God for us is truly the name of Satan" (Altizer 2006, p. 180). The God of traditional Christianity has been set aside, so that an all-encompassing, new ethos that is aggressively anti-traditional-Christian has emerged and gained salience. Altizer fully affirms the deep change in the character of Western culture, a change from being directed to the God of Abraham and Jesus (as affirmed in traditional belief) to being devoted to a focus quite other and profoundly alien from the culture of the past. A post-traditional, post-Christian Christianity has taken shape that has transformed its doctrines (e.g., affirming homosexual marriage and the ordination of priestesses) and its worship (e.g., the Roman Catholic Novus Ordo mass), so that as Altizer puts it, "Nietzsche in knowing God as the deification of nothingness could know the actuality of God more fully than any other thinker since Hegel" (Altizer 2002, p. 142). After God, a new culture cut loose from traditional Christian and traditional Jewish roots has taken shape and become dominant, whose hinge is the negation of God's presence. In this context, one can now understand why so much has changed, and so radically.

The new, fully post-traditional secular West (in which reproduction outside of marriage has become commonplace, if not a norm) is belligerently opposed to traditional Christianity and bent on recasting the character of the public space. The focus of Western public religious zeal has become anti-traditional, "anti-religious." It is an other that is both after traditional Christianity and set against traditional Christianity. The dreams of the French Revolution have finally been fulfilled. Traditional Christianity has been upended and uprooted from the public forum. There has been a transvaluation of values.

> If that apocalypse is occurring even now, it could do so only in a dark and empty mode, but that is a darkness that is finally light, a Satan that is finally Jerusalem. Is it Jerusalem who is now most deeply calling us, and even if that could occur only through the darkness of Satan, or the darkness of a total nihilism, can we nonetheless greet that calling with an ultimate affirmation and an ecstatic joy? (Altizer 2002, p. 152)

Altizer affirms Satan as the full negation of the traditional religion of Abraham that is completed in Jesus. Altizer does this in order to underscore how foundational and radical these new developments are. Altizer regards this as all being implicit in Hegel's recognition of the "death of God" now finally gaining its full force as a rational and willful affirmation. This is the case, so Altizer argues, because

> That which is simply impossible in all other philosophical thinking, the death or ending of Absolute Being itself, becomes not only possible but necessary in Hegelian thinking, and precisely because this is a genuine dialectical thinking, the only fully dialectical thinking that the West has ever known. And the "evil" that Hegel knows in God is a genuine nothingness, and a fully actual nothingness, one that is the inevitable consequence of an absolute self-negation, an absolute self-negation that is an absolute self-alienation, a self-alienation actually embodying nothingness itself (Altizer 2002, pp. 139–140).

In his often perfervid prose, Altizer underscores the dramatic implications of Hegel's acknowledgement of the death of God in the culture of the West. All of this is not to suggest that Altizer is without severe critics. Emil Fackenheim (1915–2003), for example, in speaking of Altizer's *The Gospel of Christian Athe-ism* (1966) underscores "the work's totally inadequate grasp of Hegel, more obviously even than Nietzsche its philosophical patron saint. . . . Hegel lends no support to *The Gospel of Christian Atheism*. On the contrary, he anticipates the move taken in that work and rejects it" (Fackenheim 1967, pp. 207, 208). One might be more nuanced than Fackenheim so as also to recognize that Altizer engages powerful images in order to recast Hegel in radically novel ways. Altizer sees himself as disclosing the higher truth of Hegel regarding the death of God, namely, the loss of any ultimate point of orientation.

Some of the implications of Altizer's radical transformation of theology were anticipated by Dietrich Bonhoeffer's (1906–1945) account of belief "coming of age" in his anticipation of mainline Christianity becoming a "religionless Christianity" (Bonhoeffer 1972). Bonhoeffer, in anticipating the emerging post-Christian Christianity that followed in the 1960s, pointed to a substantively different Christianity than the Christianity of traditional Christianity, what John Caputo would characterize as structured by a theology without theology (Caputo 2006). Bonhoeffer's Christianity involved a substantive recasting of Christianity into a post-transcendent form (Caputo 2006) where Christ is deconstructed into the lord of the secular world. In the *Götterdämmerung* of moral and religious commitments at the end of Hitler's Germany, Bonhoeffer affirmed a Christianity that has lost its religious soul, so that the result is a near cultural self-parody. One must in particular lament that Hitler's Germany triumphed in producing Bonhoeffer's religionless Christianity, which became the dominant Christianity of Germany. Perhaps one can make better sense of Bonhoeffer's position by recalling Alasdair MacIntyre's remarks about an analogous occurrence among the English in the mid-20th century: "The creed of the English is that there is no God and that it is wise to pray to him from time to time" (MacIntyre 1963, p. 10). The result is the realization of a space for cult that is both different from and transformative of the public space and forum that had been inherited from the traditional Christianity of the past.

> The emergence of the radical death of God theology, therefore, is set within a cultural context of ideological crisis: in the absence of universals, of world-views and value-orientations, of sanctions for social arrangements, and of prototypes for individual motivations, the new theology acquires an empirical fit and significance far broader than its sources in academic theology would suggest (Fenn 1968, pp. 171–172).

In the ruins of mainline Western Christianity, one encounters a theology after God.

These cultural transformations reflected, and in part set the stage for, the intra-Roman Catholic broad cultural changes that followed Vatican II, which radical transformations were explored in chapter 7. As a result of the complex theological and moral chaos that emerged, the collapse of mainline Western Christianity led to a major and unanticipated decline in all mainline Christian congregants and clergy. All of this, as we have seen, has been hard for many to assess because Vatican II had been heralded by many Roman Catholics as a new Pentecost. Remarkably, despite the destruction of traditional belief and piety it engendered, even in retrospect these changes were certified as a new Pentecost. Pope John XXIII invoked Pentecostal expectations in his solemn opening address for Vatican II, *Humanae salutis* (December 25, 1961). The "truth" of this expectation, for example, was then confirmed by the International Theological Commission of the Catholic Church (June 21, 2014) in reflection on what had taken place. The central question that nevertheless painfully remains and in a more emphatic tone, given the destructive forces unleashed by Vatican II: what spirit other than the Holy Spirit was it who descended on post-Vatican II Roman Catholicism and Western Christianity generally, given the radically secularizing consequences? How could the "spiritual awakening" that inspired the radically post-traditional and divisive understandings that followed Vatican II be considered Pentecostal? Astoundingly, there never before has been such a dying off of Christianity, absent radical bloodshed. The dramatic loss of clergy and congregants that occurred in the last third of the 20th century in the West was unparalleled in the past. It was a novum. Paradoxically, the Western Christian theological response to the globally remarkable and untoward happenings that followed Vatican II, the startling death of Christianity as the dominant culture of the West, has not in most quarters been to ask what went so radically wrong with and after Vatican II. Instead, there has been a commitment (particularly in Roman Catholicism) to affirm, celebrate, and embrace the transformations that have been tied to the dramatic post-Vatican II collapse of active ecclesial membership, faith, and practice. Indeed, there is a firm commitment on the part of many to declare the whole Vatican II fiasco, evidence to the contrary notwithstanding, a resounding "success," even though in its wake millions left any active involvement in Christianity. Through an ideologically driven denial of the obvious, there has been a large-scale refusal to admit what has actually taken place in the Christianity in the West during the latter part of the 20th century.

After Vatican II as Roman Catholicism's neoscholastic philosophical paradigm was abandoned, one found a cacophony of competing accounts of how to regard theology, Christianity, and indeed reality. The controversies that arose led to monumental theological challenges, indeed more bluntly to a religious cultural cul-de-sac. As a consequence of secularization and the loss of an acknowledgement of God, as well as given the collapse of the dominant philosophical paradigm that had been inherited from the Middle Ages and that had given coherence to Roman Catholicism, Western theology no longer possessed a generally plausible intellectual framework. Much more importantly, having lost a living experience of the presence of the true God, there remained only ideas and arguments set within the horizon of the finite and the immanent. Reflections on the human condition became severed from any hope of access to reality as it is in itself. Against the background of these major cultural events, the mention of theological grounds for moral beliefs became a conversation-stopper in that the dominant culture has become not just thoroughly post-Christian, but even worse, everything has become after God. The result is that in the shadow of a dominant secular culture, within the context of a dominant culture after God, religion in the West, especially after Vatican II, has been separated from a common framework of orientation. The result is that religion has been so thoroughly privatized that rather than the mention of God opening a conversation and the hearts of those in conversation as to why a God's-eye perspective must be considered, mention of God has become disruptive. Recognition of God has been driven into a very private sphere. A major retreat from any hint of a transcendent reality is coming to be enforced. One is not publicly to mention God. Rorty summarized this state of affairs within the rhetoric of his secular advocacy: "The main reason religion needs to be privatized is that, in political discussion with those outside the relevant religious community, it is a conversation-stopper" (Rorty 1999, p. 171).

Kant had thought he could have his atheism while still having a traditional Western Christian morality through the postulates of God and immortality. Hegel appreciated that this is not possible. The consequences for the dominant culture of living after God are vast. The death of God is as well the death of man. It is the death of any hope for a canonical sense of the *humanissimus vir*, of the most truly human man, and of what it is to live *humaniter* (Engelhardt 1991). Humanism is left with only an ambiguous meaning, for there is no canonical account of the truly human. Vattimo summarizes this state of affairs by paraphrasing a joke: "God is dead, but man isn't doing so well himself" (Vattimo 1988, p. 30). Among the consequences is that the humanities, including the medical humanities, have no canonical meaning. They can disclose no canonical way of being human. To Martin Heidegger's (1889–1976) question, "In what does the humanity of humans consist?"[13] there is no canonical answer. It is not just that the classical vision of the *homo humanus* was at root the *homo romanus*, highly ethnocentric, but that all visions of the normatively human are socio-historically located.[14] Again, all is adrift without an anchor in being or conclusive sound rational argument. After rationality, there is animality. What Hegel recognized in the early 19th century laid the basis for Alexander Kojève (1902–1968) and Francis Fukuyama recasting Hegel so as to talk about an end of history found in humans embracing their animality. The world after God leads to a world after humanism, and, as we have also seen, after morality.

II. The Contemporary Human Condition: A Culture Resolutely without Roots[15]

We surely have not yet experienced the full social and political consequences of the secularization of the dominant culture and the large-scale collapse of the mainline Western Christianities, along with the loss for the dominant secular culture of any anchor in reality beyond the merely socio-historically conditioned. We have not yet frankly confronted, much less experienced, what it is to live in societies fully purged of an ultimate point of orientation, having lost any hint of ultimate meaning. Supporters of liberal constitutionalism, democracy, and human rights are only beginning to acknowledge the unnerving state of affairs in which the contemporary secular culture finds itself: secular morality and secular bioethics, along with human equality, human rights, human dignity, and liberal social-democratic commitments, are elements of what turns out to be only a particular macro life-style choice, an ethnocentrism, even if this represents, as Rorty put it, an anti-ethnocentric ethnocentrism (Rorty 1991, p. 2). As we go to the future, the full implications of the lack of foundations for secular culture, secular morality, secular bioethics, clinical ethics, politics, biopolitics, liberal constitutionalism, democracy, and human rights will become ever clearer. This will happen as the dominant secular culture experiences the results of the spreading recognition of the demoralization and deflation of public morality and bioethics, along with the acknowledgement of the moral delegitimization of political authority.[16]

The character of secular societies is likely to change ever more substantially when a major portion of society is innocent of any clear remembrance of the commitments of traditional Christianity or Judaism, or even of the zeal of true-believing utilitarians, Kantians, or defenders of the liberal democratic vision who have the convictions of the Enlightenment. When the grandparents of most people will not have been raised in a traditional religion, when people are the third generation after God, raised by a post-Christian single mother, everything will feel, look, and be for them quite different. A generation will have grown up fully after God, as well as fully within the demoralization and deflation of morality and bioethics, after the delegitimization of political structures, and after the evanescence of the family as a substantive intermediate social structure. People nurtured, schooled, and directed by such a culture will increasingly in their comfortable pursuit of self-realization and self-absorption be without any nostalgia for God, metaphysics, or foundations. For them, a night of riot and pillage after the violation of some civil right or human right will appear only too "natural." This generation will have even less of an anchor in being than the pagans of the pre-Christian Roman Empire, who were nested within a framework of marginally grounded beliefs that gave testimony regarding a transcendent world.

The Christian West had survived as the public ethos in some areas of the West, even into the mid- and in some cases the late-20th century (e.g., in the American Southern Bible belt, upper Bavaria, and Ireland). The traditional Christian ethos of the West characterized the life-world of a great many, if not the majority, of the people I encountered on the streets of Italy in 1954. In contrast, the thoroughly secular generation, the generation that is after God and is still fully to come, the generation that will take for granted the demoralization and deflation of morality, as well as the moral delegitimization of public authority, will consciously feel, see, experience, and know everything within a framework of meaning radically different from that of the traditional Christianity of Italy of the 1950s. They will take for granted a life-world not only fully after Christendom, but after Christianity. Their choices regarding sexuality, reproduction, social relations, marriage, and end-of-life decision-making, their whole way of viewing morality and bioethics, will have been encompassingly transformed into a life-world of post-moral life-style and death-style choices.[17] They will live fully after sin, after any transcendently anchored sense of wrong-doing or ultimate purpose.

These people, locked within the bounds of the finite and the immanent, will gain content for their lives from that which hands can touch, noses smell, tongues taste, ears hear, eyes see, and immanent thought assess. The life-world within which they will be nourished will not support a hunger for a reality beyond the horizon of the finite and the immanent. These humans will have become, to engage a metaphor from Alexander Kojève (1902–1968), human animals. Kojève sees in the American culture of the late 1940s and 1950s the beginning of "Man's return to animality" (Kojève 1969, p. 161, Note), an entrance into a future in which "man will remain alive [but only] as animal."[18] It was an existence fully within the immanent and the finite. Kojève's Hegelian interpretation of history affirmatively looks towards history coming to an end when humans will no longer be engaged in conflicts and wars moved by ideas, much less by concerns for the transcendent. Kojève envisages a final resting point in a human animalistic mutual recognition as satisfied animals that are too well fed to riot and pillage. Then history would not start up again, nor would one once again enter into conflicts moved by ideas.

This view of history extracted from Hegel,[19] communicated to Francis Fukuyama through Allan Bloom (1930–1992), and grounded in Kojève, led Fukuyama to look for an enduring peace that would be realized once there were no longer men ready to die for ideas, but instead only to live as human animals, who would find fulfillment in immanent pleasures and satisfactions. Fukuyama in a sketchy fashion recognized that this retreat within immanence had already occurred by the early 1980s, thus implicitly predicting the collapse of the convictions that had sustained the Soviet bloc. Those living in the Soviet bloc had become more concerned with consumer goods than with the goals of international socialism. This had all led to the final nail in the coffin of the Marxist-Leninist alternative to liberal democracy. . . . nobody in that country truly believed in Marxism-Leninism any longer, and that this was nowhere more true than in the Soviet elite, which continued to mouth Marxist slogans out of sheer cynicism. . . . What has happened in the four years since Gorbachev's coming to power is a revolutionary assault on the most fundamental institutions and principles of Stalinism, and their replacement by other principles which do not amount to liberalism *per se* but whose only connecting thread is liberalism. This is most evident in the economic sphere, where the reform economists around Gorbachev have become steadily more radical in their support for free markets (Fukuyama 1989, p. 12).

The Soviet bloc was about to collapse.

That this was seen fairly clearly by Fukuyama led to the immense success of his book, *The End of History and the Last Man*. There he outlined in greater detail what he saw taking place: a cultural development that promised the end of history, the end of ideological conflicts.

The end of history would mean the end of wars and bloody revolutions. Agreeing on ends, men would have no large causes for which to fight. They would satisfy their needs through economic activity, but they would no longer have to risk their lives in battle. They would, in other words, become animals again, as they were before the bloody battle that began history. A dog is content to sleep in the sun all day provided he is fed, because he is not dissatisfied with what he is. He does not worry that other dogs are doing better than him [sic], or that his career as a dog has stagnated or that dogs are being oppressed in a distant part of the world (Fukuyama 1992, p. 311).

Hegel's account of history is thus recast in the service of offering a development of one of Hegel's key insights: the radical immanentization of morality, reality, and human flourishing. History's final intellectual standpoint is to be a liberal democratic consumerism within which the notion of the truly human is radically deflated into the merely human or animal. With humanity absorbed in the pursuit of self-satisfaction, history would not start up again; one would not again enter into wars moved by ideas.

Under such circumstances, according to Kojève and Fukuyama, there would still be various events about which there would be a historical narrative, but history as a conflict about ideas would have ceased. On this point, Fukuyama still saw "the danger that we will be happy on one level, but still *dis*-satisfied with ourselves on another, and hence ready to drag the world back into history with all its wars, injustice, and revolution" (Fukuyama 1992, p. 312). Fukuyama acknowledges that humans may always at some level recognize that there is more to life than the rich immanent satisfactions of the human animal. Fukuyama's hope is that self-indulgence, consumerism, and a fully immanent mutual recognition can ensure an enduring peace by rendering humans into satisfied animals. This would mean that the need to struggle and find recognition can be fully realized within the pursuit of a satisfying life-style. "[T]he liberal project of filling one's life with material acquisitions and safe, sanctioned ambitions appears to have worked all too well. It is hard to detect great, unfulfilled longings or irrational passions lurking just beneath the surface of the average first-year law associate" (Fukuyama 1992, p. 336). Such a well-fed dog in the sun will remain peaceful despite or perhaps even due to the struggle for better satisfactions.

To sustain its focus on the immanent, on self-indulgence, self-satisfaction, and an immanently directed mutual recognition, such a secular society will act not only to marginalize, but indeed to ban outright, any public intimation of the transcendent. Such a culture's moral and bioethical vision needs to be framed in terms of an understanding of human flourishing that is not simply innocent of any reference to the transcendent, but one that positively eschews interest in the transcendent to the point of being phobic regarding the transcendent. The transcendent will be resisted because it will threaten the reappearance of sin, shame, God, and the recognition of wrongdoing when making "improper" life-style choices. The culture will find itself committed to nourishing a faith that there is nothing transcendent. In order to maintain themselves, such secular societies will need positively to be brought to promote the view that human flourishing can be fully realized and supported within a life-world set within the horizon of the finite and the immanent. The counter-traditional rallying cry in the culture wars, "no tolerance for the intolerant" (where failure to accept the demoralization of morality as, for example, with respect to homosexual acts, will count as intolerance), will be raised to bully traditional believers into silence, to drive them from the public square, to characterize them as bigots, to marginalize them sufficiently so that they constitute no threat to the culture of humans become dogs "content to sleep in the sun" (Fukuyama 1992, p. 311).

Kojève's life-world, amplified by Fukuyama, must secure hegemony for the secular and the immanent. This life-world invites one to become lost within a consumerism and a pursuit of self-satisfaction placed within the social safety net of a substantial social-welfare system supported by democratic structures that provide for a formal mutual recognition, all within a context where "[r]eligion has ... been relegated to the sphere of private life" and then with liberalism bring the possibility of humans returning to animality (Fukuyama 1992, p. 271). All of this, Fukuyama recognizes, only becomes possible after Christendom has fallen and after the marginalization of Christianity by secularism and laicism. As Fukuyama argues, Christianity "had to abolish itself through a secularization of its goals before liberalism could emerge" (Fukuyama 1992, p. 216). Fukuyama, like Hegel and Vattimo, celebrates a post-theistic Christianity. In such circumstances, history as struggle can end.

> For if man is defined by his desire to struggle for recognition, and by his work in dominating nature, and if at the end of history he achieves both recognition of his humanity and material abundance, then "Man properly so-called" will cease to exist because he will have ceased to work and struggle (Fukuyama 1992, p. 310).

Fukuyama argued that Hegel's relocation within the immanent of all that is transcendent allows envisaging the possibility of perpetual peace, a consumer culture that can secure self-satisfaction and mutual recognition so as to realize the end of history, within which there would be no more ideas for which to fight.

In this context, in a world after God, after man, and after history, morality along with bioethics is resituated within the pursuit of the satisfaction not just of needs, but of a growing sphere of desires set within a political framework that affirms mutual recognition. This encourages a developed aesthetic of consumption, in which all are invited to aspire to the hyper-aestheticism of a consumerism that is portrayed in the *Wall Street Journal*'s weekend sections "Off Duty" and "Mansion", where the latter offers estates for the truly affluent, where one can live in (or at least fantasize about living in) opulent settings (e.g., a private island, a large ranch, a seascape, etc.) supported by outbuildings for staff, sports, private jet planes, etc., all marked by an encompassing luxury, including $200,000 closets for wardrobes. Confined within the horizon of the finite and the immanent, without any ultimate anchor, one will need distractions from the danger of confronting and recognizing ultimate meaninglessness. Such a culture tends to seek the distracting and is marked by a much reduced and truncated aesthetic divorced from epiphany and transcendence. There is often a pursuit of the bizarre in order to avoid boredom. For instance, the *Wall Street Journal* reports on fashion shows for the wealthy that reveal a desperate need to overcome boredom: "Thom Browne's [fashion] show was a theater of the absurd set in a mental asylum" (Binkley 2013, p. D1). For those of ordinary means, there will be the hope that their children can realize this abundance. In the meantime, there are rock concerts, drugs, and video games.[20] In a culture marked by the demoralization and deflation of morality, it is hard to set limits to peaceable self-indulgence. "The decline of community life suggests that in the future, we risk becoming secure and self-absorbed last men, devoid of thymotic striving for higher goals in our pursuit of private comforts" (Fukuyama 1992, p. 328).

In the latter part of the 20th century and before September 11, 2001, with the destruction of the twin towers in New York, for many the prospect of enduring peaceable self-indulgence seemed without challenge. For most, the prospect remains. The large-scale decline in commitment to the once-dominant metaphysical world-views of dialectical materialism (e.g., with the collapse of the Soviet Union) and Roman Catholicism (e.g., after its theological disarray and decline following Vatican II), along with other mainline Christianities, has left most Western societies characterized by liberal constitutional commitments, fully immersed in the pursuit of self-satisfaction, self-realization, and self-indulgence. Most are aimed at a life framed within the horizon of the finite and the immanent. In this spirit, Vattimo can approve of the West as "a synonym for consumerism, hedonism, a Babel-like pluralism of cultures, loss of center, and obliviousness to any reference to 'natural' law" (Vattimo 2002, p. 70). Yet, traditionalists such as Peter Mullen see this same state of affairs as pointing to where history may start up again: "Ours is the culture which devout Muslims rightly despise as morally bankrupt" (Mullen 2009, p. 43).[21] Until the fall of the Soviet Union, many saw the West as struggling against godless communism. It was the God-affirming West against the God-denying Soviets. But now, Muslims can aptly portray themselves in contrast to a morally decadent and officially godless West. In the West, for many this has redoubled their commitment to remain after God and after metaphysics. Over against the threat that history may restart, protection is sought from the large-scale violence that would ensue if self-indulgence fails adequately to support a satisfied consumerist welfare state, and its liberal-democratic mutual recognition, and leads instead to a "return to metaphysics."

The pursuit of weak thought, the animus against objective moral truth, translates into a strong animus against traditional Christianity. Traditional Christianity seeks to wake up the happy and satisfied dog. It seeks to re-introduce the condemnation of life-style and death-style choices known by traditional Christians to be evil. Christianity shows that particular ways of life are perverse. Traditional Christianity also discloses a reality worth dying for. This gives ground enough for the defenders of the dominant culture to be opposed to traditional Christianity. Christianity supports norms for conduct that sustain a morality along with a bioethics at odds with the contemporary dominant culture and the pursuit of peace through self-love and self-satisfaction. Traditional Christianity invites the recognition of God-required norms and a reality in conflict with Fukuyama's vision. Santiago Zabala underscores that to prevent metaphysical inclinations from re-surfacing, "Thought must abandon all objective, universal, and apodictic foundational claims in order to prevent Christianity, allied with metaphysics in the search for first principles, from making room for violence" (Zabala 2005, p. 13). All moral claims, including those on behalf of human rights and human dignity, must be located within the methodological agnostic postulate, which must govern the dominant culture in order to re-enforce the ongoing rejection of the transcendent so that the content of everyday life can remain grounded in the hedonic. The peaceable pursuit of pleasure with consenting others becomes central in the affirmation of a fully immanent account. The byword by default becomes Pope Francis's mantra, "Who am I to judge?"[22] There are no canonical secular moral standards. One is left to pursue a pan-ecumenism embracing all Christians, Jews, Muslims, Buddhists, Hindus, etc., in an endless inter-religious dialogue that obscures all matters of substantive difference or importance.

Under these circumstances, the only moral and bioethical commitments that will be tolerated by the secular culture (and these only if they are radically domesticated) will be those affirmed by a post-Christian morality that asserts a cardinal but nevertheless "weak" status for liberty, equality, and human dignity, insofar as these aid in sustaining the pursuit of self-indulgence and self-satisfaction. In a culture after God with a demoralized and deflated morality *cum* bioethics, one must even guard against a revolution on behalf of a substantive view of freedom as the source of authority (e.g., permission), as a cardinal value, or as the substance of a rational (Kantian) choice. If one is to maintain the *modus vivendi* of the happy dogs sleeping in the sun with its protection of life and property, then one is not even to advocate too stridently on behalf of a global acceptance of individual autonomy and patient rights. Instead, there is to be an embrace of immanent self-realization and self-satisfaction so as to achieve a putative final historical development that will forever set aside the bloodshed inspired by the power of ideas (not to mention concern for the transcendent). One is to maintain at all costs the hegemony of Vattimo's "weak thought."[23] One is to eschew any vision of humanity and reality that could legitimate conflict, even the immoderate pursuit of equality and democracy (e.g., a committed neo-conservative ["neo-con"] dedication to liberty and equality for all), including a fully social-democratically-framed bioethics. The zealous pursuit of justice and/or liberation, of any non-demoralized view of morality and bioethics, is to be replaced by an acquiescence in the truly human as the happy human animal, as the happy and satisfied dog. Neoconservatives who are still beset with a passion for liberty, equality, human dignity, and human rights will need to advance their cause gently, so as to preserve the dominance of the life-world of Fukuyama's satisfied, well-fed dog. Even liberal democratic commitments, as we have seen, are themselves without foundations and must also be demoralized, deflated, and weakened. The result is that liberal social-democratic moral commitments will be reinterpreted as leit-motifs that point to self-realization, the pursuit of "me." The pursuit of liberty, equality, and justice will need to be restated in terms that do not lead to a struggle of ideas.

This vision of humans fully at home within the horizon of the finite and the immanent, without any nostalgia for the transcendent, is captured by Albert

Camus (1913–1960), who speaks of the "godless summer sky" in Algiers. He experienced a sky

> with nothing tender in it, before which all truths can be uttered and on which no deceptive divinity has traced the signs of hope or of redemption. Between this sky and these faces turned toward it, nothing on which to hang a mythology, a literature, an ethic, or a religion, but stones, flesh, stars, and those truths the hand can touch (Camus 1961, p. 151).

Camus's vision of human flourishing is aggressively immanent and submerged in the sensuous. One might recall that during the week before his death in an automobile accident Camus wrote letters from his home in Provence (where he was staying with his wife and their two children), expressing affection to three different lovers (Campbell 2013, p. C6). His pursuit of self-realization and self-satisfaction was central in his life. The irony is that Camus's Algiers, this land that was supposed to be after God, was substantively *de*secularized within a half century of Camus's writing his essay "Summer in Algiers." Hunger for the transcendent reasserted itself. Has history restarted?

This new Algiers of the 21st century, marked by an acknowledgement of God's existence and shaped by a civil society with a strong presence of religion, has even come to France. The results for France and more generally for Europe have been profound. With the significant Muslim immigration from northern Africa, the expectations of Camus, indeed of the French Republic and its *laïcité*, have been brought into question. There is in particular

> the failure of the dream of "les cites"—the building blocks erected in the suburbs of cities all around France. Initially conceived as a place where everyone [in great measure Muslim immigrants] would become French and thank the generous state for the opportunity provided, they slowly became ghettos, where the lowliest people in the society are gathered. The crisis of the assimilationist state begins here in the *banlieues*. Here, religion has its strongest pull. Thus fundamentalism grows in places where the secular state wanted to erase diversity and propagate republican values. By involuntarily creating these new communities in the *banlieues*, the French state shreds its

"Rousseauist myth of a republic where there is nothing between the state and the citizen-individual in his isolation" (Zucca 2009, pp. 501–2).

The contemporary residents of France are not united in a common vision of tolerance, pluralism, and human rights, as the French Republic had promised. Muslim immigrants have instead created within France substantial moral, indeed religious exclaves from France.[24] What all this means for the survival of the secular state and liberal social democracy is far from clear.

Many simply fail to acknowledge the depth of the challenges. As Zucca notes, "After the terrorist attacks in London perpetrated by British Moslems, the reaction was clear and painful. The prime minister [Tony Blair was] reduced to insisting on British values, as if to kindle the French Rousseauist myth, hoping to install them in all of society" (Zucca 2009, p. 502). However, the Rousseauian myth of the possibility of a peaceable secular polity continues to be challenged by reality. We are entering a period of profound discord within the central fabric of most civil societies. Among other things, through the blood of their victims, Islamic terrorists are advancing moral and religious visions fundamentally at odds with the moral and political visions embraced by secular Europe, thus threatening contemporary secular Europe both physically and culturally. There is indeed, as Samuel Huntington (1927–2008) put it, a clash of civilizations (Huntington 1996). Violent opposition to the fundamentalist secular ethos of Europe is being expressed again and again, as for example in the January 7, 2015, attack in Paris on the satirical and significantly blasphemous magazine *Charlie Hebdo*. The attack, led by Muslims who were French nationals, constituted yet one more in a series of bloody rejections in Europe of the dominant secular culture of Western Europe and its commitment to the moral and political vision of a secular fundamentalist Republic. Again, the consequences were global. As was remarked following the January 7 incident, "The Paris shooting hit close to home in the U.K., which has suffered several Islamic-extremist related attacks—including the fatal stabbing of soldier Lee Rigby on the streets of London in broad daylight in [May 22,] 2013" (Troianovski & Duxbury 2015). The whole of Europe, indeed the whole of the secular world, was threatened. The project of a post-Christian Europe, which had been initiated by the violence and the blood of the French Revolution and through which secular Europeans have hoped to enjoy in peace a secular hedonic cultural public space defined as being after the transcendent, as after God, is being disconfirmed by violent Islamic acts. The European Union, the would-be light of peaceable secularity, has become beclouded by an instability at its roots. How are the defenders of the contemporary secular vision to understand their cultural context and to proceed in this quite hostile moral and political terrain? Core secular myths about social democracy collide with reality. Among the secular myths that have been undermined is the pious secular belief that we all share a sufficiently common view of morality and reality, so that citizens can on the model of a Socratic dialogue frame a deliberative democracy (Gutmann & Thompson 2004). We do not share common values or a common sense of what that would mean. As we have already seen, "citizens" at best can frame a *modus vivendi* in which, somewhat like bargainers in a market (in a market the buyer and the seller agree for that moment on a price) perhaps enough "citizens" can strike at least *pro tempore* agreements so that a *modus vivendi* can be sustained. The question remains, how long can such a secular *modus vivendi* be maintained? Is a society after God sustainable? Will a mass of unemployed and underemployed youth, often with college degrees and social-democratic passions along with access to social media, tweet their way to a succession of "democratic springs" producing repeated unrest and more unemployment (Parker 2014)?[25] Fukuyama recognizes that this state of affairs may wake the sleeping dog (Fukuyama 2013).[26] One faces the question: can the social-democratic *modus vivendi* after God continue? At the very least, the future is opaque.

Affluence, complex media distractions, social welfare (i.e., bread and complex circuses), combined with a nearly anesthetizing pursuit of self-realization and self-satisfaction have made it possible for many, often with the aid of psychotherapy and psycho-pharmacology, to live without nostalgia for metaphysics and without foundations, to live without God. Yet, the question remains (especially after comparing the Algiers of the late 1950s with that of the early 21st century): is Camus's vision of Algiers a stable resting point? As we go to the future, as the full implications of secular morality and bioethics without foundations become clearer, as we more deeply experience the demoralization and deflation of morality and bioethics, along with the concomitant moral delegitimization of public authority and the ultimate disorientation of all human projects, including

that of bioethics, as the dominant culture attempts to regard everything as ultimately meaningless, will this state of affairs be stable socially and politically?
As the demoralization and deflation of morality becomes more widespread and
pervasive, as the dominant secular culture absorbs fully the recognition that
secular morality and bioethics cannot rationally justify the conditions necessary
for rational persons to be held to have acted in ways that are praiseworthy or
worthy of happiness, how will people order their lives? When the dominant secular morality and bioethics are recognized as reflecting an ethnocentrism, will
social order be maintainable within an all-encompassing pursuit of self-realization and self-absorption? Will it be enough to attempt to raise people to be nice,
other-respecting, sympathetic, empathetic, and able to recite with conviction
the mantra of human rights while also ensuring that they are personally secure
and well off, as well as pursuing their own self-satisfaction and self-fulfillment?
Will this culture in fact be compatible with social stability?[27]

For those who are not partisans of the particular political movement whose
morality is established at law and public policy, the established morality and
bioethics will have legal governance and legal force, but no intrinsic moral force
or authority. The notion of political legitimacy will have been radically reduced,
becoming a mere legal fact of the matter. Political legitimacy will also often be a
matter of power. It will be a brute fact of the matter. The dominant secular culture may find it increasingly difficult not explicitly to recognize that the established morality and its view of human flourishing is *merely* a secular ideology
that happens to be established at law and in public policy, and that its bioethics
does not possess the traditional moral force of right-making conditions and/or
a view of the good that all should endorse. Secular morality and bioethics have
been disclosed as nothing more than macro life-style choices made within a particular cultural viewpoint, reflecting particular ethnocentrisms rendered incarnate in a particular *modus vivendi* that is sustained by a particular state's use of
indoctrination, propaganda, seduction, and coercion. That which is forwarded
as normative, as morally rational or politically reasonable, has been disclosed as
no more than one contingent perspective among a plurality of other contingent
moral perspectives. In addition, the moral point of view itself has been deflated
so that it no longer necessarily trumps personal, prudential concerns.

One is left in a secular world that is being fully exorcised of all ultimate, indeed non-contingent meaning. As Rorty puts it, we are invited to "the point where we no longer worship *anything*, where we treat *nothing* as a quasi divinity, where we treat *everything*—our language, our conscience, our community—as a product of time and chance" (Rorty 1989, p. 22). Rorty appreciates that the secular moral and political project has stepwise been despoiled of any ultimate point of orientation.

> I can crudely sum up the story which historians like [Hans] Blumenberg [1920–1996] tell by saying that once upon a time we felt a need to worship something which lay beyond the visible world. Beginning in the seventeenth century we tried to substitute a love of truth for a love of God, creating the world described by science as a quasi divinity. Beginning at the end of the eighteenth century we tried to substitute a love of ourselves for a love of scientific truth, a worship of our own deep spiritual or poetic nature, treated as one more quasi divinity (Rorty 1989, p. 22).

Rorty, however, wishes to go further. As he acknowledges, "In its ideal form, the culture of liberalism would be one which was enlightened, secular, through and through. It would be one in which no trace of divinity remained" (Rorty 1989, p. 45). Rorty correctly points to the post-Christian, post-religious world in which nothing possesses ultimate significance and in which morality has been both demoralized and deflated. The result will likely be a transformation of the public ethos so as radically to thin out the legitimacy of the state as it becomes ever clearer that rational moral argument cannot secure a particular moral vision as morally canonical or as necessarily trumping the interests of individual prudence or individual advantage.

After God, after the demoralization and deflation of morality, as well as after the delegitimization of the state, what more striking example of the worship of the creature rather than the Creator (Rom 1:22–15) can there be than the emergence of Hegel's notion of Absolute Spirit. That is the reason this chapter ends this book with so much emphasis on Hegel. By ignoring the presence of God, and by then entering into the collective solipsism of a narrative that floats free of any ultimate anchor within the horizon of the finite and the immanent, one is free to do things "my way." One turns a blind eye to the God Who shines through reality as through an icon, and one secures a seeming *carte blanche* for one's peaceable life-style and death-style choices. One enters into the soft and easy decadence realized in affluent northern Western Europe and affirmed by the European Union. One can be reassured by the high likelihood that one can live well until one dies, recognizing that even if one does have children, one may not have grandchildren on whom to expend capital. Moreover, there remains only a truncated notion of family. But again, over the long run will that be enough? The answer for some is surely yes. They can at least *pro tempore* live in a well-crafted world of passion, pleasure, and self-satisfaction that affirms themselves in their own self-absorption. But over the long run, can such a culture maintain the sovereignty of its self-appreciation as Absolute Spirit? Are enough people able to remain deaf to God? Can their life maintain a moral coherence? Will all shatter like a glass vase?

Facing the circumstance that all secular moralities and bioethics are only foundationless fabrics of moral intuitions supported by particular moral narratives, which can at best be recognized as constituting one freestanding moral position among others, will likely generate not only practical problems for societal coherence, but also a profoundly existential disorientation. What happens when ever more people realize that Judd Owen's description of the secular moral predicament is right?

> There is nothing to which we can appeal in order to settle the most profound human disagreements, and thus there is no possibility that the awesome variety of conflicting opinions about the things most important to human beings, including the best political order, can be transcended toward universal and objective knowledge (Owen 2001, p. 2).

Will it be enough to be a well-fed dog in the sun? When it is appreciated that secular bioethics and morality have been fully demoralized and deflated, why ought one to try very hard to be moral? Why should one do more than conform minimally to the particular morality and bioethics that are established at law, when disobedience is unlikely to involve the likelihood of sufficiently costly consequences? After all, the more-than-minimal state is only a *modus vivendi*. Can such a society framed by a culture after God sustain a fabric of law and order when moral authority is reduced to the mere force of the law, when one feels obliged to act "rightly," support "the good," or be "virtuous" only when someone else is looking?[28] What can one make of one's own life and any "obligation" to obey the law when all is viewed as ultimately meaningless? When all personal relationships are radically recast within a discourse of immanence, nothing any longer has ultimate meaning. What this portends for the societies of the future is far from clear.

We are in new and strange territory. Until the 20th century, there had never been a culture fully without God, without some transcendent anchor. Many persons have lived as if there were no God, but no large-scale culture has ever affirmed ultimate meaninglessness. Most hoped in some way to scry a deeper meaning, to find orientation from beyond the horizon of the finite and the immanent. The pattern of what-is-for-us was regarded as in some way tied to what-is-in-and-for-itself. The attempts of the I-Ching to disclose the mandate of heaven, or of Cicero in his office as the augurer for Rome to search for contact with the divine, all gestured beyond the finite and the immanent. Even atheistic communism invoked the final path of history. But what of a culture that wishes to eschew any hint of the divine with the result that its morality and bioethics are fully demoralized and deflated, so that in addition its political structures can claim no ultimate or final legitimization beyond the sword? After so great a God as the God of Abraham, what will it be like to have shut the door on all ultimate meaning? Under such circumstances, how will bioethics and morality be experienced? We really do not know. Will such a moral and political vacuum call the anti-Christ from the depths of Hell? Will such rise up and forthrightly confront us? As William Butler Yeats, fearing the advent of the anti-Christ in his poem "Second Coming," lamented: "Things fall apart; the centre cannot hold" (written in 1919). Can people have a stable existence as human animals? Can one really live as if all were in the end pointless? Can one over the long run make do with a fully immanentized human flourishing (e.g., as fat and happy human dogs) while holding existence to be thoroughly surd? Against the background of such an atheism or at least agnosticism, how should people live and act in the face of quotidian temptations and passions? Is such a life in the end actually livable? Are a demoralized morality and bioethics enough? Can one in the end avoid theological questions? Can one avoid reflecting on the meaning of it all? And again, there is the question raised by the transformation of Camus's Algiers, namely, whether a renewed recognition of God, of metaphysics, and of ultimate meaning will not always break in so as to disestablish the contemporary dominant secular culture, as occurred in Algiers. Can one successfully hide from God?

III. Cultural Guerrilla Wars in the Ruins of Christendom

Orthodox Christians and Orthodox Jews know that there is a God Who commands. They have moral norms and a bioethics rooted in the living God. Such Christians and Jews will remain. They know that relations to other humans are always misdirected in the absence of a rightly-directed relationship with the living God. They will increasingly be joined by traditionalist Muslims. Their normative commitments will contrast, indeed conflict with the established secular culture, along with its morality and bioethics. The tensions will be profound. The very existence of such believers will be provocative within the secular culture of the fundamentalist secular state. Their moral norms and bioethics will collide with the secular professional demands of an increasingly secular fundamentalist state. Among other things, by their difference traditional believers underscore the poverty of a moral discourse that is demoralized, deflated, "weakened," and radically secularized. Authentic Orthodox Christians will also be intransigent impediments to much secular public policy, particularly health care policy bearing on sexuality, reproduction, abortion, and end-of-life decision-making, because it will not be possible for these believers to be reconciled to a secular moral vision as well as to what its law and public policy requires. Traditional Christians with their highly politically incorrect rejection of abortion, reproduction outside of the marriage of a man and a woman, homosexual acts, and the impossibility of homosexual marriage know that their moral vision is anchored in a reality beyond the horizon of the finite and the immanent. Moreover, they understand that a transcendently grounded morality and bioethics can be worth dying for. They know and experience that the meaning of human sexuality is only found in realizing before God the union of Adam and Eve. Those who recognize the living God have anchored their normative commitments in a transcendent God Who demands their full devotion and commitment. They will not become merely human animals.

The dominant secular culture with its morality and its bioethics in contrast has located itself fully within the horizon of the finite and the immanent. Its members live within a life-world at odds with that of Orthodox Christians. Secularists and traditional Christians are moral strangers to each other. Yet, moral strangers can be affective friends. In our broken culture, persons are often married to moral strangers. They often have children who are moral strangers to them. Some are even moral strangers to themselves, holding deeply incompatible moral visions. The gulf separating the parties cannot be set aside through an appeal to secular moral rationality, secular rational game theory, and/or secular resolutions to prisoners' dilemmas that function, if at all, only for those who live fully within the horizon of the finite and the immanent, as well as affirm the same ranking of cardinal human values. On a range of issues, Orthodox Christians, Orthodox Jews, and Muslims will rather die than compromise their obligations to God. There is no common secular solution to a prisoner's dilemma problem when one of the prisoners is willing and perhaps quite glad to die as a martyr. In the ruins of Christendom, these believers will adamantly resist the demoralization and deflation of their normative commitments. Secularists and Orthodox Christians will be moral enemies, even if they may also be affective friends.[29] Even if God does not allow the committed religious as of yet to claim the field, they can and must on many points of disagreement simply resist and refuse to collaborate.

For a number of reasons, traditional religious belief, especially traditional Christian belief, will not go away. Among other things, fundamentalists tend to out-reproduce secularists.[30] Those who try to accommodate to the secular culture, including Orthodox Christians among them, will demographically die out. However, male chauvinist fundamentalists, especially those who are young women, know that not only will their children disproportionately constitute the future (i.e., they will have more children than liberal women of their cohort), but most importantly, if they raise their children to be faithful Orthodox Christians, they will be saved (I Tim 2:15). In an increasingly secular world, they will be raising missionaries and martyrs. Such women are a scandal to the secular world, for they submit to God, bind their husbands to themselves and through themselves to God, and shape the next generation. They are the mothers who bear the future. As with Hassidic Jewish women, such Orthodox Christian girls realize that they are the mitzvah girls, those who obey the commandments of God (Fader 2009). Moreover, as Orthodox Christians and Jews know, the presence of the transcendent always breaks through the horizon of the finite and the immanent. Our God lives and He speaks to us even when we want most not to hear Him.

We face a cosmic puzzle: a universe immense over space and time. What can we make of it? A universe out of a big bang some thirteen-and-a-half billion years ago? What if there may be numerous parallel universes, each with a different Max Planck constant? What, then? Can one avoid the question of the why of it all? Why is it all here? There is so much unconscious stuff about which *we* are conscious, indeed, even self-conscious. Can all be without ground for its being? It would have been so much easier, had there been nothing. But there is something. And so much of it. So much vast, surd stuff. How can all this stuff account for itself? Can unconscious stuff account for unconscious stuff, or must there be Someone self-conscious and the source of Itself (Himself) to do the accounting? Does so much, indeed *anything*, call out for an infinite, self-conscious, self-sufficient Creator? A recognition of the presence of God can begin as one experiences the principle of sufficient reason: why is there not nothing? As Gottfried Wilhelm Leibniz (1646–1716) realized, "This principle having been stated, the first question which we have a right to ask will be, 'Why is there something rather than nothing?' For nothing is simpler and easier than something" (Leibniz 1969, p. 639). The presence of anything raises the question of everything, of God's existence. Only God Himself can account for the existence of something.

The question is whether over the long run most can in the face of such a vast horizon of space and time repress a moment of puzzlement about a sufficient reason for it all, thus opening their hearts to the presence of God. Can one remain willfully blind to God? Can the committed agnostic secularist avoid God by always trying to change the subject so as not to be confronted with theological questions, questions about God's existence? And what if one looks through this immense panorama of existence, sees through it like through an icon, and noetically encounters God? What if icons weep when we pray before them? What if the myrrh from a myrrh-streaming icon is put into a closed container and the volume increases (*ex nihilo fit*)? How do we face recurring miracles?

Even without a miracle in sight, we nevertheless encounter God. At stake is not a discursive philosophical argument from evidence of God to the existence of God, but rather a noetic recognition, a knowing through the reality we confront as through an icon: an experience through the visible of the Energies of the Invisible (Rom 1:19–21). Does not God rub our faces in His existence? Even though non-believers decide to worship the creature rather than the Creator (Rom 1:18, 22–25), the presence of God persists. The transcendent always breaks in, even if we then try at once to avert our attention. Attempts to stifle any hint of the transcendent go aground as we try to think of ourselves as finite beings lost in an immense and ultimately senseless universe. Reality is always an icon disclosing the presence of *the* sufficient Ground, the Creator, God.

Knowledge of God (not just knowledge about God), as St. Paul makes clear, is not the conclusion of a discursive argument from evidence from data concerning God's existence to God's existence. This would require an inference from the finite to the infinite. Instead, what is at stake involves a perceiving of His Existence (Rom 1:19). The recognition of God's existence occurs not on the basis of conclusions from evidence used in a discursive argument that leads to proving God's existence, but a move from an encounter with His Presence to an acknowledgement of His Presence. Can the transcendent Who is God *fail* to break in? St. Paul's answer is no. God always breaks in, becomes manifest to each person through reality. Reality is always and at all times like an icon through which one can look and see God. Our response, how we react to God's presence, establishes the significance of our lives. It forms who we are. It relates us to God Who is the Ground and Judge of all created reality. St. Paul insists that agnostics, not to mention atheists, are therefore always without excuse, for they have sufficiently encountered God's Presence and have nevertheless chosen to act as if God did not exist. Atheists as well as agnostics, St. Paul also insists, are culpable for their failure to acknowledge God and then to worship Him, because there is always enough knowledge of His Presence (i.e., noetic experience of His existence), so that one is culpable for having worshipped the creature, rather than the Creator (Rom 1:20–21). But if the heart opens, everything can happen. One can see the presence of God.

IV. Looking to the Future: God Lives

Only God knows the future. Philosophers are not prophets. "[T]he owl of Minerva begins its flight only with the onset of dusk" (Hegel 1991, p. 23). The present is full of unanticipated occurrences. There are again Orthodox churches in Rome. Converts stand in the catholicon. Icons weep. Across the world, a literature of traditional Christian moral reflection and Christian bioethics is developing with a significant contribution from Orthodox Christians. In a culture after God, many know that God lives, philosophers among them (Vitz 2012). What all this will mean, no ordinary human can say. In any event, things unanticipated are taking place in the ruins of Christendom. In the meantime, we must be committed and patient, as Christians were during the rule of pagan Rome. We must remember that nearly three centuries passed before St. Constantine, Equal-to-the-Apostles, sat at the Council of Nicea (A.D. 325).

The Southern writer Walker Percy (1916–1990) in various ways called attention to the survival of traditional belief, indeed to the presence of the sustaining power of God. After a lecture, Percy's hosts once asked to take him to a restaurant, inquiring what kind of food he would like. His response ran somewhat in this fashion: "Thank you; please take me to a Hittite restaurant." After some confusion, the hosts responded that there were no Hittite restaurants. Percy then asked, feigning surprise, "Then please take me to a Jewish restaurant." The point is that the Hittites had been a mighty people with a developed culture who possessed an extensive empire. Their empire and culture seemed enduring. However, the Hittites are now all gone, lost in the past. In their midst was Abraham and his small band of believers in the true God (Gen 23:3–20). The Jews were seemingly insignificant. However, they were the icon of the living God. Orthodox Jews remain. They are still an icon of God's presence,Whose presence is fully in the synagogue of the Messiah, Who is Jesus Christ. The Orthodox Church, the synagogue of the Messiah Who rose from the dead and will come again, shall endure until He comes. Even in the face of secularization, committed true belief will not evanesce, because God is on our side.

Notes

[1]This chapter developed in part from a lecture, "Bioethics after Foundations: Feeling the Full Force of Secularization," delivered at the Centro Evangelico di Cultura "Arturo Pascal" and the Consulta di Bioetica ONLUS, Turin, Italy, January 31, 2012.

[2]There is a considerable literature concerning the death of God in contemporary culture. For a small sampling, see Altizer 2006; Altizer & Hamilton 1966; Caputo & Vattimo 2007; Peterson 2005; Robinson 1963; and Williams 2012.

[3]As to Kant's postulates of practical reason, "These postulates are those of immortality, of freedom affirmatively regarded (as the causality of a being insofar as he belongs to the intelligible world), and of the existence of God" (Kant 1956, p. 137, AK V.133).

[4]For Kant, in our lives God serves a moral, not a religious purpose, all without Kant's actually affirming the existence of a transcendent God. In the process, Kant construes Christian norms in terms of his rationally grounded morality.

> The Christian principle of morality is not theological and thus heteronomous, being rather the autonomy of pure practical reason itself, because it does not make the knowledge of God and His will the basis of these laws but makes such knowledge the basis only of succeeding to the highest good on condition of obedience to these laws; it places the real incentive for obedience to the law not in the desired consequences of obedience but in the conception of duty alone, in true observance of which the worthiness to attain the latter alone consists (Kant 1956, pp. 133–34, AK V 129–30).

Kant embraces the rationalist horn of Euthyphro's dilemma.

[5]As elsewhere in this book, the term *post-modernity* is used to identify the cultural recognition that secular rationality cannot provide: a canonical, universal narrative, grammar, or account of reality and/or of morality that can substitute for God. Such a universal canonical account had been the hope of modernity. It had been promised by the moral-philosophical project of the West. Indeed, it was taken for granted. Modernity had faith that reason was one, as God had been recognized as One. The Enlightenment was built on this faith. In post-modernity, this faith in reason is shown to be, and is acknowledged to be, unfounded. What was always the case regarding secular accounts of morality, bioethics, and reality, namely, the intractable plurality of such accounts, is finally openly admitted.

[6]Frederick Beiser defends the view that Hegel did not make a radical break from traditional Christianity. Beiser interprets Hegel's remarks regarding the death of God as a reference to "Johann Rist's [1607–1667] hymn 'O grosse Not! Gott selbst ist tod. Am Kreuz ist er gestorben' (Oh, great need! God himself is dead. He has died on the cross)" (Beiser 2005, p. 138). My position, along with others such as Walter Kaufmann and Horst Althaus, is that Hegel was an atheist, or at least an agnostic, and that he set out radically to transform the meaning of Christianity and therefore the meaning of being a Lutheran (Kaufmann 1966; Althaus 2000).

[7]There has been a fair amount of puzzling concerning the death of God in the early 19th century. See, for example, Amengual 2003; Brinkmann 2006; Desmond 2005 and 2003; Franke 2007; Hodgson 2005; Houlgate 2005; Lauer 1982; Nichols 2005; and Olson 1992.

[8]Art, religion, and philosophy, the major categories of Absolute Spirit, are different shapes, *Gestalten*, through and in which one knows materially the same content. See, for example, Part Three of Hegel's *Encyclopedia of the Philosophical Sciences: The Philosophy of Mind*, especially §§556, 564, and 572.

[9]As already noted, a non-metaphysical reading of Hegel is advanced in this volume. Nevertheless, there are defenders of a metaphysical reading of Hegel's God, who would even make Hegel out to be a theist. One might consider the position taken by Quentin Lauer.

> The philosophy of which Hegel speaks has turned out to be startlingly—for some, perhaps, frighteningly—theological, and yet, for all that it is not less but all the more philosophical. If it is possible to identify God with infinite "Reason," absolute "Spirit," then it must be said that God, in what he *is* and what he *does*, is supremely rational, that he is infinite "rationality." To know God, then, is man's rational goal, and to be thoroughly rational is to know God. But this can make sense only if human reason is somehow "divine," continuous with "infinite" Reason, since "reason" is one, not many (Lauer 1982, pp. 323–24).

See also, for example, Hodgson 2012. For another defense of a non-metaphysical reading, see Pinkard 1996.

[10]John Rawls takes a position similar to Rorty's in characterizing some comprehensive doctrines as "mad" (Rawls 1993, p. xvii).

[11]Reflections on kenosis take their point of departure from a passage in Philippians. "Let the same mind be in you that was in Christ Jesus, who, though he was in the form of God, did not regard equality with God as something to be exploited, but emptied himself [*ekenōsen*], taking the form of a slave, being born in human likeness. And being found in human form, he humbled himself and became obedient to the point of death—even death on a cross" (Philippians 2:5–8).

[12]Martin Buber's account of the eclipse of God is a complex diagnosis of the contemporary age. "In our age the I-It relation, gigantically swollen, has usurped, practically uncontested, the mastery and the rule. . . . This selfhood that has become omnipotent, with all the It around it, can naturally acknowledge neither God nor any genuine absolute which manifests itself to men as of non-human origin. It steps in between and shuts off from us the light of heaven" (Buber 1952, p. 129). Buber makes clear that the eclipse of God is no death of God. "Something is taking place in the depths that as yet needs no name. To-morrow even it may happen that it will be beckoned to from the heights, across the heads of the earthly archons. The eclipse of the light of God is no extinction; even to-morrow that which has stepped in between may give way" (Buber 1952, p. 129).

[13]The original reads, "Doch worin besteht die Menschlichkeit des Menschen?" Heidegger 1976, vol. 9, p. 319.

[14]The socio-historically embedded character of the truly human is recognized by Christians who know that the God Incarnate is a man with a particular genealogy born in Palestine during the reign of Caesar Augustus (27 B.C.–A.D. 14).

[15]The subtitle of this section, "A Culture Without Roots," may recall to the reader the book co-authored by Joseph Ratzinger, later Pope Benedict XVI, with Marcello Pera, *Without Roots* (Ratzinger & Pera 2006). On some points, I agree with Benedict XVI's appreciation of the rootless character of the contemporary post-Christian culture of the West. However, my account of what is at stake, as well as of the proper response to our condition, differs profoundly from, and is much more radical than, that offered by Ratzinger. In his portions of *Without Roots*, Ratzinger in great measure attributes the rootlessness of the contemporary age to the failure of philosophical rationality to connect contemporary culture with objective truth, a failure he holds can be remedied by philosophy. As I have argued, Ratzinger's faith in philosophical reason is unjustified, indeed misguided. Ratzinger's account falls short of the mark by failing to recognize the depth and the character of the crisis in foundations, the absence of an anchor in being, or in sound rational argument for Western European civilization. He does not appreciate that there is not only no hope to establish a secular vision of a canonical morality, but he fails to see what is essential to restoring a Christian culture, namely, a return to right worship and right belief, in particular through re-embracing the ascetical disciplines of the Church of the Apostles and the Fathers, which aid in turning one from self-love to the transcendent God and to a noetic experience of His Will.

[16]For a study of the emerging appreciation of bioethics as biopolitics in the sense of being a political movement with a particular political agenda, see Engelhardt 2012.

[17]Those who recognize God tend to be committed to raising a new generation of pious young men and women who will beget and raise further generations of rightly-directed worshippers of God. For an account of the Hasidic Jewish view, see Fader 2009.

[18]Even as a philosopher participating in the higher truth of Absolute Spirit, one is still not necessarily more than one of Kojève's and Fukuyama's human animals, insofar as one is disposed to enjoy one's ease and is *not* disposed to die for ideas.

[19]Kojève's and Fukuyama's account of Hegel's view of history is not *sensu stricto* congruent with what Hegel actually argued. This Fukuyama himself concedes (p. 144). For a critique of Fukuyama's account of Hegel (especially Fukuyama's assertion that "Hegel declared that history had ended after the Battle of Jena in 1806" [Fukuyama 1992, p. 64]), as well as of the views of Kojève, see Grier 1990. Such criticisms to the contrary notwithstanding, Kojève and Fukuyama correctly saw a higher truth of what Hegel actually argued, at least as it bears on the character of our age. Once all is regarded within the horizon of the finite and the immanent, there are no transcendental goals, only immanent satisfactions to be sought.

[20]Psychotropic drugs associated with rock concerts have become an ordinary element of life with the dominant secular culture. See, for example, Campo-Flores & Elinson 2013.

[21]Although Fukuyama wrote after the establishment of Ayatollah Khomeini's (1900–1989) Iran in 1979, he does not recognize Islam as having a constellation of ideas that could drive history—i.e., restart history. Fukuyama dismisses the significance of Islam on the grounds *inter alia* that it "has no resonance for young people in Berlin, Tokyo, or Moscow" (Fukuyama

1992, p. 46). Fukuyama rather sees the contemporary success of fundamentalist Islam as lying in resentments due to the persistent economic failures of Islamic countries, as well as to what he terms slights of history suffered by those countries. Nevertheless, young Europeans and Americans convert to fundamentalist Islam.

[22]The statement "Who am I to judge?" made by Pope Francis while returning from Brazil on July 29, 2013, has become a battle cry against the remoralization of life-style choices and has even spawned a T-shirt.

[23]For a definition of "weak thought", consider:

> The theses that I and other Italian post-Heideggerian philosophers have called "weak thought" have become very popular in a certain part of Italian Catholic thought because they have been interpreted, though with a degree of partiality, as a pure and simple confession of reason's weakness. True, the demise of the metanarratives is a recognition of weakness in this sense (Vattimo 2002, p. 20).

[24]The presence of Muslim communities in France has brought the country's dominant self-image as a laicist republic into question (Laborde 2009). "Islam seems to call into question the very identity of the country, or at least the nature of its institutions. People mobilize for the defense of 'republican values' and 'laïcité'" (Roy 2007, p. 1). These challenges are tied as well to the intractability of inequality (Clark et al. 2014) and to what appears to be increasing inequality (Piketty & Saez 2014).

For Europe as a whole, the presence of large Muslim communities may prove transformative, as Christopher Caldwell has argued.

> Europe's basic problem with Islam, and with immigration more generally, is that the strongest communities in Europe are, culturally speaking, not European communities at all. . . . Islam is a magnificent religion that has also been, at times over the centuries, a glorious and generous culture. But, all cant to the contrary, it is in no sense Europe's religion and it is in no sense Europe's culture.
>
> It is certain that Europe will emerge changed from its confrontation with Islam. It is far less certain that Islam will prove assimilable. . . . When an insecure, malleable, relativistic culture meets a culture that is anchored, confident, and strengthened by common doctrines, it is generally the former that changes to suit the latter (Caldwell 2009, p. 349).

The consequences will likely challenge those who have celebrated Europe as the embodiment of liberal democratic aspirations (Rifkin 2004).

[25]"Democratic Springs" driven by a relatively secularized, college-educated, underemployed "middle class" can be destructive. As David Goldman observes,

> The so-called Arab Spring was not a leap into democracy but a swoon into societal failure. . . . Wael Ghonim, the Google employee who became the poster-boy for the Egyptian revolution, toured the United States accepting book deals and public service awards while Egypt plunged into deep economic distress. The *punditeska* barely had weeks to drool over these Nile apparitions of Western coolness before mourning their disappearance (Goldman 2011, pp. 2, 3).

Matters are more complex than Goldman recognizes. The so-called Arab Spring had roots in a deep frustration with a failure to guarantee basic property and market rights.

It is widely known that the Arab Spring was sparked by the self-immolation in 2011 of Mohamed Bouazizi, a 26-year-old Tunisian street merchant. But few have asked why Bouazizi felt driven to kill himself—or why, within 60 days, at least 63 more men and women in Tunisia, Algeria, Morocco, Yemen, Saudi Arabia and Egypt also set themselves on fire, sending millions into the streets, toppling four regimes and leading us to today's turmoil in the Arab world. . . .

These suicides, we found, weren't pleas for political or religious rights or for higher wage subsidies, as some have argued. Bouazizi and the others who burned themselves were extralegal entrepreneurs: builders, contractors, caterers, small vendors and the like. In their dying statements, none referred to religion or politics. Most of those who survived their burns and agreed to be interviewed spoke to us of "economic exclusion." Their great objective was "*ras el mel*" (Arabic for "capital"), and their despair and indignation sprang from the arbitrary expropriation of what little capital they had. . . .

I asked Bouazizi's brother Salem if he thought that his late sibling had left a legacy. "Of course," he said. "He believed the poor had the right to buy and sell." As Mehdi Belli, a university information-technology graduate working as a merchant at a market in Tunis, told us, "We are all Mohamed Bouazizi" (de Soto 2014, p. C2).

[26]Fukuyama recognized the danger of the bored lower-middle class even before the advent of social media. He advanced, for example, the following assessment of the French *evénéments* of 1968.

Those students who temporarily took over Paris and brought down General de Gaulle had no "rational" reason to rebel, for they were for the most part pampered offspring of one of the freest and most prosperous societies on earth. But it was precisely the *absence* of struggle and sacrifice in their middle-class lives that led them to take to the streets and confront the police (Fukuyama 1992, p. 330).

[27]Already in the mid-1990s, Samuel Huntington became concerned regarding the stability of Fukuyama's society of well-fed dogs lying in the sun.

Far more significant than economics and demography are problems of moral decline, cultural suicide, and political disunity in the West. Oft-pointed-to manifestations of moral decline include:

1. increases in antisocial behavior, such as crime, drug use, and violence generally;
2. family decay, including increased rates of divorce, illegitimacy, teen-age pregnancy, and single-parent families;
3. at least in the United States, a decline in "social capital," that is, membership in voluntary associations and the interpersonal trust associated with such membership;
4. general weakening of the "work ethic" and rise of a culture of personal indulgence;

5. decreasing commitment to learning and intellectual activity, manifested in the United States in lower levels of scholastic achievement (Huntington 1996, p. 304).

[28]For an example of a society whose members by and large obey the law only when someone is looking, one might consider Banfield's classic study of the dysfunctional character of the Italian commune of Chiaromonte in Basilicata (population 3,400), where although there was nominal belief in God and the presence of intact families, there were few effective extrafamilial norms. As Banfield describes the state of affairs,

> In a society of amoral familists, the law will be disregarded when there is no reason to fear punishment. Therefore individuals will not enter into agreements which depend upon legal processes for their enforcement unless it is likely that the law will be enforced and unless the cost of securing enforcement will not be so great as to make the undertaking unprofitable (Banfield 1958, p. 90).

One should note, however, that cultural determinants are significant. For example, Nordics have done well in maintaining a stable society after God (Zuckerman 2008).

[29]After I gave a paper in German in a German-speaking country, a Muslim professor at the institution asked if I had any grandchildren. He had stereotyped me as a typical non-reproducing European. (None of my European intellectual friends has grandchildren.) I responded by listing my grandchildren. The most recently born at that time was Stefan Daniel. I explained that he was named after St. Stefan the Great, warrior-king of Romania, who had won 47 battles against the Muslims. He looked at me in silence for a moment. Then he said, "The rest of the people here only worship ideas. We both worship God and know that it is good to die fighting for Him."

[30]Data indicate, as Phillip Longman has observed, that male chauvinist fundamentalist religions out-reproduce liberal ones (Longman 2004a, 2004b, and 2006).

References

Althaus, Horst. 2000. *Hegel: An Intellectual Biography.* Cambridge: Polity Press.

Altizer, Thomas. 2006. *Living the Death of God: A Theological Memoir.* Albany: State University of New York Press.

Altizer, Thomas J. J. 2002. *The New Gospel of Christian Atheism.* Aurora, CO: Davies Group Publishers.

Altizer, Thomas J. J. 1966. *The Gospel of Christian Atheism.* Philadelphia: Westminster.

Altizer, Thomas & William Hamilton. 1966. *Radical Theology and the Death of God.* Indianapolis: Bobbs-Merrill.

Amengual, Gabriel. 2003. Nihilismus und Gottesbegriff, in *Hegel-Jahrbuch* (pp. 38–44). Berlin: Akademie Verlag.

Banfield, Edward C. 1958. *The Moral Basis of a Backward Society*. New York: Free Press.

Beiser, Frederick. 2005. *Hegel*. New York: Routledge.

Berger, Peter L. (ed.). 1999. *The Desecularization of the World*. Grand Rapids, MI: Wm. Eerdmans.

Binkley, Christina. 2013. Styles and stunts of fashion week, *Wall Street Journal* CCLXII.62 (September 12): D1, D4.

Blamires, Harry. 1963. *The Christian Mind*. London: S.P.C.K.

Blom, Philipp. 2008. *The Vertigo Years: Change and Culture in the West, 1900–1914*. New York: Basic Books.

Bonhoeffer, Dietrich. 1972. *Letters and Papers from Prison*, ed. Eberhard Bethge. New York: Macmillan.

Brinkmann, Klaus. 2006. Panthéisme, panlogisme et protestantisme dans la philosophie de Hegel, in *Les Philosophes et la question de Dieu*, ed. Luc Langlois (pp. 223–38). Paris: Presses Universitaires de France.

Buber, Martin. 1952. *Eclipse of God*. New York: Harper & Bros.

Bultmann, Rudolf. 1984. *New Testament & Mythology and Other Basic Writings*, trans. Schubert M. Ogden. Philadelphia: Fortress Press.

Burrough, Bryan. 2015. *Days of Rage*. New York: Penguin.

Caldwell, Christopher. 2009. *Reflections on the Revolution in Europe: Immigration, Islam, and the West*. New York: Doubleday.

Campbell, James. 2013. Betwixt and between, *Wall Street Journal* (May 4–5): C5–C6.

Campo-Flores, Arian & Zusha Elinson. 2013. Club drug takes deadly toll: Billed as pure ecstasy, 'Molly' often gets laced with more-dangerous substances, *Wall Street Journal* (Sept. 25): A3.

Camus, Albert. 1961. *The Myth of Sisyphus and Other Essays*, trans. Justin O'Brien. New York: Alfred A. Knopf.

Caputo, John D. 2006. *The Weakness of God: A Theology of the Event*. Bloomington: Indiana University Press.

Caputo, John & Gianni Vattimo. 2007. *After the Death of God*. New York: Columbia University Press.

Clark, Gregory. 2014. *The Son Also Rises: Surnames and the History of Social Mobility*. Princeton, NJ: Princeton University Press.

Cox, Harvey. 1965. *The Secular City*. New York: Macmillan.

Danto, Arthur C. 1980. *Nietzsche as Philosopher*. New York: Columbia University Press.

Desmond, William. 2005. Hegel's God, transcendence, and the counterfeit double: A figure of dialectical equivocity? *Owl of Minerva* 36.2: 91–110.

Desmond, William. 2003. *Hegel's God. A Counterfeit Double?* Aldershot: Ashgate.

De Soto, Hernando. 2014. The capitalist cure for terrorism, *Wall Street Journal* (October 11): C1–C2.

Dupré, Louis. 1993. *Passage to Modernity*. New Haven: Yale University Press.

Dworkin, Ronald. 2013. *Religion Without God*. Cambridge, MA: Harvard University Press.

Engelhardt, H. T., Jr. (ed.). 2012. *Bioethics Critically Reconsidered: Having Second Thoughts*. Dordrecht: Springer.

Engelhardt, H. T., Jr. 2010a. Religion, bioethics, and the secular state: Beyond religious and secular fundamentalism, *Notizie di Politeia* 26.97: 59–79.

Engelhardt, H. T., Jr. 2010b. Political authority in the face of moral pluralism: Further reflections on the non-fundamentalist state, *Notizie di Politeia* 26.97: 91–99.

Engelhardt, H. T., Jr. 1991. *Bioethics and Secular Humanism*. Philadelphia: Trinity Press International.

Fackenheim, Emil L. 1967. On the self-exposure of faith to the modern-secular world: Philosophical reflections in the light of Jewish experience. *Daedalus* 96.1 (Winter): 193–219.

Fader, Ayala. 2009. *Mitzvah Girls: Bringing up the Next Generation of Hasidic Jews in Brooklyn*. Princeton, NJ: Princeton University Press.

Fenn, Richard. 1968. The death of God: An analysis of ideological crisis, *Review of Religious Research* 9.3 (Spring): 171–181.

Franke, William. 2007. The deaths of God in Hegel and Nietzsche and the crisis of values in secular modernity and post-secular postmodernity, *Religion and the Arts* 11.2: 214–41.

Fukuyama, Francis. 2013. The middle-class revolution, *Wall Street Journal* (June 28). http://online.wsj.com/news/articles/SB10001424127887323873904578571472700348086 [accessed November 20, 2015].

Fukuyama, Francis. 1992. *The End of History and the Last Man*. New York: Free Press.

Fukuyama, Francis. 1989. The end of history? *The National Interest* (Summer): 3–18.

Goldman, David P. 2011. *It's Not the End of the World, It's Just the End of You.* New York: RVP Publishers.

Grier, Philip T. 1990. The end of history, and the return of history, *The Owl of Minerva* 21.2: 131–144.

Gutmann, Amy & Dennis Thompson. 2004. *Why Deliberative Democracy?* Princeton, NJ: Princeton University Press.

Habermas, Jürgen & Joseph Ratzinger. 2006. *The Dialectics of Secularization.* San Francisco: Ignatius Press.

Hamilton, William. 1961. *The New Essence of Christianity.* New York: Association Press.

Hartmann, Klaus. 1972. Hegel: A non-metaphysical view. In *Hegel,* ed. Alasdair MacIntyre (pp. 101–124). Garden City, NY: Anchor Books.

Hegel, G.W.F. 1991. *Elements of the Philosophy of Right,* ed. Allen W. Wood, trans. H. B. Nisbet. Cambridge: Cambridge University Press.

Hegel, G.W.F. 1977. *Faith & Knowledge,* trans. Walter Cerf and H.S. Harris. Albany: State University of New York Press.

Hegel, G.W.F. 1971. *Hegel's Philosophy of Mind,* trans. William Wallace. Oxford: Clarendon Press.

Hegel, G.W.F. 1970. *Hegel's Philosophy of Nature,* vol. 1, ed. & trans. M. J. Petry. New York: Humanities Press.

Hegel, G.W.F. 1968. *Jenaer kritische Schriften,* in *Gesammelte Werke,* vol. 4. Hamburg: Meiner.

Hegel, G.W.F. 1910. *The Phenomenology of Mind,* trans. Sir James Baillie. London: George Allen & Unwin.

Heidegger, Martin. 1976. Brief über den 'Humanismus' in *Wegmarken* (*Gesamtausgabe,* vol. 9). Frankfurt/Main: Vittorio Klosterman.

Hodgson, Peter C. 2012. *Shapes of Freedom: Hegel's Philosophy of World History in Theological Perspective.* New York: Oxford University Press.

Hodgson, Peter C. 2005. Hegel's God: Counterfeit or real? *Owl of Minerva* 36.2: 153–63.

Houlgate, Stephen. 2005. Hegel, Desmond, and the problem of God's transcendence, *Owl of Minerva* 36.2: 131–52.

Huntington, Samuel P. 1996. *The Clash of Civilizations and the Remarking of World Order.* New York: Simon & Schuster.

Kant, Immanuel. 1956. *Critique of Practical Reason,* trans. Lewis White Beck. Indianapolis: Bobbs-Merrill.

Kaufmann, Walter. 1966. *Hegel: A Reinterpretation*. Garden City, NY: Anchor Books.

Kojève, Alexander. 1969. *Introduction to the Reading of Hegel*, ed. Alan Bloom, trans. James H. Nichols, Jr. New York: Basic Books.

Kreines, James. 2007. Between the bounds of experience and divine intuition: Kant's epistemic limits and Hegel's ambitions, *Inquiry* 50: 306–334.

Kuhn, Thomas. 1962. *The Structure of Scientific Revolutions*. 2nd ed. enlarged, 1970. Chicago: University of Chicago Press.

Küng, Hans. 1966. *Freedom Today*. New York: Sheed & Ward.

Laborde, Cécile. 2008. *Critical Republicanism: The Hijab Controversy and Political Philosophy*. Oxford: Oxford University Press.

Lauer, Quentin. 1982. *Hegel's Concept of God*. Albany: State University of New York Press.

Leibniz, Gottfried Wilhelm. 1969. *G.W. Leibniz: Philosophical Papers and Letters*, 2nd ed., trans. Leroy Loemker. Dordrecht: Reidel.

Longman, Phillip. 2006. The return of patriarchy, *Foreign Policy* 153 (March/April): 56–65.

Longman, Phillip. 2004a. *The Empty Cradle*. New York: Basic Books.

Longman, Phillip. 2004b. The global baby bust, *Foreign Affairs* 83.3 (May/June): 64–79.

MacIntyre, Alasdair. 1963. God and the theologians. *Encounter* 21.3 (September): 3–10.

Macquarrie, John. 1961. *The Scope of Demythologizing: Bultmann and His Critics*. New York: Harper & Brothers.

Mascall, Eric L. 1966. *The Secularization of Christianity*. New York: Holt, Rinehart, & Winston.

Mullen, Peter. 2009. Make your own hope, in *The Nation that Forgot God*, eds. Edward Leigh & Alex Haydon (pp. 37–52). London: Social Affairs Unit.

Murray, Charles. 2012. *Coming Apart*. New York: Crown Forum.

Nichols, Craig M. 2005. The eschatological theogony of the God Who may be: Exploring the concept of divine presence in Kearney, Hegel, and Heidegger, *Metaphilosophy* 36.5: 750–61.

Novak, Michael. 1967. Christianity: Renewed or slowly abandoned? *Daedalus* 96.1 (Winter): 237–266.

Ogden, Schubert. 1961. *Christ without Myth: A Study Based on the Theology of Rudolf Bultmann*. Dallas: SMU Press.

Olson, Alan M. 1992. *Hegel and the Spirit*. Princeton: Princeton University Press.

Owen, J. Judd. 2001. *Religion and the Demise of Liberal Rationalism*. Chicago: University of Chicago Press.

Parker, Emily. 2014. *Now I Know Who My Comrades Are*. New York: Farrar, Straus & Giroux.

Peterson, Daniel J. 2005. Speaking of God after the death of God, *Dialog: A Journal of Theology* 44.3: 207–26.

Piketty, Thomas & Emmanuel Saez. 2014. Inequality in the long run, *Science* 344.6186 (May 23): 838–843.

Pinkard, Terry. 2012. *Hegel's Naturalism: Mind, Nature, and the Final Ends of Life*. New York: Oxford University Press.

Pinkard, Terry. 1996. What is the non-metaphysical reading of Hegel? A reply to F. Beiser, *Bulletin of the Hegel Society of Great Britain* 34: 13–20.

Ratzinger, Joseph & Marcello Pera. 2006. *Without Roots*, trans. Michael F. Moore. New York: Basic Books.

Rawls, John. 1993. *Political Liberalism*. New York: Columbia University Press.

Rifkin, Jeremy. 2004. *The European Dream*. New York: Penguin.

Robinson, John A. T. 1963. *Honest to God*. Philadelphia: SCM Press.

Rorty, Richard. 1991. *Objectivity, Relativism, and Truth*. New York: Cambridge University Press.

Rorty, Richard. 1989. *Contingency, Irony, and Solidarity*. New York: Cambridge University Press.

Rorty, Richard & Gianni Vattimo. 2005. *The Future of Religion*, ed. Santiago Zabala. New York: Columbia University Press.

Roy, Olivier. 2007. *Secularism Confronts Islam*, trans. George Holoch. New York: Columbia University Press.

Rubenstein, Richard L. 1966. *After Auschwitz: Radical Theology and Contemporary Judaism*. Indianapolis: Bobbs-Merrill.

Taylor, Mark C. 2006. Foreword: The last theologian, in Thomas J. J. Altizer, *Living the Death of God* (pp. xi–xviii). Albany: State University of New York Press.

Troianovski, Anton & Charles Duxbury. 2015. Paris shooting attack poses new challenge for European leaders, *Wall Street Journal* (January 7). http://www.wsj.com/articles/paris-shooting-attack-poses-new-challenge-for-european-leaders-1420654140 (accessed November 20, 2015)

Vahanian, Gabriel. 1961. *The Death of God: The Culture of Our Post-Christian Era*. New York: Braziller.

Van Buren, Paul. 1963. *The Secular Meaning of the Gospel.* New York: Macmillan.

Vattimo, Gianni. 2004. *Nihilism and Emancipation,* ed. Santiago Zabala, trans. William McCuaig. New York: Columbia University Press.

Vattimo, Gianni, 2002. *After Christianity,* trans. Luca D'Isanto. New York: Columbia University Press.

Vattimo, Gianni. 1999. *Belief,* trans. Luca D'Isanto & David Webb. Stanford, CA: Stanford University Press.

Vattimo, Gianni. 1988. *The End of Modernity,* trans. Jon R. Snyder. Baltimore: Johns Hopkins University Press.

Vitz, Rico (ed.). 2012. *Contemporary Philosophers and the Ancient Christian Faith.* Yonkers, NY: St Vladimir's Seminary Press.

Williams, Robert W. 2012. *Tragedy, Recognition, and the Death of God: Studies in Hegel and Nietzsche.* Oxford: Oxford University Press.

Zabala, Santiago. 2005. A religion without theists or atheists, in Richard Rorty and Gianni Vattimo, *The Future of Religion* (pp. 1–27), ed. Santiago Zabala. New York: Columbia University Press.

Zucca, Lorenzo. 2009. The crisis of the secular state—A reply to Professor Sajó, *International Journal of Constitutional Law* 7.3: 494-514.

Zuckerman, Phil. 2008. *Society Without God: What the Least Religious Nations Can Tell Us About Contentment.* New York: New York University Press.

Index